Emergency War Surgery

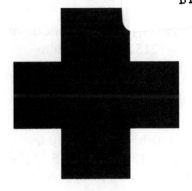

Second United States Revision
The Emergency War Surgery NATO Handbook

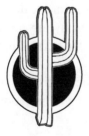

Desert Publications
El Dorado, AR 71731-1751 U. S. A.

Emergency War Surgery

Second United States Revision
Emergency War Surgery
NATO Handbook
1988

© 1992 by Desert Publications
215 S. Washington
El Dorado, AR 71731-1751
870-862-2077

ISBN 0-87947-410-6
12 11 10 9 8 7 6
Printed in U. S. A.

Desert Publication is a division of
The DELTA GROUP, Ltd.
Direct all inquiries & orders to the above address.

Foreword

The success of any military health care system in wartime is directly related to the number of casualties adequately treated and returned to duty with their units. This must be accomplished as soon and as far forward in the theater of operations as possible.

The Second Battle of Bull Run near Manassas, Virginia, was one of the major engagements of the United States Civil War. Three days after that great battle, three thousand wounded men still lay on the field. Relatives travelled to the front and took their loved ones home for treatment rather than leave them to the uncertainties of military medicine. We have made phenomenal progress in the century since that battle occurred.

I have had the privilege of being a physician for nearly forty years. Half of that time was spent on active duty in the military services and the other half was spent in the civilian sector. I have participated in the delivery of health care in every conceivable setting: in a battlefield tent in Korea; on a hospital ship; in an air squadron; from austere county and state hospitals to large, glossy high technology institutions. I have seen people strive for, and achieve, excellence in all those settings. I see it now in the military health care system, and no one is more proud than I of the accomplishments and the quality of that system and of the special type of men and women who make the system work. Our system is not without its problems and its frustrations. It takes a long time for equipment to be delivered; the personnel system doesn't always provide the proper mix of people in a timely manner to get the job done; but with rare exceptions, the medical mission is accomplished in exceptional fashion.

This handbook should serve as a constant reminder that ours is a high calling. We are here to save lives, not to destroy them. We are committed to the future, not the past, and to the primary mission of military medicine, which is to keep the soldiers, sailors, airmen and marines alive and whole: in the words of Abraham Lincoln, to minister to "him who has borne the brunt of battle."

This revised edition represents the contributions of talented and gifted health professionals from the military services as well as from the civilian sector. All who contributed have the grateful appreciation of the editorial board for the enthusiasm, dedication, and perseverance which made this revision possible.

William Mayer, M.D.

WILLIAM MAYER, M.D.
Assistant Secretary of Defense
(Health Affairs)

Preface

This edition of the Emergency War Surgery Handbook is written for and dedicated to the new generation of young, as yet
untested surgeons, who may be given the opportunity and the
honor of ministering to the needs of their fallen fellow coun-
trymen. What is the likelihood that you will be called to serve? The
ancient Plato provided the answer: "Only the dead have seen the
end of war!"

Will you be adequate, will you be successful in salvaging the lives
and limbs of those comrades by applying the principles of the
lessons hard-learned by countless generations of combat surgeons
that have preceded you? The answer is a resounding yes, for "I
would remind you how large and various is the experience of the
battlefield and how fertile the blood of warriors in the rearing of
good surgeons" (T. Clifford Albutt).

What sort of wounds will you be expected to manage? The
Wound Data and Munitions Effectiveness Team (WDMET) data
derived from the Vietnam battlefield provide some insight into
the types of wounds and the casualty mix that might be expected.
The WDMET data indicate that 100 combat casualties, who survive long enough to be evacuated from the field, could be
statistically expected to present the following casualty mix:

Thirty casualties with minor or superficial wounds, minor
burns, abrasions, foreign bodies in the eye, ruptured ear drums,
and deafness.

Sixteen with open, comminuted fractures of a long bone, of
which several will be multiple and several will be associated with
injury of named nerves.

Ten with major soft tissue injury or burns requiring general
anesthesia for debridement. Several will have injury of named
nerves.

Ten will require laparotomy, of which two will be negative and
several will involve extensive, complicated procedures.

Six with open, comminuted fractures of the hand, fingers, feet or toes.

Five will require closed thoracostomies and soft tissue wound management; at least one will have a minithoracotomy.

Four will have major multiple trauma, i.e., various combinations of craniotomies, thoracotomies, laparotomies, amputations, vascular reconstructions, soft tissue debridements, or fracture management.

Three will be major amputations (AK, BK, arm, forearm). In three out of four, the surgeon will simply complete the amputation.

Three craniotomies. Two will be craniectomies for fragments and one will involve elevation of a depressed fracture.

Three vascular reconstructions, half involving femoral arteries. One-half will have associated fractures, or venous or nerve injuries.

Three major eye injuries, one of which will require enucleation.

Two amputations of hands, fingers, feet or toes.

Two maxillofacial reconstructions. Half will have mandibular injuries and most of the remainder will have maxillary injuries.

One formal thoracotomy.

One neck exploration (usually negative).

One casualty statistically is delivered up by the computer as "miscellaneous."

If this surgical handbook is on the mark in achieving its objective, we will have provided you with specific guidelines or general principles governing the management of the foregoing 100 randomly selected battle casualties.

There are some who, as they study the chapters that follow, will perceive this handbook guidance as overly regimented, too rigid or prescriptive, and leaving too little room for the individual surgeon's judgment. On the contrary, these lessons and countless others have had to be learned and relearned by generations of surgeons pressed into the combat surgical environment. These very standardized approaches are necessitated by the echeloned management of casualties by many different practitioners at several different sites along a diverse evacuation chain, as opposed to the civil sector in which an individual surgeon can hold and manage an individual patient throughout that patient's entire course. Historically, these standardized approaches have repeatedly provided the highest standard of care to the greatest number of casualties.

Several chapters have been completely rewritten and two new chapters have been added to this edition. In an attempt to maintain perspective and continuity between this and the First United States Edition of the Emergency War Surgery NATO Handbook, Professor T.J. Whelan was asked to write a "bridge" between his and this edition. The advice, counsel, and contributions of this outstanding soldier, surgeon, and citizen are truly appreciated. His prologue to the Second United States Edition follows forthwith.

THOMAS E. BOWEN, M.D.
Editor
Brigadier General, U.S. Army

Prologue

This is a handbook of war surgery. Its lessons have been learned and then taught by combat surgeons — "young men who must have good hands, a stout heart and not too much philosophy; he is called upon for decision rather than discussion, for action rather than a knowledge of what the best writers think should be done."

In a world where multinational forces may be thrown together on one side in a large war, a need was clearly seen for standardization of equipment and techniques among nations expected to fight as allies. In 1957, SHAPE (Supreme Headquarters Allied Powers Europe) published the first Emergency War Surgery Handbook, familiarly known as the NATO Handbook. This was the product of a committee of the surgical consultants of the United Kingdom, France, and the United States, chaired by Brigadier General Sam F. Seeley of the United States. In 1958, the handbook was issued in the United States following suitable amendments. In April, 1959, the NATO Military Agency for Standardization promulgated NATO Standardization Agreement (STANAG) 2068, which retrospectively placed a stamp of approval on the Emergency War Surgery Handbook of 1957 by agreeing that NATO Armed Forces would standardize emergency war surgery according to its contents and tenets. This handbook, in addition to being issued to all active duty medical officers in the U.S. Armed Forces Medical Departments, was also forwarded to medical school surgical departments and libraries. At that time the MEND (Medical Education for National Defense) program war active. This was an excellent program, instituted in all university medical schools by the universities and the armed forces, in which a faculty representative, normally a surgeon, was selected to be briefed on a regular basis by the medical departments of the armed forces and, in turn, to teach principles of care of military casualties at their respective schools. Much of the early exposure of these individuals dealt with the concept of mass casualties and thermonuclear warfare.

In 1970, Dr. Louis M. Rousselot, Assistant Secretary of Defense for Health and Environment, an outstanding surgeon himself, realizing that, during the Korean and Vietnam conflicts, new surgical information had been learned or relearned and that this new information required broad exposure, tasked the Army Surgeon General to update the Emergency War Surgery Handbook. The editorial board for the new U.S. edition consisted of Rear Admiral Edward J, Rupnick, MC, US Navy; Colonel Robert Dean, MC, USAF; Colonel Richard R. Torp, MC, USA; and Brigadier General Thomas J. Whelan, Jr., MC, USA, who chaired the board. Chapters were rewritten, and the format changed to include chapters on aeromedical evacuation, mass casualties in thermonuclear warfare, and reoperative abdominal surgery. The final paragraphs on mass casualties in each chapter of the original handbook were excluded. At the same time, a NATO Handbook Revision Committee chaired by Colonel Tommy A. Pace, RAMC, and with representatives from the United Kingdom, France, the Federal Republic of Germany, the Netherlands, and Greece has been proceeding with minor chapter changes. The U.S. committee felt that the NATO committee might welcome the more extensive changes. Therefore, in 1973 the completed revision of the U.S. Handbook was presented to the committee. Within 48 hours there was a unanimous decision to accept the new U.S. edition with certain minor modifications and to use it as the basis of a new edition for NATO nations. These modifications were proposed by the representative from France; they related to a description of an external fixation device for use in open fractures and to a minor change in the management of chest injuries. It seems certain that no NATO accord ever came so swiftly or easily. The goodwill on both sides was exemplary and heartening. In 1975, the new U.S. edition was published, and in 1977 it became the guide for all NATO forces, pursuant to a reissue of STANAG 2068. Now it is time for a third edition.

War surgery represents no crude departure from accepted surgical standards. A major responsibility of all military surgeons is to maintain these principles and practices as fully as possible, even under adverse physical conditions. The physical requirements are, however, relatively simple:

1. Experienced surgeon, anesthetist, and operating room personnel.

2. Simple X-ray facilities.

3. Good lighting and water supplies.

4. Reasonable accommodations under shelter.

5. Well-trained nurses and other professional administrative staff.

6. Ability to retain post-operative patients in the hospital for at least a few days to allow stabilization.

7. Simple surgical equipment, supplemented by a few items of specialized equipment, such as Bovie units, defibrillators, ventilators, blood gas machines, anesthesia delivery equipment, and vascular and orthopedic instruments.

There are, however, differences betwen war surgery and surgery in the civilian setting:

1. The tactical situation may impose major constraints upon the performance of the indicated operation, and threats to the safety of the patient and medical personnel may make appropriate care inconvenient, if not impossible.

2. The high-velocity weapons of war may produce tremendously greater tissue destruction than the low-velocity weapons producing civilian wounds.

3. There are few civilian wounds which resemble the multiple fragment wounds of artillery or mortar shells, bombs, booby traps, and landmines.

4. Wounds are cared for by many surgeons along an evacuation chain that extends from combat zone to home, rather than by one surgeon and his house staff throughout all phases of wound repair.

5. Casualties are frequently received in large numbers over a short time in combat hospitals. Although an occasional catastrophe of similar magnitude has occurred in a few metropolitan civilian hospitals, this is a commonplace occurrence in forward combat hospitals.

6. During aeromedical evacuation, the casualty will require long flights during which lowered air pressure may complicate abdominal, chest, eye, head, and spinal wounds. The cabins of high-altitude aircraft are pressurized only to about 4,000-8,000 feet above sea level, and not to sea level pressures.

We are now faced with a fast-moving, highly mobile, remote control type of warfare which will require major changes in philosophy and management of war casualties. It may, for instance, be necessary to evacuate casualties much earlier than the organism's physiologic responses to injury dictate as optimal. The initial definitive surgery may be required aloft or on shipboard. Or because of noxious fumes or radioactive dust, we may find it necessary to emulate the mole, remaining underground for protracted periods. We must not ever expect that the protected hospital environments of the Korean or Vietnam conflicts, bought with very necessary air superiority, will necessarily be present in future conflicts. Plans for the care of the wounded must be laced with a generous sprinkling of multiple alternatives and options, ranging from immediate air or surface evacuation with delayed suboptimal definitive surgical care to the more standard, early definitive treatment in a combat hospital with a 4-10 day retention period prior to further evacuation. The latter is optimal; the former, however, may be forced by the tactical situation.

As in any medical endeavor, prevention is far more efficacious than treatment. This is true for wounds sustained in war. Unfortunately, there is no precedent to suggest that man and nations have learned to coexist without armed conflict. Although I, personally, and most military men, who "above all other people pray for peace, for they must suffer and bear the deepest wounds and scars of war" (quoted from General Douglas MacArthur's oration "Duty, Honor, Country"), would be profoundly grateful if this handbook might become superfluous, redundant, and unnecessary, it nonetheless continues to serve a useful purpose in these times. Furthermore, a reasonably standard, phased method of treatment of war wounds, to be enunciated in the remainder of this handbook, is imperative when many surgeons, of multiple national extractions, along long evacuation chains, care for those wounded in combat.

Thomas J. Whelan, Jr.

THOMAS J. WHELAN, JR.
Brigadier General (RET)
Medical Corps, U.S. Army

Acknowledgements

Appreciation is expressed to those authors who provided manuscripts for the second United States revision of the *NATO Handbook on Emergency War Surgery.* Some chapters are entirely new and some have been substantially revised, while a few chapters from the previous edition required only very minor changes. To avoid implying authorship of those first U.S. edition chapters that required only minimal revision, all contributors are cited alphabetically rather than in association with a specific chapter.

Robert A. Albus, COL, MC, US Army
Peter J. Barcia, COL, MC, US Army
Roberto H. Barja, COL, MC, US Army
Ronald F. Bellamy, COL, MC, US Army
George P. Bogumill, COL, MC, US Army (RET)
Thomas E. Bowen, BG, MC, US Army
Scott H. Burner, MAJ, MC, US Army
Richard A. Camp, COL, MC, US Army
Frank A. Cammarata, COL, MSC, US Army
William G. Cioffi, CPT, MC, US Army
Howard B. Cohen, COL, MC, US Army (RET)
George J. Collins, Jr., COL, MC, US Army (RET)
Brian F. Condon, COL, MC, US Army
James J. Conklin, COL, MC, US Air Force (RET)
Donald T. Crump, National Institutes of Health
Howard P. Cupples, CPT, MC, US Navy (RET)
Rudolph H. de Jong, Former COL, MC, US Army
Teodoro F. Dagi, LTC, MC, US Army
Eran Dolev, BG MC (RET) Israeli Defense Force
Martin L. Fackler, COL, MC, US Army
David A. Gaule, MAJ, MSC, US Army
Eugene D. George, COL, MC, US Army
Geoffrey M. Graeber, LTC, MC, US Army
Theresa A. Graves, CPT, MC, US Army
Robert G. Grossman, MD, Baylor University

John H. Hagmann, MAJ, MC, US Army
Murray E. Hamlet, DVM, DAC
Ben T. Ho, CAPT, MC, US Navy
John H. Hutton, Jr., COL, MC, US Army
Joseph P. Jackson, Jr., COL, MC, US Army (RET)
Mark R. Jackson, CPT, MC, US Army
Darrell A. Jaques, COL, MC, US Army (RET)
John J. Kearney, COL, MC, US Army
David G. Kline, MD, Louisiana State University
Francis G. La Piana, COL, MC, US Army
Manfred W. Liechtmann, COL, MC, US Army (RET)
Douglas Lindsey, COL, MC, US Army (RET)
Judson C. Lively, CPT, MC, US Army
John E. Major, MG, MC, US Army
Arthur D. Mason, MD, DAC
David G. McLeod, COL, MC, US Army
William F. McManus, COL, MC, US Army
Paul R. Meyer, Jr., COL, MC, US Army Reserve
William J. Mills, Jr., RADM, MC, US Naval Reserve (RET)
Stanley J. Pala, COL, MC, US Air Force (RET)
Yancy Y. Phillips, LTC, MC, US Army
Basil A. Pruitt, Jr., COL, MC, US Army
William J. Reynolds, COL, MC, US Army Reserve
Norman M. Rich, COL, MC, US Army (RET)
James M. Salander, COL, MC, US Army
John R. Saunders, Jr., COL, MC, US Army Reserve
Carlton G. Savory, COL, MC, US Army (RET)
Lloyd A. Schlaeppi, COL, MSC, US Army
David Shelton, COL, DC, US Army (RET)
Stephen A. Sihelnik, MAJ, MC, US Army
Michael B. Strauss, CAPT, MC, USNR-R
Ray E. Stutzman, COL, MC, US Army (RET)
Jack K. Tippens, COL, MC, US Army
Richard I. Walker, CDR, MC, US Navy
Thomas J. Whelan, Jr., BG, MC, US Army (RET)
Paul V. Whitmore, COL, MC, US Army (RET)
Joan T. Zajtchuk, COL, MC, US Army

Special thanks to Ms. Coleen M. Treser for typing the manuscripts.

Contents

CONTENTS

CONTENTS

Illustrations

Tables

CHAPTER I

General Considerations of Forward Surgery

Military surgery, a subset within the art and science of surgery, is designed to carry out a specialized and highly significant mission under the adverse conditions of war. The mission of military surgery differs from civil sector surgery in that it is limited to emergency surgery that is performed on a mass production basis in what may amount to severely limiting circumstances. Stated another way, the military medical officer does what must be done rather than what could be done to the casualty before either returning him to his unit or rendering him transportable to the next higher echelon of medical care. To achieve these objectives, the military surgical care system depends upon an organized prehospital treatment and medical evacuation system and utilizes somewhat different and successively staged techniques to treat the penetrating, perforating, and blast injuries of the battlefield. These wounds and their method, of management differ from those of a community practice in which the preponderance of surgery is elective and the majority of trauma is blunt. The additional necessity of haste in caring for the continuous flow of battle casualties does not mean that military surgery is carried out in an atmosphere of confusion and disorder or that standard principles of treatment are abandoned. On the contrary, as all past military history shows, intelligent planning and appropriate training in anticipation of the needs of the battlefield have resulted in enviable ånd ever-improving military medical results.

The currently employed, phased concept of wound management was developed, to a large extent, by Colonel Edward Churchill during World War II. *Initial surgery*, if necessary, rendered the casualty *transportable* via rapid evacuation to a rear hospital for *reparative surgery*. The initial surgical effort at the forward facility, by definition, was not complete surgery, but rather "that initial effort required to save life and limb, prevent infection and render

1

the casualty transportable.... Surgical procedures not essential to wound management at that time may make a transportable patient non-transportable and are to be avoided." This concept of wound management allowed forward hospitals to be more mobile and concentrated more resource-intensive casualty care far to the rear in secure base areas where evacuation hospitals were not required to move with changing tactical situations. This phased approach to the management of war wounds has withstood the test of time. However, the newer technologies of warfare will inevitably increase the depth and breadth of the modern battlefield. Fundamental changes in the nature of warfare will dictate certain alterations in the way medical assets accomplish their missions.

What are the missions of the combat commander's medical assets? And what are the relative priorities of those medical missions? The conservation of the army's fighting strength is clearly the primary goal. This goal is achieved by accomplishing several interwoven goals, listed not necessarily in rank order of importance: the maintenance of the health of the command, the prevention of loss of the fighting strength to disease, the very positive contribution to high morale and promotion of the individual soldier's willingness to fight by establishing a visibly creditable medical system, the provision of timely and efficient evacuation of casualties from the battlefield, and the preservation of life and limb.

How one structures his combat medical care delivery system will depend in large measure upon the nature of the war, the quantitative and qualitative aspects of the casualty load and the medical personnel, logistical and physical plant capabilities. If the nature of the war allows, sophisticated medical facilities can be positioned very near the wounded soldier. If not, the soldier must be moved considerable distances to the well-equipped, relatively immobile "state-of-the-art" surgical hospital. As a general rule, as the medics increase their technical capabilities, they do so at the price of increased requirements for complex equipment, which in turn requires increased lift. These increased cube and gross weight medical airlift requirements compete with combat arms lift requirements. Combat hospitals are already large, bulky, and difficult to move. Highly sophisticated hospitals in the battle zone could encumber the combat commander, restrict his freedom of movement, and at times become a liability rather than an asset. A battlefield medical system must be a compromise between what is best for the soldier and what is best for the conduct of the battle. The basic objective is the realistic minimization of the loss of life and limb.

Examples of two different approaches to combat casualty care can be drawn from World War II. The medical system of the German Army in Russia in 1941 was designed to evacuate the seriously wounded well to the rear and to care for the lightly wounded at the divisional level. This approach required only half as many medical personnel and achieved higher return-to-duty rates than did the U.S. Army's system in France in 1944, because the German system was intentionally designed for return to duty. The American system, on the other hand, returned proportionately fewer casualties to their combat units, but salvaged many more lives because of the capability to perform lifesaving surgery further forward. The ideal system for the modern battlefield must be optimized to maximize return to duty without sacrificing life or limb.

In the event of a sudden, so-called "come-as-you-are" war, medical channels that return soldiers to duty may be the only functional personnel replacement system during the first few weeks of a lightning war. In this sort of scenario, it is of critical importance to the war effort that lightly wounded soldiers who do not require hospitalization be treated at or returned to their divisional areas if they can be held there without encumbering their combat commanders. We refer here to soldiers who are mobile and quite capable of defending themselves, but not yet ready to return to the fire fight. These valuable personnel assets are already trained, are battle-hardened, and are quickly available as opposed to untried replacements who must be transported from a distant homeland. The combat medical system of the short, lightning war must not be allowed to become a giant evacuation conduit through which trained, blooded soldiers pour out of the theater. The medical officer must "fix forward," for as has been said, "The farther a wounded soldier is evacuated from the combat zone, the greater will be his number of noneffective man-days and the less will be his motivation to return to combat duty." In the near-chaos of the mass casualty situation, medical officers must be ever-vigilant in their search for the lightly wounded, but heavily bandaged, casualty who can be returned to his unit rather than further retrograded through medical evacuation channels.

As alluded to earlier, advances in technology are changing the nature of modern warfare. The battlefield of the future will be broader, deeper, more fluid, more destructive, and more resource-hungry. The concepts of phased wound management and initial and reparative surgery will certainly persist but the distances between echelons may be significantly increased. Resource-intensive facilities that are staffed to perform reparative surgery will, of tactical necessity, be deployed considerably further to the rear. The same could pertain, although to a lesser extent, to facilities that perform initial wound surgery. The same technology that increases the depth of the battlefield and of necessity forces fixed surgical capabilities further to the rear may also provide practical solutions. A new tiltrotor aircraft, with the vertical take-off and landing capabilities of a conventional helicopter is currently undergoing flight testing. This twin-engined craft, in the air ambulance configuration, is capable of picking up and moving twelve litter cases plus three medical attendants at speeds of up to 300 nautical miles/hour with a range of 1,000 nautical miles.

It is not inconceivable that on a highly mobile battlefield, initial wound surgery may have to be performed very far forward under extremely austere, even primitive, conditions within enveloped enclaves. Surgical teams carrying their equipment in rucksacks on their backs may be tasked to perform only that emergency life-saving surgery required to make the casualty transportable. Surgical teams of this sort would be assigned to airborne or air assault units that habitually operate in isolation for short periods of time. Other surgical capabilities would be brought forward and deployed as the situation requires and permits.

Another aspect of the recently envisioned "fix forward" approach to combat casualty care is the two-track flow of casualties. This system would divide the casualty flow at the division-level medical facility (Figure 1).

Casualties who are not expected to return to duty within the time constraints of the theater evacuation policy are passed through a chain of evacuation hospitals and out of the theater as rapidly as their conditions will permit. Only that surgery which is necessary to permit transport to the next hospital in the chain—generally planned as six-hour bed-to-bed moves—would be performed. These hospitals would serve as trauma centers and be equipped and staffed to stabilize casualties for transport back to a secure base. If that secure base were in the continental United States, the last hospital in the theater evacuation chain would do

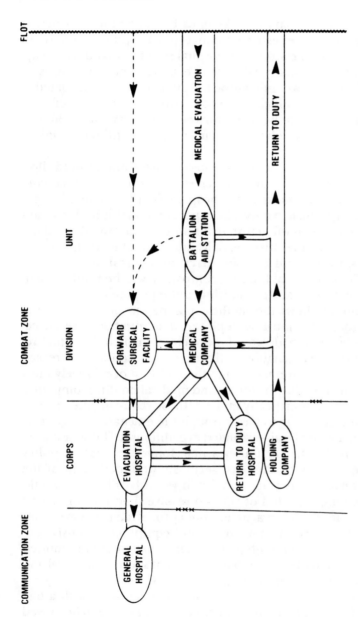

FIGURE 1.—Generic organizational diagram for combat casualty care. Width of pathway is proportional to size of casualty populations. Broken line indicates potential for aeromedical evacuation from the field of the critically injured. Triage identifies three groups of casualties: 1) those needing urgent surgery, 2) those likely to have an early return to duty, and 3) those requiring evacuation from the combat zone.

whatever was necessary for a 24-hour bed-to-bed move. Current evacuation doctrine restricts combat zone hospital stays to seven days and communication zone hospital stays to thirty days. If it appears that the casualty will require more than seven days of hospitalization in a combat zone hospital, he will be evacuated as rapidly as is safely possible to a communications zone facility. If that casualty will not be ready for return to duty within 30 days at this level, he is expediently evacuated to the continental United States.

Casualties on the other track (those whose wounds would allow return to duty within the theater evacuation policy time constraints) would be moved to a hospital facility intended to encourage early return to duty. The expectation in this facility would be that each patient will return to his unit and the war. When these soldiers no longer require the daily attention of medical officers or nurses, they would be transferred to medical holding companies. These medical holding companies will be minimal self-care facilities with austere staffing and equipment.

This model allows the medical planner to better tailor the medical force that must be deployed. The number of resource-intensive hospital beds would more closely match the actual requirements. The evacuation policy timeframe could be increased with the only requirement being the addition of relatively inexpensive return-to-duty hospitals and medical holding companies to the theater. The critically injured (those requiring the greatest care) would continue to pass through the evacuation or general hospital chain and be air-evacuated expeditiously. Those casualties retained in the theater under a new, longer evacuation policy would necessarily be the least seriously wounded or ill of the population formerly evacuated. Their wounds or illnesses would require a longer period of time to resolve than those retained under the old, shorter evacuation policy timeframe; however, they would not require the personnel- and equipment-intensive environment of evacuation-type hospitals. They would be shunted to and treated in the return-to-duty (combat support) hospital and convalesce in medical holding companies.

The medical planner of the future may be faced with a battlefield of such great depth that casualties may have to be moved very great distances to reach secure base areas where reparative surgery can be performed. The feasibility of safely accomplishing prolonged moves of fresh casualties has been demonstrated several times in the recent past. In the 1973 Arab-Israeli War, more than 4,000 stable casualties were evacuated approximately 150 miles from the Sinai to central Israel for definitive care. Most arrived within 24 hours of being wounded. In the Falklands Campaign, the British evacuated more than 500 casualties to the United Kingdom by way of Uruguay and the Ascension Islands. This 8,000 mile trip required 20 hours. The majority of casualties arrived within 48-72 hours of wounding. Following the 1983 terrorist bombing of the U.S. Marine Barracks in Lebanon, 55 casualties were evacuated directly to USAF medical facilities in West Germany within hours of injury. Although there was some criticism of this move, an examination of patient outcomes suggest that the results would probably have been the same had they been taken to closer medical facilities.

ECHELONS OF MEDICAL CARE

A basic characteristic of the organization of modern military medical services is the distribution of medical resources and medical capabilities to facilities at various levels of location and function, which are referred to in formal military parlance as "echelons". Echelonment is a matter of principle, practice, and organizational pattern, not a matter of rigid prescription. Scopes of function may be expanded or contracted on sound indication; one or more echelons may be bypassed on grounds of efficiency or expediency, and formal organizational structure will differ with time and among various armed forces. The following general pattern; however, is usually apparent.

ECHELONS OF COMBAT MEDICAL CARE

1. At the first echelon (Level 1) a "buddy" (or the trained medical aidman) provides first aid and conveys or directs the casualty to the battalion aid station. The U.S. Army, in an effort to upgrade "buddy aid", provides all basic trainees with 16 hours of first aid training. A more recent initiative identifies one member of each crew-served weapon system (air crew, tank crew, mortar crew, weapons team, etc.) with 40 additional hours of first aid training. Because of the proximity of the aid station to the battlefield, its mission is simply to provide essential emergency care allowing the

return of the soldier to duty or the preparation of the casualty for evacuation to the rear. In the former case, this care would be minimal, whereas in the latter case care might include the establishment of an airway, the control of hemorrhage, the application of field dressings, the administration of an analgesic, or the initiation of intravenous fluid administration.

2. Second echelon care (Level 2), depending on the circumstances, is rendered at an assembly point, a clearing station, or the brigade medical company. Here the casualty is examined, and his wounds and general status are evaluated to determine his priority, as a single casualty among other casualties, for return to duty or continued evacuation to the rear. Emergency care, including beginning resuscitation, is continued and, if necessary, additional emergency measures are instituted, but they do not go beyond the measures dictated by the immediate necessities. This function is performed typically by company-size medical units organic to the brigade or division. These units have the capability to hold and treat the most lightly wounded.

3. At the third echelon of care (Level 3), the casualty is treated in a medical installation staffed and equipped to provide resuscitation, initial wound surgery, and postoperative treatment. Casualties whose wounds make them nontransportable receive surgical care in a hospital close to the clearing station. Those whose injuries permit additional transportation without detriment receive surgical care in a hospital farther to the rear.

4. In the fourth echelon (Level 4) of medical care, the casualty is treated in a general hospital staffed and equipped for definitive care. General hospitals are located in the communications zone, which is the support area to the combat zone or army area. The mission of these hospitals is the rehabilitation of casualties to duty status. If rehabilitation cannot be accomplished within a predetermined holding period, these casualties are evacuated to the Zone of Interior (Level 5) for reconstructive surgery and rehabilitation.

It is important to remember that there is a logistical problem in the care of all battle casualties. Military medical facilities must always be in a state of readiness to receive an influx of fresh battle casualties or to move according to the dictates of the tactical situation, though this necessity in no way lessens the responsibility of the medical service for providing for the medical care and disposition of casualties. Despite the exceedingly unfavorable circumstances of war, movement of casualties from echelon to echelon in the forward area is usually accomplished within a matter of hours. Distances, which are usually measured in terms of ground transportation or flight time, vary with the local tactical situation, but as a general rule, casualties are moved a distance of many miles between the battlefront and a hospital.

Because the individual who has been wounded in combat is cared for by multiple surgeons at different echelons of medical care and because hospitals at different echelons are usually separated by great distances, the consultant system has been developed. Certain individuals, selected as consultants because of their expertise in a given specialty field, have been utilized to evaluate and correlate end results noted in hospitals of the communication zone with initial surgical care provided in the combat zone. The responsibility for evaluating the effectiveness of combat surgery and for feedback to the individual surgeons in forward hospitals resides with these consultants. To augment the consultant system, professional meetings of practicing surgeons from both the combat and the communication zone hospitals have been utilized to evaluate the results and to exchange views on methods of surgical care. During the Vietnam conflict, annual War Surgery Conferences were held to bring American surgeons at all levels and from all branches of the armed services up to date on the latest information and results in the care of the wounded.

PART I

Types of Wounds and Injuries

CHAPTER II

Missile-Caused Wounds

INTRODUCTION

Previous contributions to earlier editions of this handbook devoted considerable effort to differentiating between the magnitude of injury caused by "ordinary" versus "high" velocity missile wounds. To a certain extent, as a result of experience gained in recent conflicts and to a greater extent based on wound ballistic research performed over the past decade, new and somewhat different concepts are evolving. One very fundamental concept is that the high-velocity wound is not necessarily a totally different entity, as had been previously thought.

Certain misconceptions continue to be associated with the high-velocity projectile. One misconception concerns the very development of high-velocity weapons. The explanation usually encountered is that these weapons were developed to deliver greater wounding power and higher lethality. Proponents offer the kinetic energy formula in support of their position. Weapons developers state that the real reason that certain countries shifted to low-weight, high-velocity projectiles was that their soldiers (who were not the best marksmen) tended to conserve their ammunition and were not discharging their weapons until the enemy was close at hand. It was reasoned that an automatic weapon would obviate some of these shortcomings. From a practical standpoint, the automatic weapon, with its increased requirement for ammunition, necessitated lighter weight ammunition. To compensate for the loss in missile mass, if wounding power was to be maintained, it was necessary to increase missile velocity. These tradeoffs resulted in considerably less recoil, making it easier to maintain the sight picture on repetitive shots, resulting in increased accuracy. The lighter cartridge allowed the individual infantryman to carry the increase in basic load of ammunition (more rounds, same weight) and allowed the maneuver element to present the enemy with greater and more sustained firepower.

These are important considerations as the spectrum of warfare shifts more to the left, such as with guerilla-type warfare in which small units engage one another at isolated points, usually at considerable distances from strong points that offer safe haven and resupply. In circumstances such as these, the ability to carry double or triple the basic ammunition load allows small units to take advantage of the increased and sustained firepower that lighter, higher velocity missiles offer. It was for this reason that the current generation of high-velocity weapons was designed, rather than to develop a weapon that inflicts a more severe wound.

It is vigorously affirmed by some that velocity, almost to the exclusion of mass, is the operative factor in wounding power. From a theoretical standpoint, velocity can be the dominant determinant of kinetic energy (KE); doubling the mass only doubles the KE, whereas doubling the velocity quadruples the KE. However, from a practical standpoint, doubling the velocity is very difficult to achieve. The M-16 represents only a 10% increase in velocity over the M-14 it replaced. On the other hand, quadrupling the mass is easy. Switch from a .22 to a .44 caliber projectile and you immediately square the mass; then double the length of the projectile so that it flies straighter and you now have an eightfold increase in KE at the same velocity.

There are some who mistakenly believe that only the more modern, higher velocity projectiles produce temporary cavitation. The 1870-1890 Vetterli deforming bullet, typical of the military rounds utilized at that time, is depicted in Figure 2. It should be noted that in spite of its relatively low velocity, only 1,357 ft/sec, a very substantial temporary cavity is produced. The formation of a temporary cavity is not a new phenomenon associated with modern high-velocity weapons.

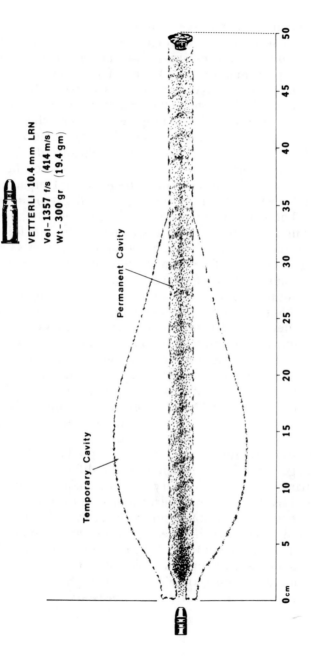

FIGURE 2.—*Wound Profile.* This large lead bullet, used by the Swiss and Italian Armies (1870-1890), is typical of the projectiles used by military forces in the latter half of the 19th century. It produces a very substantial temporary cavity despite its "low" velocity.

Some maintain that a larger-exit-than-entry wound is evidence of the devastating potential of increases in velocity. While this in fact may be the case (and exit wounds are larger than entry wounds in about 60 percent of the cases), the difference in the size of the wound of entry and exit is not per se directly attributable to velocity since the velocity is greater at the smaller entry wound and lesser at the greater exit wound. The larger exit wound, when present, is caused by projectile yaw, by projectile fragmentation, or as a result of multiple secondary bone fragment projectile. Projectile yaw represents a deviation of the longitudinal axis of the bullet from its line of flight. Rifling within the gun barrel impacts a spin to the bullet, which stabilizes the projectile's flight in air, preventing yaw. The stability imparted by rifling is not enough to prevent yaw in tissues or when the missile passes through foliage or other intermediate objects. Tumbling simply represents yaw that has progressed to a full 180°, at which point the center of mass results in stabilized base-forward flight.

The point to be borne in mind is that while the high-velocity projectile has the potential for higher energy transfer with subsequent greater tissue disruption, this may not always be the case. Whereas the military surgeon should have some familiarity with wound ballistics and the "worst case" result of high-velocity missile wounds, the surgeon is better advised to concern himself with the individual wound that confronts him rather than with the variable potential of the weapon. On the other hand, wounds of the brain, liver, and heart caused by high-velocity projectiles are catastrophic in nature.

The study of wound ballistics attempts to predict and to analyze the damage that will be sustained by the different tissue types when struck by missiles of varying sizes, shapes, weights, and velocities. Missiles that penetrate the human body disrupt, destroy, or contuse tissue, invariably resulting in a contaminated wound. Subsequent triage and treatment decisions are based upon an estimation of the type of wound, the location of the wound, and the amount of tissue disruption. Objective data from the physical examination and appropriate roentgenographic studies of the casualty provide the information necessary to make these decisions.

MECHANISMS OF WOUNDING

The penetrating missile or fragment destroys tissue by *crushing* it as it punches a hole through the tissue (Figure 3). This hole or missile track represents the so-called *permanent cavity*. The cross-sectional area of the missile track is comparable to the presenting area of the missile and its dimensions are roughly the same for all soft tissues.

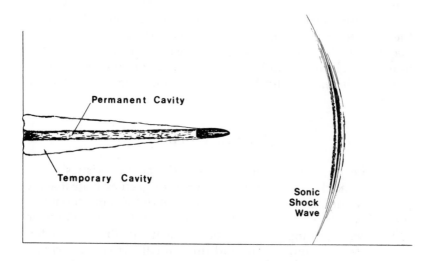

FIGURE 3.—The sonic shock wave and temporary cavity. Diagram of bullet passing through tissue showing sonic shock wave and the formation of a temporary cavity by outward stretch of the permanent cavity.

After passage of the projectile, the walls of the permanent cavity are temporarily stretched radially outward. The maximum lateral tissue displacement delineates the *temporary cavity*. Any damage resulting from temporary cavitation is due to *stretching* of the tissue. Resistance or vulnerability to stretch damage depends mostly on tissue elasticity. The same stretch which causes only moderate contusion and minor functional changes in relatively elastic skeletal muscle, can cause devastating disruption of the liver. The result of temporary displacement of tissue is analogous to a localized area of blunt trauma surrounding the permanent cavity left by the projectile's passage.

The typical wounding potential of a given missile can be assessed by measuring the two types of tissue disruption it produces.

A method developed by U.S. Army researchers captures the entire path of missiles fired through gelatin tissue-simulant blocks. Measurements taken from the gelatin are used to illustrate the location and the extent of both crush and stretch types of tissue disruption on a drawing or "Wound Profile". The scale included on each profile can be used to measure the extent of tissue disruption at any point along the path of the projectile. This method allows comparison of the wound profiles of different wounding agents.

The sonic shock wave seen at the far right of Figure 3 precedes the projectile's passage through the tissue. Although the magnitude of the sonic wave may range up to pressures of 100 atmospheres, its duration is so brief, about 2 microseconds, that it does not displace tissue. It has no detectable harmful effect on tissues.

PROJECTILES

The following is a compendium of the characteristics of the more commonly encountered small arms projectiles. Note that the projectiles depicted in Figures 4-9 do not deform upon passing through soft tissues, whereas those in Figures 10-14 either deform or fragment, forming secondary bullet fragments. Projectile deformation, fragmentation, yaw and individually or collectively increase the resultant degree of tissue disruption.

45 AUTOMATIC—This full-metal-jacketed military bullet (Figure 4) is one of few that does not yaw (turn the long axis in relation to direction of travel) significantly in soft tissue. Lack of yaw, coupled with the large mass of this bullet, results in deep penetration. The crush tissue disruption remains nearly constant throughout the bullet path. Temporary cavity stretch is maximal near the point of entry, gradually diminishing with penetration, but with this bullet type and velocity the temporary cavity is too small to show a stretch wounding effect.

22 LONG RIFLE—This commonly used rimfire bullet (Figure 5) yaws through 90° and ends up traveling base forward for the last half of its tissue path. The crush tissue disruption increases with yaw angle, reaching its maximum when the bullet is traveling sideways. Temporary cavity stretch increases with increasing bullet yaw, much the same as a diver hitting the water makes a

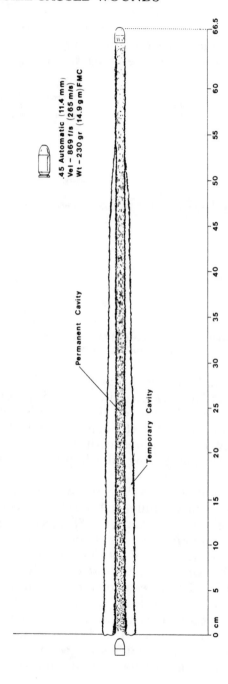

FIGURE 4.—45 Automatic. This was the standard U.S. Army pistol until recently. The short, round-nosed, full-metal-cased bullet does not deform or yaw significantly in tissue but penetrates deeply.

larger splash as his body angle to the water surface increases. Even at the point of maximum bullet yaw, the temporary cavity produced remains too small to add a detectable stretch wounding effect.

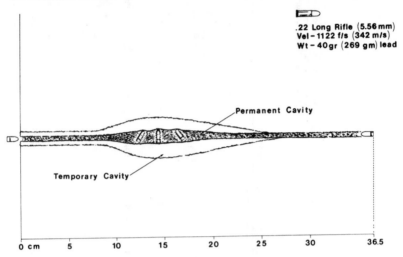

.22 Long Rifle (5.56 mm)
Vel – 1122 f/s (342 m/s)
Wt – 40 gr (269 gm) lead

Permanent Cavity

Temporary Cavity

0 cm   5   10   15   20   25   30   36.5

FIGURE 5.—*22 Long Rifle.* This solid lead round-nosed bullet yaws through 90° and travels base-forward for the last half of its tissue path.

38 SPECIAL—This round-nosed lead bullet (Figure 6), like the 45 Automatic (Figure 4) and the 22 Long Rifle (Figure 5), produces its wounding almost solely by the crush tissue disruption mechanism. Although still too small to show an observable stretch wounding effect, the maximum temporary cavity is of 20% greater diameter than that made by the 22 Long Rifle despite the fact that its velocity is 40% less.

9 MM PARBELLUM—This bullet is widely used in both pistols and submachine guns. As with the full-metal-jacketed bullet type, it produces a profile that resembles that of the .38 Special (Figure 6), but the maximum temporary cavity is about 2 cm larger in diameter and will show some *stretch* effects (radial splits) in less elastic, more susceptible tissues such as those of the liver.

7.62 NATO FMC—FMC is the abbreviation for full-metal-cased, which is a synonym of full-metal-jacketed. This refers to the harder metal covering of the bullet core. This full-metal-jacketed military bullet (Figure 7) shows the characteristic behavior in tissue observed in non-deforming pointed bullets. It yaws through 90° and, after reaching the base-forward position, continues the rest

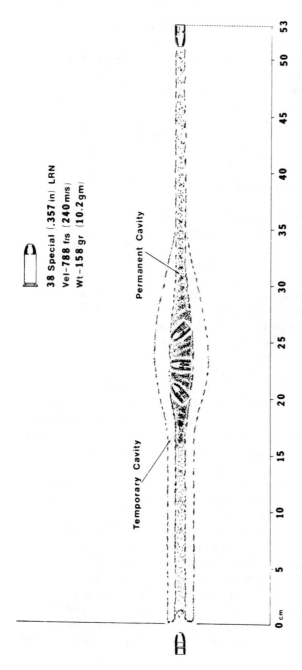

38 Special (.357 in) LRN
Vel–788 f/s (240 m/s)
Wt–158 gr (10.2 gm)

Permanent Cavity

Temporary Cavity

0 cm 5 10 15 20 25 30 35 40 45 50 53

Figure 6.—*38 Special lead, round-nosed bullet*Seven out of ten of these bullets yawed through 90° and traveled base forward for the latter part of their tissue paths as shown. Three shots yawed to about 80°, then straightened out and traveled point-forward for the remainder of their paths.

of its path with little or no yaw. The bullet is stable traveling base first in tissue, since this position puts its center of mass forward. The rotation imparted to the bullet by the rifled gun barrel is sufficient to cause point-forward travel in air, but not in tissue where such factors as bullet shape and location of center of mass outweigh rotation effects. The tissue disruption in the first 15-18 cm of bullet penetration, during which the streamlined bullet is still traveling point forward, is minimal. At 20-35 cm, however, in which bullet yaw is marked, a large temporary cavity is produced. If the bullet path is such that this temporary cavity occurs in the liver, this amount of tissue disruption is likely to make survival improbable.

AK-47—The Russian Assault Rifle's full-metal-cased military bullet (Figure 8) travels point forward for 25-27 cm in tissue prior to beginning significant yaw. Wounds from this rifle are familiar to surgeons who served in Vietnam and have been documented by the WDMET study of wounds from that conflict.

AK-74—This new generation, smaller caliber Russian Assault Rifle (Figure 9) follows the example set by the USA with the M-16. The full-metal-cased bullet designed for this weapon has a copper-plated steel jacket, as does the bullet of its predecessor, the AK-47. A unique design feature of the AK-74, however, is an air-space (about 5 mm long) inside the jacket at the bullet's tip. The speculation that this air-space would cause bullet deformation and fragmentation on impact proved to be unfounded, but the air-space does serve to shift the bullet's center of mass toward the rear. This bullet yaws after only about 7 cm of tissue penetration, assuring an increased temporary cavity stretch disruption, even in many extremity hits. The typical exit wound from a soft-tissue thigh wound (12 cm thick) is stellate, with skin split measuring from 9-13 cm across. The underlying muscle split is about half that size. The bilobed yaw patterns shown in the profiles of the AK-47 and the AK-74 represent what is seen in four-fifths of test shots. In the rest, the bullet reaches 90° of yaw and continues to 180° or the base, forward position, in one cycle. Whether there are one or two yaw cycles does not influence the point of prime clinical relevance—the distance the bullet travels point forward before yaw. The bilobed yaw pattern depicted in Figures 8 and 9 results from initial bullet yaw returning to zero yaw (first lobe), but then yawing a second time (second lobe) to 180° where the center of mass

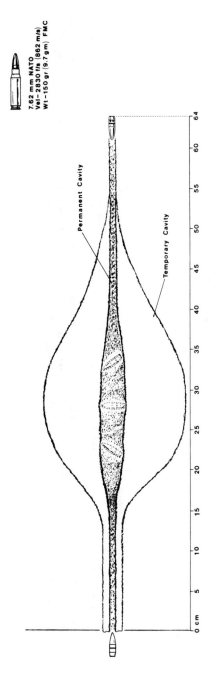

7.62 mm NATO
Vel – 2830 f/s (862 m/s)
Wt – 150 gr (9.7 gm) FMC

Permanent Cavity

Temporary Cavity

FIGURE 7.—*762 NATO cartridge with full-metal-cased military bullet.* This was the standard U.S. Army rifle until the adoption of the M-16 in the 1960's. It is still used in snipers' rifles and machine guns. After about 16 cm of penetration, this bullet yaws through 90° and travels base forward. A large temporary cavity is formed and occurs at point of maximum yaw.

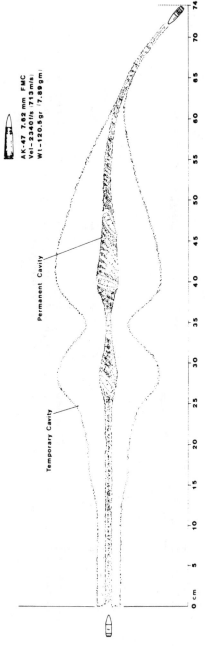

FIGURE 8.—*AK 47.* This was the standard rifle used by the communist forces in Vietnam and is used today very widely throughout the world. The long path through tissue before marked yaw begins (about 25 cm) explains the clinical experience that many wounds from this weapon resemble those caused by much lower velocity handguns.

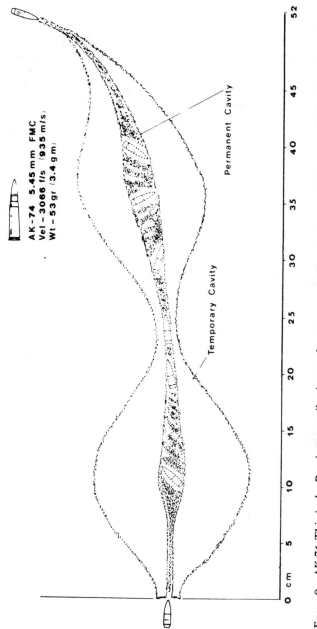

AK-74 5.45 mm FMC
Vel – 3066 f/s (935 m/s)
Wt – 53 gr (3.4 g m)

Permanent Cavity

Temporary Cavity

0 cm 5 10 15 20 25 30 35 40 45 52

FIGURE 9.—*AK 74.* This is the Russian contribution to the new generation of smaller caliber assault rifles. The bullet does not deform or fragment in soft tissue but yaws early (after about 7 cm of penetration). As this bullet strikes soft tissue, lead flows forward filling the air space inside the bullet's tip. X-rays of recovered fired bullets show that this "internal deformation" produces an asymmetrical bullet which may explain the unusual curve of close to 90° made by the bullet path in the latter part of its penetration.

stabilizes the projectile in base forward travel.

357 MAGNUM JSP—The jacketed soft-point bullet (Figure 10) and the jacketed-hollow-point bullet flatten their tips on impact. This "expansion" or "mushrooming" (in which the final bullet shape resembles a mushroom) results in a doubling of effective bullet diameter in tissue, and allows the bullet to crush four times as much tissue (π times radius squared equals the cross section area of the bullet which impacts tissue). This conversion of the bullet to a non-aerodynamic shape causes the same sort of increased temporary cavity tissue stretch as does the yawing of a bullet. The maximum temporary cavity produced by the expanding bullet occurs at a shallower penetration depth than that caused by the full-metal-jacketed military type bullet. This soft-point pistol bullet is typical of the type most commonly used by law enforcement agencies in the USA. Its decreased penetration depth, as compared to the depth of penetration of the nondeforming bullets depicted in Figures 2 and 4, decreases the likelihood of the bullet perforating a criminal and going on to injure an innocent bystander.

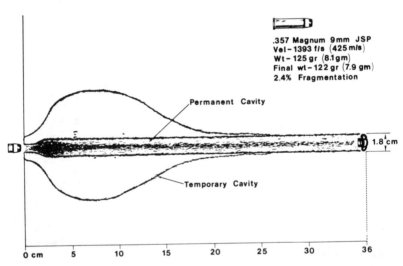

.357 Magnum 9mm JSP
Vel – 1393 f/s (425 m/s)
Wt – 125 gr (8.1 gm)
Final wt – 122 gr (7.9 gm)
2.4% Fragmentation

Permanent Cavity

1.8 cm

Temporary Cavity

0 cm   5   10   15   20   25   30   36

FIGURE 10.—*357 Magnum jacketed soft-point pistol bullet.* This expanding bullet is typical of those used by the majority of law enforcement agencies in the USA.

7.62 SP (SP is the abbreviation for soft-point) The same cartridge case shown in Figure 7, when loaded with a soft-point bullet, produces the wound profile shown in Figure 11. Changing only the variable of bullet construction causes massively increased tissue disruption compared to that of the full-metal-cased bullet (Figure 7). Bullet expansion occurs on impact as seen with the 357 Magnum pistol bullet (Figure 10); however, the crush in the tissue that results from bullet expansion accounts for only a small part of the large permanent cavity. As this bullet flattens, pieces break off and make their own separate paths of crushed tissue. These bullet fragments penetrate up to 9 cm radially from the bullet path. The following temporary cavitation stretches muscle that has been weakened by multiple perforations. The fragment paths act to concentrate the force of the stretch, increasing its effect and causing pieces of muscle to be detached. This synergistic effect, resulting in the large tissue defect shown in Figure 11, is seen only with bullets that fragment. The 7.62 NATO soft-point is a popular big game hunting bullet, and although shooting accidents are not infrequent with such rounds, they are rarely seen in the hospital since few victims of torso shots survive.

22 CAL FMC—This is the M-193 bullet shot from the M-16A1 Assault Rifle (Figure 12). The large permanent cavity shown in the profile was observed by many surgeons who served in Vietnam, but the tissue disruption mechanism responsible was not clear until the importance of bullet fragmentation as a cause of tissue disruption was worked out. This military round is full-metal-jacketed and, as with other bullets of this type, it causes little tissue disruption so long as it remains traveling point forward through tissue. Its average distance of point-forward travel is about 12 cm, after which it yaws to 90°, flattens, and breaks at the cannelure (groove around bullet mid section). The bullet point remains a flattened triangular piece, retaining about 60% of the original bullet weight. The rear portion breaks into many fragments that penetrate up to 7 cm radially from the bullet path. The temporary cavity stretch, its effect increased by perforation and weakening of the muscle by fragments, then causes a much enlarged permanent cavity by detaching muscle pieces. The degree of bullet fragmentation decreases with increasing shooting distance, as striking velocity decreases. At a distance of 80 meters, the bullet breaks in half, forming two large fragments. At ranges in excess of 180 meters, this projectile does not break in two and the wounding capacity and mechanisms are essentially the same as those of the AK-74.

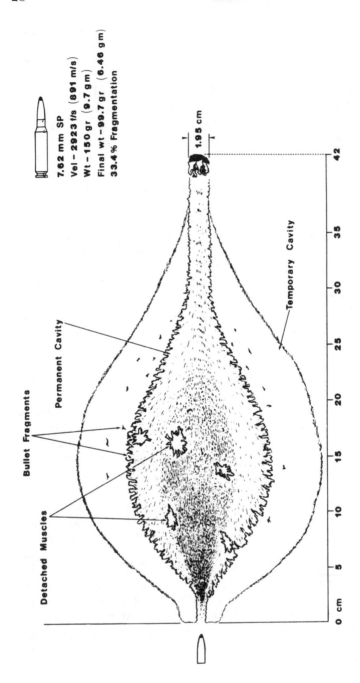

7.62 mm SP
Vel – 2923 f/s (891 m/s)
Wt – 150 gr (9.7 g m)
Final wt – 99.7 gr (6.46 g m)
33.4% Fragmentation

1.95 cm

Temporary Cavity

Permanent Cavity

Bullet Fragments

Detached Muscles

FIGURE 11.—7.62 Soft-point bullet. The fragmentation of this bullet is largely responsible for the massive tissue disruption, compared to that produced by the nondeforming military bullet fired from the same cartridge. (Figure 7).

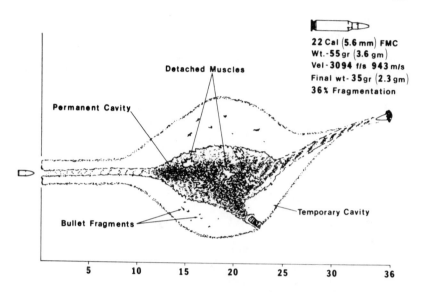

22 Cal (5.6 mm) FMC
Wt.-55gr (3.6 gm)
Vel-3094 f/s 943 m/s
Final wt-35gr (2.3 gm)
36% Fragmentation

Detached Muscles

Permanent Cavity

Temporary Cavity

Bullet Fragments

5   10   15   20   25   30   36

FIGURE 12.—*22 Caliber full-metal-cased (M-16 rifle firing M-193 bullet).* This is the standard weapon of the U.S. Armed Forces, although it is soon to be replaced by a new rifle using the same caliber and cartridge but with a longer and slightly heavier (62 grain) bullet.

M-855 22 CAL FMC—The slightly heavier M-855 bullet shot from the M-16A2 Assault Rifle will eventually replace the M-193 bullet shot as the standard bullet for the U.S. Armed Forces. The wound profile is similar to that produced by the M-193, although the tip generally does not remain in one piece. The temporary cavity size and location are about the same and any difference in wounds caused by the two would be difficult to recognize.

The smaller bullets of the new generation Assault Rifles (M-193, AK-74, M-855) are susceptible to deflection and disturbance of their point-forward flight by intermediate targets such as foliage. This was not the case with the previous generation of larger and slower projectiles. This can result in large yaw angles at impact and a shallower location in the body of maximum tissue disruption. For these bullets that rely on yaw in tissue for their maximum effect, the wound profiles show the average penetration depth at which this yaw occurs.

.224 SOFT-POINT—This 50 grain soft-point bullet is designed for maximum deformation and fragmentation. To produce the wound profile shown in Figure 13, it was shot from the M-16 cartridge case (known as the 223 Remington in civilian shooting parlance). The amount and type of damage caused is about the same as that caused by the military M-193 (M-16) bullet, but the location of the maximum disruption is at a shallower penetration depth.

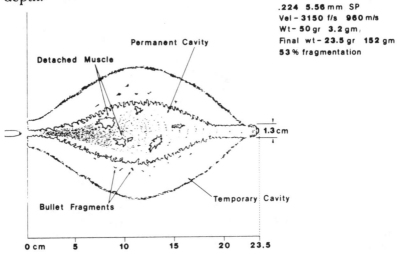

FIGURE 13.—*.224 Soft-point bullet.* This is a typical 22 caliber center-fire hunting bullet (.224 inches is actual bullet diameter) fired from the same cartridge as the military M-16.

12 GAUGE SHOTGUN #4 BUCKSHOT—Loaded with 27 pellets of #4 Buckshot (Figure 14), the 12 gauge shotgun at close range (3 meters in this case) causes massive crush type tissue disruption. At this short range, soft-tissue impact deforms the individual pellets, increasing their original 6 mm cross section to about 10 mm with concomitant increase in tissue crush or hole size. The 27 perforations of this size in a 7-8 cm diameter area result in severe disruption of anatomy by direct crush and in disruption of blood supply to tissue between the multiple wound channels.

The foregoing wound profiles portray an estimate of the maximum soft-tissue disruption expected at short ranges (under 25 meters). A gradual decrease in the amount of bullet deformation, fragmentation, and maximum size of the temporary cavity occurs with distance as the striking velocity of the projectile decreases. When bone is struck by the penetrating projectile, the result is predictable and easily verified on X-ray. Total penetration depth

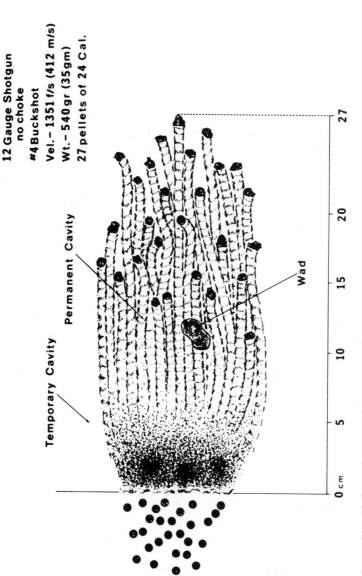

FIGURE 14.—12 Gauge shotgun with #4 size buckshot. This load is used by the military and by law enforcement groups for special situations.

will be less; however, the degree of tissue disruption will be greater
due to increased projectile deformation and the creation of secondary bone fragment missiles.

FRAGMENTS FROM EXPLOSIVE DEVICES

The great majority of fragments from explosive devices are of
blunt or irregular shape, distinctly not aerodynamic, and of steel
or less dense material. This causes them to lose velocity rapidly
in air with resultant decreases in tissue penetration depth compared to the denser streamlined rifle bullets. Although initial fragment velocities in the 5,900 ft/sec (1800 m/sec) range have been
reported for some of these devices, the wounds observed in survivors indicate that striking velocities were less than 1900 ft/sec
(600 m/sec). For this reason, body armor affords much better protection against these fragments than against the rifle bullet. The
crush type of tissue disruption predominates in the injury pattern caused by the individual fragment from these devices, with
little evidence of temporary cavity stretch. The projectile track
made by the fragment is consistent with its size and generally remains constant throughout its path. It is analogous to the wound
from a single shotgun pellet. In cases where a survivor was close
enough to the device to be struck by multiple fragments in a
localized area, such as stepping on a landmine, the injury pattern
is similar to that produced by #4 buckshot at close range (Figure
14). In this situation, the crush mechanism results in the massive
tissue disruption one encounters when many permanent wound
paths in close proximity to one another totally destroy anatomic
integrity.

DISCUSSION

It becomes apparent from observing of data on the Wound Profiles that a projectile's striking velocity and mass determine only
the *potential* for tissue disruption. For example, a shot through soft
tissue of the average human thigh by a 7.62 NATO round loaded
with the soft-point bullet (Figure 11) could result in an exit wound
up to 13 cm in diameter with massive tissue loss. The same potential is available in the 7.62 NATO FMC military bullet (Figure 7),
but the exit wound it causes in a comparable shot would most likely not exceed 2 cm in its largest dimension.

If one presented at the average large city hospital with a gun-shot wound in the thigh (entrance and exit holes of less than 1 cm in diameter) and gave the history of being shot with a 22 Long Rifle bullet, the surgical treatment rendered would be minimal. The same would probably apply if the history were of a wound from a 38 Special or a 45 Automatic. If, however, the history was given that the wound had been made by an M-16, the victim would most likely be subjected to an excision of the entire bullet track and possibly even several cm of tissue on all sides of the track. Comparing *the first 12cm of penetration* on the M-16 wound profile (Figure 12) with that of the other examples mentioned (Figures. 4-6), shows that *in such a wound the M-16 is unlikely to cause any more tissue disruption than the 22 Long Rifle.* The reason for this is that the M-16 round does not fragment or yaw in the first 12 cm of soft tissue it traverses, nor does it develop its very significant temporary cavitation effects prior to 12 cm of penetration. The widespread belief that each and every wound caused by "high-velocity" pro-jectiles must be treated by "radical debridement" is incorrect and results from failure to recognize the role of other variables, such as bullet mass and construction, in the projectile-tissue interaction.

Serious misunderstanding has been generated by looking upon "kinetic energy transfer" from projectile to tissue as a mechanism of injury. In spite of data to the contrary, many assume that the amount of "kinetic energy deposit" in the body by a projectile is directly proportional to the damage it does. Such thinking stops short of delving into the actual interaction of projectile and tissue that is the crux of wound ballistics. Wounds that result in a given amount of "kinetic energy deposit" may differ widely. The nondeforming rifle bullet of the AK-74 (Figure 9) causes a large temporary cavity which can cause marked disruption in some tissues (liver), but considerably lesser disruption in others (mus-cle, lung, bowel wall). The temporary cavitation produced by the M-16 (Figure 12), acting on tissue that has been perforated by bullet fragments, causes a much larger permanent cavity in tissues such as muscle and bowel wall and a similar disruption to that caused by the AK-74 in liver. A large slow projectile will crush a large amount of tissue (permanent cavity), whereas a small fast missile *with the same kinetic energy* will stretch more tissue (tem-porary cavity) but crush a proportionately smaller volume of tissue.

The "temporary cavity/energy deposit mystique" has spilled over into the field of weapons development and evaluation, where one large study rates handgun bullets based upon the unfounded assumption that the degree of incapacitation a bullet causes in the human target is directly proportional to the size of the temporary cavity produced by the bullet. Many soft tissues (muscle, skin, bowel wall, lung) are flexible and elastic, having the physical characteristics of a good energy absorber. The assumption that tissue *must* be damaged by the temporary displacement of cavitation makes no sense physically or biologically. Not surprisingly, law enforcement agencies are finding increasing numbers of cases in which handgun bullets chosen on the basis of such studies fail to perform as predicted.

In the missile-wounded combat casualty, determination of the missile's path through the body is a major concern. Since the majority of penetration projectiles follow a relatively straight course in tissue, an estimate of the missile's path can be made from the location of the entrance wound and the location of the exit wound or the position at which the expended projectile comes to rest within the body. In most cases, physical examination and biplanar X-rays establish these two points and allow clinical estimation of structures that might have been damaged. In some cases, oblique X-ray views will be needed and it may be impossible to determine with certainty whether penetration of a body cavity has occurred. When the question arises as to whether or not the peritoneal cavity has been perforated by abdominal wall wounds, experience has clearly demonstrated that it is better to look and see (by laparotomy) than to wait and see.

Bullet fragmentation and its correlative severe permanent tissue disruption (Figures 11 - 13) are especially useful roentgenographic signs. Rifle wounds of the chest wall in which a large disruption has occurred in the muscles of the shoulder girdle (M-16, AK-74, or AK-47 if it strikes bone) may be expected to have pulmonary contusion even without penetration of the pleural cavity. This may not be evident on X-rays taken shortly after wounding. The surgeon must be aware of this potentially life-threatening situation and assure adequate follow-up observation and treatment. This is one of the more common situations in which occult damage from temporary cavity "blunt trauma" results in a clinical problem.

A point worth reiterating is that the surgeon is best advised to treat the wound and not the weapon!

CHAPTER III

Burn Injury

Extensive use of the various fuels needed to provide both ground and air mobility for the present-day armed forces increases the risk of thermal burns in military personnel. During times of conflict, the possibility of the unintended ignition of these fuels is greatly increased, as is the chance of thermal injury from antipersonnel and other weapons. The development of thermonuclear devices has created the possibility of virtually instantaneous generation of large numbers of burn patients, creating not only medical but also severe logistical problems.

Even under the best conditions, the simultaneous arrival of many extensively burned patients at any hospital disrupts the activities of the professional and paramedical staff and places heavy demands upon the logistical system of that treatment facility. Recent laboratory developments and the clinically demonstrated efficacy of topical chemotherapy have resulted in general acceptance of simplified burn treatment techniques readily adaptable to the combat surgery environment.

The first priority in the management of the burn patient is given to maintenance of the airway, control of hemorrhage, and prompt institution of resuscitative therapy. The presence of associated traumatic wounds in patients with burn injuries may complicate the management of their burns and vice versa. The essence of the successful treatment of burn patients, with or without other traumatic injuries, is effective triage, timely diagnosis, accurate assessment of surgical priority, and appropriate resuscitation.

ETIOLOGIC AGENTS

Ignition of gasoline and other fuels accounts for the greatest number of thermal injuries. Flame or flash burns may be caused by various other agents contained in explosive devices. Casualties with chemical burns and burns from white phosphorus require immediate wound care in contrast to those with "conventional" burns. Thermal injury created by electric current also deserves separate consideration because of special treatment requirements.

Even in the combat zone, burns resulting from carelessness outnumber those resulting from hostile action. The enforcement of safety procedures and existing regulations will reduce such occurrences. The use of gloves, goggles, protective headgear, and flame-retardant clothing by personnel at high risk will also minimize, if not prevent, thermal injury in those individuals. This equipment is particularly important to fire-rescue personnel, and the use of these items should be strictly enforced, even (within limits) at the expense of personal comfort.

MAGNITUDE OF INJURY

The severity of thermal injury is dependent upon the depth and extent of the burn. These two factors determine not only mortality and initial treatment requirements, but also morbidity, metabolic consequences of injury, character of healing, and the ultimate functional result.

The extent of the body surface burned can be estimated by employing the "rule of nines." The distribution of surface area by anatomical part in the adult is illustrated in Figure 15, showing the percentage of total skin surface represented by each body part to be: head and neck, 9%; anterior trunk, 18%; posterior trunk, 18%, upper extremities, 9% each; lower extremities, 18% each; and genitalia and perineum, 1%.

To estimate the extent of irregularly disposed burns one can make use of the fact that one surface of the casualty's hand represents approximately 1% of his total body surface. Patients with burns of more than 15% of the body surface typically require some resuscitative treatment and, in most situations, are best cared for in the hospital. Young soldiers tolerate thermal injury best, while older casualties (above 50) and the very young have greater mortality rates for a given extent of burn. The location of the burn influences not only prognosis but also the need for hospitalization. Small burns of the face, hands, feet, or perineum may require hospitalization, even if these limited areas are the only sites of burn injury.

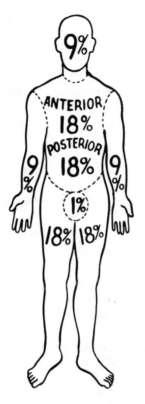

FIGURE 15.—Rule of nines, showing distribution of body surface area by anatomical part in the adult.

DEPTH OF INJURY

The depth of thermal injury can be determined with certainty only by histologic examination. However, the clinical criteria in Table 1 will permit an initial, usually quite accurate differentiation between second- and third-degree burns. The total percentage of skin surface involved in second-degree and third-degree burns is the primary concern during resuscitation. Differentiation between second-degree and third-degree burns is more important later in the postburn course as related to the duration of hypermetabolism, the anticipated functional result, and the ultimate need for autograft closure of the burn wound.

TABLE 1.—*Diagnosis of depth of burns*

Criteria	Second-degree Burns	Third-degree Burns
Cause	Hot liquids, flashes of flame	Flame, electricity, chemicals
Color	Pink or mottled red	Dark brown or black charred, translucent with thrombosed superficial veins visible, pearly white ±
Surface	Vesicles or weeping	Dry and inelastic
Pinprick	Painful	Anesthetic

Those areas of thermal injury that are waxy-white, soft and pliable, yet nonpainful formerly were regarded as full-thickness injuries, but in actuality are deep, partial-thickness burns; they frequently heal without the need for grafting if protected from invasive infection by topical chemotherapy. Charring with thermal injury of subcutaneous and deeper tissues is infrequent, but may occur in the unconscious victim, in individuals trapped by burning debris or in a burning vehicle, or in individuals with high-voltage electric injury. Injuries of less than partial thickness, that is, first-degree burns (erythema of intact epidermis) , are important only so far as patient comfort and vasomotor lability are concerned and are, with few exceptions, treated symptomatically without need for resuscitation.

The depth of thermal injury after a thermonuclear explosion is dependent upon the intensity and duration of the thermal pulse, but burns also may be sustained from ignition of clothing or burning debris. These burns do not differ from burns of other etiology except for the associated effects of ionizing radiation, which decrease survival for a given size burn.

PATHOPHYSIOLOGY

Thermal injury, regardless of the etiologic agent, results in cell death by coagulation necrosis. In areas of cell death and cell damage, capillary permeability is increased with the loss of integrity of the vascular system and the escape of the nonformed blood elements. This is manifested clinically by edema, which forms most rapidly in the immediate postburn period and reaches a maximum in the second postburn day. Thereafter, as vascular integrity is restored and fluid resorption begins, edema slowly resolves. This increase in capillary permeability results in a decrease in blood volume and an increase in blood viscosity, causing an increase in peripheral resistance and a decrease in cardiac output. Fluid resuscitation is carried out in the immediate postburn period to minimize these changes by maintaining blood volume at a level adequate for organ perfusion.

FIRST AID

The first consideration is removal of the source of thermal injury from the patient. Burning clothing should be extinguished and removed, and the patient should be removed from a burning vehicle or building. In electric injury, the patient should be removed from the point or points of contact, with the rescuing personnel taking care to avoid contact with the power source. Chemical agents should be washed immediately from the skin surface by copious water lavage. First aid should be reduced to a minimum, and nothing must be done that could prejudice subsequent treatment. All constricting articles, such as rings, bracelets, wristwatches, belts, and boots must be removed, but the patient is not undressed unless the injury has been caused by a chemical agent, in which case all contaminated clothing must be removed. The patient should be covered with a clean sheet and a blanket, if appropriate, to maintain body temperature and prevent gross contamination during transport to a treatment facility. If available, burn dressings can be used for such initial wound coverage.

Patency of the airway should be assured, hemorrhage should be controlled, and fractures should be splinted. If at all possible an intravenous pathway should be established in an unburned area and in an upper extremity vein if there are associated abdominal wounds. Resuscitation may be safely begun with electrolyte solution alone, and should be continued before and during movement to an installation where definitive medical care is available. An intravenous cannula is preferable in all situations

since large volumes of fluid are required for patients with extensive burns, and patient restlessness, transportation, or edema may
dislodge an intravenous needle. Patients with injuries from white
phosphorus should have the burns dressed with saline-soaked
dressings to prevent reignition of the phosphorus by contact with
the air.

Pain is seldom a major problem in patients with severe burns,
but patients with extensive partial-thickness burns may have considerable discomfort, which can be relieved by appropriate doses
of morphine or meperidine administered intravenously. Subcutaneous or intramuscular injections of analgesics will not be
mobilized during the period of edema formation and will be in-
effective in pain control. A patient who has received multiple subcutaneous or intramuscular doses of an analgesic may later
mobilize them simultaneously and develop severe respiratory
depression, which must be treated promptly.

On the day of injury, after hemorrage is controlled, ventilatory
stability achieved, and urinary output established, one should
promptly move the extensively burned patient to a definitive treatment facility. Intravenous fluid administration should be maintained throughout transportation and, if any question exists as to
adequacy of the airway, a tracheostomy should be performed or,
preferably, an endotracheal tube placed and secured.

INITIAL TREATMENT OF EXTENSIVE BURNS

At the definitive treatment facility, control of hemorrhage and
airway adequacy again must be insured. Initial consideration of
the burn patient includes a complete physical examination following removal of the patient's clothing. Once a secure intravenous
pathway has been established, one then must estimate the
resuscitation fluids to be given to the burned patient.

TABLE 2.—*Formula for estimating fluid requirements in burn patients*

First 24 hours postburn:
  Adult: 2 ml lactated Ringer's solution/kg body weight/% burn
  Child: 3 ml lactated Ringer's solution/kg body weight/% burn

Second 24 hours postburn:
  Adult and child:
      Colloid: Estimated deficit and replace with a plasma
              equivalent, e.g., albumin diluted to physiologic con-
              centration in normal saline or fresh frozen plasma
          (a) 30-50% burn: 0.3 ml/kg body weight/% burn
          (b) 50-70% burn: 0.4 ml/kg body weight/% burn
          (c) >70% burn: 0.5 ml/kg body weight/% burn

  5% Dextrose in water: Volume necessary to maintain urinary
  output.

Several formulas exist for calculation of the fluid requirement of the burn patient. They are based upon body weight and extent of the burn. Clinical success has been reported for each such formula and, in a civilian setting with unlimited amounts of the full spectrum of intravenous fluids available, the attending physician's preference can certainly dictate the resuscitation regimen employed. In a combat situation, logistical considerations speak strongly for simplicity of resuscitation using readily available fluids in a volume sufficient to prevent renal or other organ failure, yet avoid later complications of fluid overload. Extensive clinical and laboratory studies have demonstrated that: (1) in the first 24 hours postburn, colloid has no specific restorative effect on cardiac output beyond that of electrolyte-containing fluids and is retained within the vascular compartment to no greater extent than an equal volume of electrolyte-containing fluid, and (2) in the second 24 hours postburn, capillary integrity is largely restored so that fluid and salt loading can be minimized by using colloid-containing fluid to correct any persistent plasma volume deficit. These studies have led to a revision of the Brooke formula, simplifying the logistics of initial resuscitation (only electrolyte-containing fluid is administered in the first 24 hours postburn) and reducing fluid and salt loading (no electrolyte-free water is administered in the first 24 hours postburn and no electrolyte-containing fluid is administered in the second 24 hour period postburn). The formula, which is detailed in Table 2, should be modified according to the individual patient's response in terms of urinary output, vital signs, and general condition. The fact that children have a greater cutaneous surface area per unit body mass and therefore form a relatively greater amount of edema per unit body surface burn necessitates that their initial electrolyte fluid resuscitation needs be estimated on the basis of 3 ml/Kg of body weight multiplied by the percentage of body surface burned. One should plan to administer one-half of the total fluid volume estimated for the first 24 hours postburn within the first 8 hours following injury, the time of most rapid edema formation. The actual rate of administration is adjusted according to the patient's response as noted below. If the casualty is not received immediately following burn injury, the first half of the resuscitation fluid should be administered in the time remaining prior to 8 hours postburn. The remaining half of the estimated fluid should be administered, ideally at a uniform rate, in the succeeding 16 hours of the first 24 hours postburn. Patients with massive burns (greater than 70% of the body surface) and those in whom initiation of resuscitation has been delayed may require considerably more than the estimated volume of resuscitation fluid. Such patients require frequent observation and examination, and one must not hesitate to increase the volume or infusion rate of resuscitation fluids, or to otherwise alter therapy to obtain the physiologic response desired. Even in these patients, the proposed formula should be used to plan fluid therapy, keeping in mind that it is safer to add fluid as necessary than to deal with the complications of excessive fluid administration. Only in this manner can treatment be properly supervised and individualized.

The electrolyte-containing solution should be lactated Ringer's, which contains a more physiologic concentration of the chloride ion, but isotonic saline may be employed if the former is not available. Even though red blood cell destruction occurs after thermal injury, whole blood is not administered as a portion of the resuscitation fluids, since loss of the plasma, due to increased capillary permeability and intravascular retention of the red cells, would further elevate the patient's hematocrit and adversely affect the rheological properties of the blood. The colloid solution administered during the second 24 hours postburn can be fresh frozen plasma or albumin, with each 25 gram bottle of that material diluted with normal saline for administration as a 5% solution.

Potassium supplements are not needed and may be deleterious during the first 48 hours, since the serum potassium is commonly elevated as a result of the destruction of red blood cells and other tissue. Potassium, lost from injured cells, appears in the blood at a time when renal function may be depressed. From the third postburn day onward, potassium supplements should be added to the intravenous fluids if renal function is unimpaired. Average daily potassium requirements range from 60-200 meq per day.

From the third postburn day onward, an adequately resuscitated burn patient commonly has a normal and, in some instances, a supranormal plasma volume, so that further administration of salt- or colloid-containing fluids is usually unnecessary and should be carried out with great caution. In patients treated by the exposure technique, the burn wound acts essentially as a free-water surface with considerable evaporative losses (that is, 6-8 liters per day in patients with very extensive burns), following the third postburn day and until it is healed or grafted. Evaporative water losses can be estimated according to the formula: evaporative water loss in ml/hr = (25 + percent of body surface burned) x total body surface in square meters. This formula estimates evaporative water loss at the low end of the observed range, and replacement of the evaporative water loss should be guided by assessing the adequacy of hydration, which can be determined by careful monitoring of patient weight, serum osmolality, and serum sodium concentration. In patients treated with occlusive dressings, evaporative water loss is considerably less. Following resuscitation, salt-containing fluid need be given only for the treatment of symptomatic hyponatremia. Following elimination of the resuscitation-related salt and water load, salt-containing fluid should be administered in the amount needed to maintain a "normal" serum sodium concentration. Later in the postburn course, whole blood should be administered to maintain the hematocrit between 30-35%.

URINARY OUTPUT

The most readily available clinical guide to the adequacy of resuscitation is the hourly urinary output, which should be maintained between 30-50 ml in patients weighing more than 30 kilograms and 1 ml/kg/hr in patients weighing less than 30 kilograms. In patients who require fluid resuscitation, an indwelling urethral catheter should be placed and the hourly urine output should be measured and recorded. Except possibly in patients with electric injury, oliguria in the first 48 hours postburn is rarely caused by acute renal failure and is treated by increasing fluid administration rather than by decreasing fluid administration or giving a diuretic.

Three categories of patients may require an osmotic diuretic: (1) those patients with significant electric injury in whom liberated hemochromogens increase the risk of acute renal failure, (2) those patients with associated crush or other injuries with extensive tissue death and large hemochromogen loads in the urine, and (3) those patients with large burns to whom one has given considerably more than the estimated fluid requirement but in whom oliguria persists. Osmotic diuretics, such as mannitol, will insure an adequate urinary output, but one must remember that this will occur at the expense of blood volume even in hypovolemic patients. Urinary output in patients who have received a diuretic is no longer a guide to the adequacy of resuscitation. Other diuretics, such as furosemide and ethacrynic acid, also have been used in burn patients.

ENDOTRACHEAL INTUBATION

The indications for endotracheal intubation are essentially those that exist in any other surgical patient: namely, acute laryngeal or upper airway edema or obstruction, inability to handle secretions, and associated chest wall injury. Severe smoke inhalation with respiratory insufficiency is another indicator for endotracheal intubation. The presence of inhalation injury and the adequacy of the airway should be assessed by direct examination of the oropharynx and the upper airway using a fiberoptic laryngoscope or bronchoscope.

If the burn patient is to be evacuated and the adequacy of the airway is at all questionable, the caregiver should perform endotracheal intubation or tracheostomy before movement rather than risk the possibility of acute airway obstruction in transit. Three categories of patients are most apt to require endotracheal intubation on the basis of the indications listed: (1) patients with severe head and neck burns, (2) patients with steam burns of the face, and (3) patients burned in a closed space who have inhaled smoke or other noxious products of incomplete combustion.

The severe chemical tracheobronchitis which results from inhalation injury may cause acute respiratory insufficiency. Such patients may have marked hypoxemia persisting for several weeks. Marked bronchospasm and frequent bouts of coughing are common and the patient may raise sputum containing carbonaceous material, confirming the diagnosis of inhalation injury. Conservative therapy with administration of humidified air or oxygen and nasotracheal aspiration, as indicated, is employed initially. The ability of the patient to clear the tracheobronchial tree and the quantity of endobronchial debris will determine whether bronchoscopy is necessary and the frequency with which it should be employed. Endotracheal intubation should be performed for the indications previously noted. Tracheostomy should be carried out only if prolonged mechanical ventilation is necessary or if the endobronchial toilet cannot be adequately performed through an endotracheal tube. Daily chest roentgenograms must be obtained of all patients with significant inhalation injury, with endobronchial cultures obtained if pneumonic infiltrates appear. Antibiotic treatment is guided by the results of the microbiology reports of those cultures. Mucolytic agents and bronchodilators may also be useful. Mechanical ventilatory assistance may be necessary in the treatment of those patients who have severe bronchospasm, profound hypoxemia, or significant hypercarbia.

Steroids in large doses are employed only in those patients with unrelenting bronchospasm, and such treatment should be terminated at the earliest possible time to minimize the increased risk of infection attendant upon their use.

ESCHAROTOMY

Circumferential full-thickness burns of the limbs may impair the circulation to distal and underlying unburned tissue. To prevent secondary ischemic necrosis of these tissues, an escharotomy may be necessary to relieve constriction caused by edema beneath the inelastic, unyielding eschar. The adequacy of the circulation of a burned limb must be assessed on a scheduled basis, e.g., hourly. The most reliable assessment of the circulation can be made by using an ultrasonic flowmeter to detect pulsatile flow in the distal palmar arch vessels in the upper limb and the pedal vessels in the lower limb. Absence of pulsatile flow or progressive diminution of flow on sequential flowmeter examinations is an indication for escharotomy. If a flowmeter is not available, the caretaker must depend upon the less reliable clinical signs of circulatory compromise. Swelling and coldness of the distal unburned parts are not indications for escharotomy, but cyanosis, impaired capillary refilling, and signs of neurologic dysfunction, such as relentless deep tissue pain and progressive paresthesia, are. Should evidence of vascular impairment be present, escharotomy should be promptly performed. The procedure can be carried out in the ward or emergency room without anesthesia, since it is performed through insensate full-thickness burn. An initial escharotomy incision is placed in the midlateral line of the involved extremity and, if this does not improve distal blood supply, a second escharotomy incision is made in the midmedial line in the longitudinal axis of the limb. The escharotomy incision should be carried throughout the entire length of full-thickness burn to ensure adequate release of vascular compression. The incision must cross involved joints, since in those areas the paucity of subcutaneous tissue permits ready compression of vessels and nerves. The escharotomy incision is carried through the eschar and the immediately subjacent thin connective tissue to permit expansion of the edematous subcutaneous tissue. When performed in this manner, blood loss from the escharotomy incision is not excessive and is readily controlled by either electrocoagulation or brief application of pressure.

Fasciotomy is rarely necessary for relief of vascular compromise in a limb with conventional thermal injury. Fasciotomy may be required in patients with high voltage electric injury, in other patients with burns involving deep tissues, or in patients with associated traumatic injuries (i.e., patients in whom edema is present below the investing fascia). Fasciotomy should be performed in the operating room using appropriate anesthesia.

Patients with circumferential truncal burns may also require escharotomies in the anterior axillary line to relieve restriction of chest wall movement by the eschar and permit a more satisfactory ventilatory exchange. This is particularly important in children with truncal burns who may be rapidly exhausted by the increased respiratory effort required. These patients frequently will be restless, agitated, and hypoxemic before escharotomy and will show prompt clinical improvement as well as improved ventilatory exchange and blood oxygenation following escharotomy. An incision along the lower margin of the rib cage may be necessary in those patients with deep burns extending onto the upper abdominal wall (Figure 16).

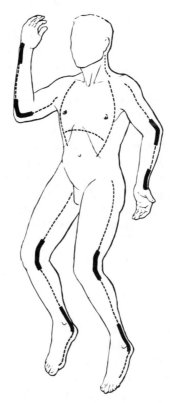

FIGURE 16.—The dashed lines indicate the preferred sites for escharotomy incisions. The solid segments of the lines emphasize the importance of extending the incisions across involved joints.

ADJUVANT TREATMENT

The burn patient who has been actively immunized against tetanus should be given a booster dose of tetanus toxoid. Those patients who have not received prior active immunization should receive hyperimmune human antitetanus serum as well as an initial dose of tetanus toxoid, with active immunization continued at weekly intervals until complete.

Unless specifically contraindicated, penicillin is administered to all burn patients for the first 5 days postburn to prevent beta-hemolytic streptococcal burn wound infection. Thereafter, antibiotics are administered only on the specific indication of clinical infection supported by positive bacteriologic cultures.

As previously noted, restlessness and agitation frequently can be relieved by insuring adequate oxygenation. The need for analgesia is usually minimal except in those patients with extensive partial-thickness burns. Analgesia, when required in the first 3 days postburn, should be administered intravenously in appropriately small dosages.

Ileus is a common accompaniment of thermal injury involving 20% or more of the total body surface, and nasogastric intubation and drainage to prevent emesis and aspiration are critically important in these patients. It is also important to maintain nasogastric intubation in all patients who are to undergo air evacuation, not only in the early postburn period but also later, if evidence of gastrointestinal dysfunction exists.

WOUND CARE

Attention is directed to the burn wound only after hemodynamic stability and the previously mentioned aspects of patient care have been accomplished. General anesthesia is not required for burn wound debridement; in fact, during this period of vascular instability and hypovolemia, it is ill-advised. Intravenous analgesia will suffice for pain control during such a procedure. The body hair is shaved from the area of thermal injury and well back from the margins. The burns are gently cleansed with a surgical soap solution, and nonviable epidermal remnants are debrided. Bullae are excised, since the proteinaceous fluid contained within them is an ideal culture medium for bacteria. After this initial debridement, the patient may be placed in bed, on surgically clean sheets. During the period of active wound exudation, placing bulky dressings beneath the burned parts to absorb the serious exudate has been found helpful. These dressings

should be changed as necessary and patients with circumferential burns should be turned on a scheduled basis to expose the
burned areas on an alternating basis and to prevent maceration.

Patients with burns of the buttocks, perineum, and thigh do not
require colostomy. The frequency of anal stricture is greatly increased by performance of such a procedure. Even when an abdominal operation is required to treat associated injuries, performing a colostomy is unwise solely for the treatment of buttock,
perineal, or upper thigh burns. If a colostomy is indicated for
other reasons, daily anal dilations are mandatory.

Fractures associated with thermal injury are best treated by
skeletal traction or external fixation to permit exposure of the
burns and their treatment with topical chemotherapy. The application of a cast over an area of thermal injury promotes suppuration and enhances the possibility of the development of invasive burn wound infection. Nevertheless, plaster is acceptable
over areas of burn in preparation for and during evacuation, if
the cast is bivalved and removed promptly when the patient arrives at the definitive treatment installation.

ELECTRIC INJURY

Although the pathologic change resulting from electric injury
is coagulation necrosis, the extent and severity of such injury may
initially be seriously underestimated. Limited areas of cutaneous
necrosis may be evident at points of entry, exit, or arcing, yet be
associated with extensive, subcutaneous, deep tissue involvement,
leading to an inappropriate estimation of resuscitation fluid requirements. This "iceberg" effect also may necessitate the performance of fasciotomy rather than escharotomy to insure viability
of distal unburned parts. The prophylactic use of an osmotic
diuretic may be indicated because of extensive muscle necrosis
with consequent liberation of hemochromogens. The presence of
brawny, deep induration in a limb involved in electric injury, with
signs of vascular impairment, indicates a need for fasciotomy. Approximately one-third of all patients with significant electric injury of the extremities will require amputation. This procedure
should be delayed until resuscitation has been completed unless
signs of systemic toxicity develop. Amputations in this situation
as in any thermal injury should be consistent with conservative

principles of limb salvage and should be carried out by disarticulation without opening a narrow cavity in the presence of the contaminated burn wound. Because of the difficulty of accurately distinguishing viable and nonviable tissue at the time of initial debridement, patients with high-voltage electric injury should be returned to the operating room 24 hours or, at the most, 48 hours following initial debridement. At the time of reoperation, further debridement is carried out as is necessary or, if no further necrotic tissue is identified, the wound may be loosely closed over tissue drains.

CHEMICAL BURNS AND WHITE PHOSPHORUS INJURY

The depth and severity of chemical burns are related to both the concentration of the agent and the duration of contact with the tissues. These are the only burn injuries which require immediate care of the burn wound. The offending agent must be washed from the body surface as soon as possible. Full-thickness, third-degree injury of the skin caused by strong acids may result in tanning or bronzing of the skin which will be waxy, yet pliable to the touch, leading the unwary to underestimate the extent of burn.

Many antipersonnel weapons employed in modern warfare contain white phosphorus. Fragments of this metal, which ignite upon contact with the air, may be driven into the soft tissues; however, most of the cutaneous injury resulting from phosphorus burns is due to the ignition of clothing, and is treated as conventional thermal injury. First aid treatment of casualties with imbedded phosphorus particles consists of copious water lavage and removal of the identifiable particles, following which the involved areas are covered with a saline-soaked dressing and kept moistened until the patient reaches a definitive treatment installation. If transfer will require more than 12 hours, the involved areas should be covered by a liberal application of topical antimicrobial agent to prevent microbial proliferation and the reignition of retained phosphorus particles.

At the site of definitive treatment, the wounds containing imbedded phosphorus particles may be rinsed with a dilute (1%) freshly mixed solution of copper sulfate. This solution combines with the phosphorus on the surface of the particles to form a blue-black cupric phosphide covering which both impedes further oxidation and facilitates the identification of retained particles. If sufficient copper is absorbed through the wound to cause intravascular hemolysis, acute renal failure may result. To avoid this potential complication, copper sulfate solution should never be applied as a wet dressing, and all wounds must be lavaged thoroughly with saline following a copper sulfate rinse to prevent absorption of excessive amounts of copper. As an alternative to the use of a copper sulfate rinse, a Woods lamp can be used in a darkened operating room, or the lights in the operating room may be turned off to identify retained phosphorescent particles during debridement. The extracted phosphorus particles must be immersed in water to avoid their ignition in the operating room. Inflammable anesthetic agents should not be used with these cases.

Combustion of white phosphorus results in the formation of phosphorous pentoxide, a severe pulmonary irritant. The ignition of phosphorus in a closed space may result in the development of concentrations of phosphorous pentoxide sufficient to cause acute inflammatory changes in the tracheobronchial tree. The effects of this gas can be minimized by placing a moist cloth over the nose and mouth to inactivate the gas and prevent endobronchial irritation. Hypocalcemia and hyperphosphatemia have been described as effects of white phosphorus injury and have been associated with electrocardiographic changes and sudden deaths. Hypocalcemia associated with cardiac arrhythmia should be corrected by the administration of calcium.

VESICANT GASES

Patients with cutaneous injuries due to vesicant gases are treated as are patients with other chemical injuries by personnel appropriately protected from the gaseous agent. All contaminated clothing must be removed and all skin exposed to the agent immediately lavaged with copious amounts of water. Vesicles should be debrided while being lavaged during the cleansing procedure to prevent injury to contiguous areas by serous vesicle fluid containing the vesicant. Subsequent treatment of the cutaneous injury is as for any burn, with emphasis placed on prevention of infection by the use of topical chemotherapy. Inhalation injury can also be produced by vesicant gases, and the previously described endoscopic examination of the airway should be carried out in such patients to determine the need for tracheal intubation and mechanical ventilatory support.

TOPICAL CHEMOTHERAPY

If the burn patient can be moved to a definitive treatment installation within 48-72 hours, no specific topical antimicrobial therapy need be employed in the field. However, if either the tactical or logistical situation is such that treatment must be continued at a relatively forward area, topical chemotherapy should be begun once the patient has become hemodynamically stable. There are three topical antimicrobial agents which are commonly employed for burn wound care in civilian practice. Each agent has specific advantages and limitations with which the clinician must be familiar to provide optimum wound care. Both mafenide acetate and silver sulfadiazine are available in the form of topical creams which are commonly applied directly to the burn wound twice a day and do not require the twice or thrice daily application of occlusive dressings, as does the 0.5% silver nitrate soak treatment regimen.

Sulfamylon burn cream is an 11.1% suspension of mafenide acetate in a water dispersible base. The active ingredient, mafenide acetate, is water soluble and diffuses freely in the eschar to establish an effective antibacterial concentration throughout the eschar and at the viable/nonviable tissue interface where bacteria characteristically proliferate prior to invasion. Because of this characteristic, Sulfamylon is the best agent for use if the patient to be treated has heavily contaminated burn wounds or is received several days postburn and a dense bacterial population already exists on and within the eschar. The side effects of Sulfamylon burn cream are: (1) hypersensitivity reactions (usually responsive to antihistamines) in 7% of patients, (2) pain or discomfort of 20-30 minutes duration when applied to partial-thickness burns (seldom a cause for discontinuing Sulfamylon application), and (3) inhibition of carbonic anhydrase. The inhibition of carbonic anhydrase may produce both an early bicarbonate diuresis and an accentuation of postburn hyperventilation. The resulting reduction of serum bicarbonate levels renders such patients liable to a rapid shift from an alkalotic to an acidotic state, if pulmonary complications supervene, even with a measured pCO_2 at levels ordinarily considered to be normal. If acidosis should develop during Sulfamylon therapy, the frequency of application of Sulfamylon burn cream should be reduced to once a day, or dosage omitted for a 24-48 hour period, with buffering employed as necessary and efforts made to improve pulmonary function.

Silver sulfadiazine burn cream is a 1% suspension of silver sulfadiazine in a water-miscible base. As a consequence of poor water solubility, the active agent shows only limited diffusion into the eschar. Silver sulfadiazine burn cream is most effective when applied to burn wounds immediately after thermal injury to prevent bacterial colonization of the burn wound surface as a prelude to intraeschar proliferation. This agent has the advantages of being painless when applied to the wound and being free from acid-base and electrolyte disturbances. The limitations of silver sulfadiazine burn cream include neutropenia, which usually relents when application is discontinued; hypersensitivity, which is rare; and ineffectiveness against certain strains of Pseudomonas organisms and virtually all strains of Enterobacter cloacae.

The characteristics of silver sulfadiazine burn cream recommend it for initial wound treatment at the first echelons of medical care, while the characteristics of Sulfamylon burn cream, especially its more efficient and broader spectrum of antimicrobial action, mandate that it be available for the care of patients with extensive burns at the definitive level of surgical care.

Either Sulfamylon R or silver sulfadiazine burn cream should be applied in a layer one-eighth inch thick to the entire burn wound with a sterile gloved hand immediately following initial debridement and wound care. Twelve hours later, to ensure continuous topical chemotherapy, a one-eighth inch coat of cream should be reapplied to those areas of the burn wound from which it has been abraded by the bed clothes. The topical cream should be gently cleansed once each day from all of the burn wound and the wound inspected by the attending physician. Daily debridement should be carried out to a point of bleeding or pain without the use of general anesthesia. Following the debridement, the wound is again covered by the topical cream.

If topical antimicrobial creams are not available, multilayered occlusive gauze dressings, saturated with a 0.5% solution of silver nitrate, can be used. These soaks are changed two or three times each day and moistened every two hours to prevent evaporation from raising the silver nitrate concentration to cytotoxic levels within the soaks. Transeschar losses of sodium, potassium, chloride, and calcium should be anticipated and appropriately replaced. Silver nitrate soak therapy, as in the case of silver sulfadiazine burn cream therapy, is best used for bacterial control in burn patients who are received immediately after injury before significant microbial proliferation has occurred. Silver nitrate is immediately precipitated upon contact with proteinaceous material, does not penetrate the eschar, and consequently is in-effective in the treatment of established burn wound infection.

BURN WOUND EXCISION

Surgical excision of the burned tissue, commonly performed in civilian practice, has no place in the care of burn patients in the theater of operations. The extensive blood loss associated with a burn wound excision, up to 9% of circulating blood volume per each 5% of body surface area excised, would impose a prodigious and unnecessary need on the military blood supply system, and the surgical manpower expended on lengthy excisions would divert such personnel from the care of other casualties in whom surgical treatment could directly influence survival. The time re-quired for skin graft maturation, permitting return to active du-ty, even precludes excision for patients with third-degree burns of limited extent in the theater of operations.

TRIAGE

Triage is an important aspect of military burn care to ensure that available medical care resources are matched to the severity of burn injury and the number of burn casualties. In civilian prac-tice, with optimum resources available, every burn patient receives emergency care. Thereafter, care at a facility with optimum resources, i.e., a burn unit or burn center, is recommended for adults with second-degree burns of more than 25% of the body surface, for all patients with third-degree burns of 10% or more of the total body surface, and for all patients with significant burns involving the hands, face, feet, and perineum. Similarly, all burn patients with significant inhalation injury, significant high-voltage electrical burns, and with associated fractures or other major trauma, should be cared for in a facility with special expertise. Those patients with moderate, uncomplicated burn injury (that is, those with second-degree burns of 15-25% of the total body surface area and with third-degree burns of less than 10% of the total body surface area without the associated complications or associated injury, as noted above) should be cared for in a general hospital. Patients with less extensive uncomplicated burn injuries can commonly be cared for on an outpatient basis.

In the combat setting, the tactical situation, logistical limitations, or limited availability of health care personnel may necessitate reduction in the upper limits of these categories. In the best of circumstances, optimum treatment results in salvage of approximately 50% of patients whose burns involve 60-70% of the total body surface. With limited resources, burn care resources should be applied to that group of patients in which greatest benefit will be realized, with less attention given to those with lesser burns or those with more extensive burns. In a situation with resource restrictions or large numbers of casualties, hospital care can be delayed for those patients with burns of 20% or less of the total body surface. Similarly, expectant care should be applied to those patients with burns which exceed 70% of the total body surface and the available care facilities and resources applied to those with burns of from 20-70% of the total body surface. With even greater restriction of health care availability, the upper limit of the maximum treatment group should be reduced by stepwise decrements of 10% until the surgical workload matches available resources. Triage modifiers include significant coexisting inhalation injury and associated mechanical injury, each of which lowers the upper limit of the maximum treatment group by 10%. Conversely, burns of the hands, face, feet, and perineum, occurring in patients with lesser total body surface burns, will increase the medical care necessary for such patients.

EVACUATION

The burn patient best tolerates movement by either ground or air in the early postburn period; that is, after hemodynamic and respiratory stabilization and before the development of septic complications which may make movement particularly hazardous. Patency of the airway must be insured throughout the evacuation procedure, and continued appropriate fluid administration via a secure intravenous pathway is essential. Nasogastric intubation with adequate gastric decompression is also necessary during patient movement in the early postburn period if any gastrointestinal dysfunction exists. Bulky dressings may be used effectively during evacuation.

It is essential that adequate documentation of the patient's premovement and in-flight course be maintained and accompany the patient so that continuity of medical care is ensured. Particularly important in this regard is an adequate record of administered fluids, urinary output, medications administered, and any other features of the patient's course that will require serial evaluation, such as neurological deficit. During evacuation, the seriously ill, extensively burned patient should be accompanied by trained surgical personnel familiar with the exigencies of patient movement during the early postburn course.

CHAPTER IV

Cold Injury

HISTORICAL ASPECTS

Although cold injury is seen only sporadically in the population in peacetime, it can be of paramount importance to an Army. Cold injury has played a major role in the outcome of a number of military operations throughout history. Larrey's description of the loss of over 250,000 soldiers of Napoleon's Army in Russia in 1812 identified cold as the major force in the defeat of this Grand Army. In the Crimean war (1852-1856), 309,000 French troops experienced 5,215 cases of frostbite, of which 1,178 were fatal. In just two nights, in Sevastopol, 2,800 cases of frostbite occurred, 900 of which were fatal. In World War I, the British incurred 115,000 trenchfoot or frostbite injuries. In one six-week period in one hospital in Rouen, there were 1,131 casualties with frostbite. In the Dardenelles, in the winter 1915-1916, there were 14,584 admissions for cold injury. U.S. Army cold injury losses in World War I amounted to 2,061 admissions, which translated to a total of 97,200 man-days lost. In just two months in World War II, December 1941 and January 1942, the German army suffered 100,000 cold injuries requiring 15,000 amputations. That was a major factor in their defeat on the eastern front. U.S. experience in World War II and Korea reveals that fully 10% of the wounded casualties (90,000 in World War II and 9,000 in Korea) were cold injuries. Recent British experience in the Falklands listed trenchfoot as the major medical problem in that conflict. Argentine amputations in the same conflict exceeded 200. Clearly, the impact that cold injury can have on military operations is a lesson that seems to have to be learned and relearned in each successive conflict.

Any force that is poorly fed, poorly clothed, or in retreat is more likely to sustain serious cold injury. Adding to the problems of command prevention of cold injuries, the medical personnel who provide care are often unaware of the seriousness of the threat and have little or no experience in dealing with these types of injuries.

CLASSIFICATION

Cold is the primary etiologic agent in producing these injuries, although wetness, duration of exposure, and other associated injuries may add to the severity or eventual outcome of a particular cold exposure. Long-term exposure in wetlands, even in tropical rice paddies, swamps, and jungles, with its prolonged cooling of the feet and constant wetness can produce an immersion-type injury. These injuries represent a continuum of insult making the definition between one type and another somewhat artificial. The spectrum of cold injury in order of increasing seriousness includes chilblain, trenchfoot, immersion foot, frostbite (including high-altitude frostbite), and systemic hypothermia.

All of these conditions represent progressive degrees of a fundamental pathologic process, which, irrespective of environmental and other modifying factors, are all related to the common factor of cold. Although the distinctions among the various types of cold injury are often artificial, particularly the distinction between trenchfoot and immersion foot, the following definitions are in fairly general use:

1. Chilblain, which frequently affects the hands as well as the feet, may result from exposure to air temperatures from just above freezing to as high as 60°F (16°C); is more likely to occur in dry, cold, windy air; but can also be associated with high humidity. It is not of major clinical significance in military operations.

2. Immersion foot implies an injury caused by exposure, usually in excess of 12 hours, to water at a temperature of about 50°F (10°C). This injury is common in wet jungles and in exposed life rafts.

3. Trenchfoot, which may also occur in the hands, results from prolonged exposure to cold at temperatures ranging from just above freezing to 50°F (10°C), often in a damp environment, and usually in connection with immobilization and dependency of the extremities. The blunt trauma of walking on wet feet hastens this injury.

4. Frostbite implies the crystallization of tissue fluids in the skin

or subcutaneous tissues after exposure to temperatures of 32°F (0°C) or lower. Depending upon the ambient temperature and wind velocity, the exposure necessary to produce frostbite varies from a few minutes to several hours. Frostbite may occur at various altitudes. Special attention has been given to high-altitude frostbite. The ambient temperature decreases approximately 3.5°F (2°C) for every 1,000 feet of increase in altitude. The temperature becomes stable at about -67°F (-55°C) at an altitude of 35,000 feet or higher, and exposure to these very low temperatures may instantaneously result in severe injuries to exposed parts of the body.

5. Systemic Hypothermia is a condition associated with a drop of the core temperature below 94°F (34.4°C). This life-threatening, non-freezing cold injury is usually the result of either long-term exposure to cold air or immersion in cold water. It should be noted that freezing temperatures are not necessary to produce hypothermia, because wind, rain, and cool temperatures increase body heat loss significantly.

PATHOGENESIS

Trenchfoot, frostbite, immersion foot, and hypothermia are the cold injuries of greatest military significance. It is believed that frostbite will continue to be the cold injury of major importance, but the use of rubberized, insulated footwear and specific training techniques and procedures will limit the trenchfoot injuries in future combat settings. It is noted that the introduction of the insulated vapor-barrier boot to U.S. forces in Korea almost eliminated cold injury as a reason for hospital admission. This insulated vapor-barrier boot revolutionized footwear for combat soldiers and played the key role in preventing of cold injury of the feet. The type of cold injury incurred is dependent upon the exposure temperature, the duration of exposure, and other environmental factors, such as wind and water, which intensify the effect of the temperature. On exposure to cold, there is an initial peripheral vasoconstriction in an attempt to conserve core heat. This vasoconstrictive episode, which is of short duration, is overcome by a physiologic protective mechanism termed cold-induced vasodilation (CIVD). CIVD intervenes to cause arteriovenous shunting to the skin. This allows relatively large volumes of blood to flow through cold extremities. Repeated cold exposures are said to improve this CIVD response, but it may be suppressed or absent when the individual is chilled, frightened, exhausted, or malnourished. This mechanism appears to be blunted in blacks and perhaps in other races.

Trenchfoot and immersion foot are essentially the same injury, the major differences being the temperatures involved and the duration of exposure. The colder it is, the shorter the duration necessary to produce trenchfoot, whereas the longer the duration and the warmer the temperature, the more likely one is to develop an immersion foot injury. The average duration of exposure in trenchfoot is three days, but the exposure may range from a few hours to many days, with individual susceptibility apparently playing a considerable role. The average duration of exposure in frostbite is ten hours, but this varies with ambient temperature, moisture, clothing, activity, and other factors which will be discussed below.

PATHOLOGIC PROCESS

Although a number of physiologic changes induced by cold may explain tissue loss, it is doubtful that they all play a significant part in clinical cold injury. Intracellular molecular changes due to hyperosmolarity, direct metabolic impairment secondary to the cold, and cellular structural damage from the mechanical effect of ice crystals seem far less important than impairment of nutritional blood flow as a final determinant of tissue injury after thawing. Vascular stasis following thaw from freezing injury has been well documented. Clinical and experimental data indicate the importance of capillary blood flow as the determinant of reversibility in tissue freezing.

Alterations in capillary permeability are evident from experimental data and, clinically, from the edema and bleb formation that occur soon after thawing. Endothelial disruption may be responsible for the progressive capillary stasis, plugging, and thrombosis that eventually occur.

EPIDEMIOLOGY FACTORS

The military community responds to cold trauma according to accepted epidemiologic principles. The specific causative agent is cold. Moisture is closely related because it speeds the loss of body heat, although it alone cannot cause cold injury. Cold produces injury by increasing the rate of body-heat loss. This rate is determined not only by the ambient temperature, but also by other factors such as moisture and wind. Moisture increases the rate of heat loss by conduction and evaporation, wind by convection.

A variety of environmental and host factors combines in the total causation of cold injury and influences the incidence, prevalence, type, and severity of the injury, though these influences vary from situation to situation. The most important environmental factors in cold injury are weather, clothing, and type of combat action.

Weather is a predominant influence in the causation of cold injury. Temperature, humidity, precipitation, and wind modify the rate of loss of body heat. Low temperatures and low relative humidity favor the development of trenchfoot. Wind velocity and low temperatures act synergistically, expressed as chill factor, to accelerate the loss of body heat under conditions of both wet and cold.

The type of combat action is apparently the most important environmental factor. Units in reserve or in rest areas have few cases. Units on holding missions or on static defense, in which exposure is greater, show a moderate increase in incidence. Factors which modify the incidence in relation to the rate of combat action include immobility under fire; prolonged exposure; lack of opportunity to warm the body, change clothing, or carry out measures of personal hygiene; fatigue; fear; and state of nutrition. In warfare, in which exposure under conditions of stress may be prolonged, adequate clothing becomes essential to welfare and survival.

HOST FACTORS

The following are host factors that may or may not influence the development of cold injury:

1. Age. There is no convincing evidence that age is a significant epidemiologic factor in cold injury among combat troops.

2. Smoking. There is very clear evidence that the vasoconstrictor action of nicotine causes increased cooling of the extremities and an increased likelihood of frostbite. A significant number of severe injuries in military populations occur in heavy tobacco users.

3. Previous Cold Injury. Individuals with previous cold injuries are at a higher-than-normal risk of subsequent cold injury. The

fact that such repetitive injury does not usually occur at the same site suggests that this relates to the individual's lower resistance to cold rather than as a result of the previous injury.

4. Branch of Service. Trenchfoot, immersion foot, and frostbite have a high selectivity for frontline riflemen, especially for riflemen of lower ranks. In World War II, approximately 90% of all casualties from cold occurred in riflemen.

5. Fatigue. Both physical and mental weariness contribute to apathy which leads to neglect of all acts except those vital to survival. Fatigue is most evident in troops who are not rotated and must remain exposed and in combat for prolonged periods of time. Three days of being cold and wet appears to be a prudent timeframe within which to consider rotation of troops.

6. Racial Susceptibility. In all studies from World War II, Korea, and recent experiences in Alaska, blacks had four to six times the incidence of cold injury of their white counterparts, matched for geographic origin, training, and education. This increased susceptibility is related to two factors: (a) differences in anatomic configuration, and (b) differences in physiologic response to cold. Because long, thin fingers and toes cool more rapidly than short, fat ones, blacks' hands tend to cool faster than those of whites. However, more importantly, once cold, blacks stay cold longer because of a less potent CIVD response to their extremities. This does not say, however, that blacks themselves must be more vigilant in cold exposure and must take measures sooner to protect themselves from cold injury. Place of origin has a significant role in cold injury susceptibility. Individuals raised in northern-tier states (i.e., cold climates) have a more protective CIVD response. This response also improves in blacks from northern climates. This is not only a physiologic improvement in response to cold but a behavioral response as well. Knowing what clothes to wear, knowing when one's extremities are too cold, not being frightened of the cold, and knowing how to deal with cold extremities all add up to make cold-experienced individuals less likely to have cold injuries. Individuals with labile vasomotor conditions, such as Raynaud's, are also susceptible to cold injury.

7. Psychological Factors. Cold injury tends to occur in passive, negative individuals. Such persons show less muscular activity in situations in which activity is unrestricted and are careless about precautionary measures when cold injury is a threat. Fear also may increase the incidence of cold injury by reducing the spontaneous rewarming known as CIVD.

8. Other Injuries. Concomitant injuries that result in a reduction of circulating volume or a localized reduction in blood flow predispose the individual to cold injury. In addition, immobilization associated with a concurrent injury increases the risk of frostbite in cold environments if adequate additional insulating protection is not provided. Poor hydration and hypovolemia decrease perfusion of the extremities.

9. Drugs and Medication. Any drug modifying autonomic nervous system responses, altering sensation, or modifying judgment can have disastrous effects on an individual's performance and survival in the cold. These factors must be impressed upon medical officers involved in the care of troops in cold environments and must be impressed upon individual unit commanders and their men. In the civilian community, alcohol use is the single most common factor associated with hypothermia.

DISCIPLINE, TRAINING, AND EXPERIENCE

Cold injury is preventable. Well-trained, fit, disciplined soldiers can be protected from cold injury even in adverse, pinned-down positions if they are knowledgeable concerning the hazards of cold exposure and informed regarding the importance of personal hygiene, care of the feet, exercise, and the rational use of clothing. Such discipline and training are a command and not a medical responsibility and reinforcement of these principles throughout the field operations is essential to the goal of protection from cold injury. Although cold injury is preventable, commanders may be faced with circumstances that are likely to lead to large numbers of casualties, and a decision may have to be made to accept a certain number of cold injuries to win the battle. The need for a major offensive in a cold, wet environment, or a retreat when faced by an overwhelming foe, may prompt a commander to accept cold injuries to change the tide of battle. The highest levels of command must be aware of the medical implications of such decisions. The combination of fit, disciplined soldiers, trained for cold weather operations, plus the provision of dry clothing, adequate food, water, and shelter will minimize the number of cold injuries.

CLINICAL MANIFESTATIONS

Patients generally describe initial feelings of cold discomfort in their extremities, followed by varying periods of pain and mild discomfort along with a cyclic, dull ache. These symptoms subside into a period of anesthesia. From there, cold injury progresses in a painless fashion. Patients often describe a sensation of walking on a wooden limb. Because of the anesthetic nature of cold injury, patients often say they were unaware that they were developing an injury. The hypothermia victim retreats inward psychologically; has dulled senses, a stumbling gait, muscle incoordination, and slurred speech; and is universally unaware of the insidious decrement in his capability.

In a cold, wet environment, trenchfoot often appears. Anesthesia of the limb in trenchfoot injury comes on rapidly. Pain which does not respond to analgesia limits the deployment of soldiers with normal-appearing extremities. Most patients are unaware of or do not care about the potential severity of their injury. The first physical manifestation of frostbite injury is reddening of the skin, which later becomes pale, waxy white, and hard. Lack of mobility of skin over joints is a common finding. In hypothermia, shivering is a clear indication of loss of body temperature. Shivering varies with age, physical condition, degree of hypothermia, and amount of ingested drugs. Shivering can significantly limit an individual's performance of specific military tasks, including sighting targets, reading maps, and manipulating small dials and radios. It is a form of involuntary exercise that produces heat. When shivering stops, the patient is at the mercy of the environment. CNS involvement appears to be the most common outward manifestation of hypothermia. Decreased dexterity and coordination, speech and memory impairment, and the eventual loss of consciousness indicate progressive loss of neurologic function. Dysarthria is a specific early indication of hypothermia and is often one of the first recognizable signs of the loss of deep body temperature.

Judgment of the degree of frostbite has historically involved a retrospective grading system involving four categories. It is more useful and realistic, however, to determine two major categories: superficial and deep. Because frostbite is a continuum of events, the differentiation between first, second, third, and fourth degrees is often clouded and may take some days or weeks to become completely obvious.

In first-degree injuries, erythema and edema, along with transient tingling or burning, are early manifestations. The skin becomes mottled blue/grey and red, hot, and dry. Swelling begins within two or three hours and persists for ten days or more, depending upon the seriousness of the injury. Desquamation of the superficial epithelium begins in 5-10 days and may continue for as long as a month, but no deep tissue is lost. Parathesias, aching, and necrosis of the pressure points of the foot are common sequelae. Increased sensitivity to cold and hyperhydrosis may appear, especially with repeated first-degree injuries. It should be noted that it is difficult to differentiate first-degree frostbite from abrasion produced by the insulated vapor barrier boot. Medical personnel must be cognizant of the difference as both injuries occur in the same clinical setting.

Second-degree cold injury starts as does first-degree, but progresses to blister formation, anesthesia, and deep color change. Edema may form, but it disappears within days. Vesicles appear within 12-24 hours. They generally appear on the dorsum of the extremities, and when these vesicles dry they form an eschar. Blisters are a good clinical sign as long as they are filled with clear fluid. If the fluid is hemorrhagic, they are not a good sign. As these vesicles dry, they sluff cleanly with pink granulation tissue beneath or they form black eschars. Throbbing and aching pain occurs 3-10 days after this injury. Hyperhydrosis is apparent at the second or third weeks. Early rupture of the blisters with subsequent infection often occurs in second-degree cold injury. This infection significantly increases the severity of the frostbite injury.

Third-degree injury involves full skin thickness and extends into the subcutaneous tissue. Vesicles are smaller and may be hemorrhagic. Generalized edema of the extremity may occur, but it usually abates within 5-6 days. Subfacial pressure increases and compartment syndromes are common in third- and fourth-degree cold injuries. If pressure rises significantly with loss of distal blood flow, faciotomy along with vasodilators is indicated for therapy. The skin forms a black, hard, dry eschar, usually thicker and more intense than that of the second-degree injury. When it finally demarcates, sloughing with some ulceration occurs if there is no complicating infection. The average healing time is 68 days. Patients often complain of burning, aching, throbbing, or shooting pains beginning on the fifth day and usually lasting through four or five weeks. Hyperhydrosis and cyanosis appear later and extreme cold sensitivity is a common post injury sequela.

In fourth-degree injury, there is destruction of the entire thickness of the part, including bone, resulting in extensive loss of tissue. After rewarming, tissue is cyanotic and insensitive, and blister formation, if present, is hemorrhagic. Severe pain on rewarming, along with a deep cyanotic appearance, regularly occurs. In rapidly-frozen extremities or the freeze-thaw-refreeze injury, dry gangrene progresses quickly with mummification. With slower freeze, there is some early swelling and deep pain, and demarcation takes much longer to occur. The line of demarcation becomes obvious at 20-36 days and extends into the bone in 60 or more days.

MANAGEMENT

A major deterrent to evaluation of therapy has been the inability to predict the outcome in any given cold injury early in the post-thaw period. Because of this, nuances of clinical management have been very difficult to evaluate. Since the extent of injury to the tissue is related to temperature and the duration of exposure, rapid rewarming is of primary importance. Other therapeutic programs, including anticoagulant therapy, administration of low molecular weight dextran or similar agents, or surgical or pharmacologic sympathectomy, while theoretically sound and supported in some instances by experimental data, have not had controlled clinical trials sufficient to encourage their general use.

In the light of most clinical experience, it should be emphasized that meddlesome manipulations, rubbing, application of unguents, or exposure to excessive temperatures should be guarded against carefully. As soon as cold injury is recognized, every effort should be made to avoid compounding the effects of cold with physical injury.

In military operations, the treatment of cold injuries is influenced by (1) the tactical situation, (2) the availability of evacuation to a fixed facility, and (3) the fact that most cold injuries are encountered in large numbers, during periods of intense combat, at the same time that many other wounded casualties are generated. Highly individualized treatment under these circumstances may be impossible. Examination and treatment of more life-endangering wounds must take precedence over this injury (lives versus limbs).

As a practical matter, any specific therapy designed to modify the physiologic changes in cold injuries must be instituted very early after thawing. Since, in many cases, the injury is not seen until some time after thawing, contemplation of therapy is purely academic and the major emphasis must be on protection from further injury, avoidance of premature surgery that might sacrifice otherwise viable tissue, early identification and control of infections, attention to maintenance of extremity function through early physiotherapy, and generalized nutritional support.

FIRST AID

The emergency treatment of cold injury is as follows:

1. All casualties with involvement of the lower extremities should be treated as litter cases if feasible.

2. Carefully assess concomitant injury or complicating systemic problems.

3. All constricting items of clothing, such as boots, gloves, and socks, should be removed, but only when adequate protection from further cold exposure is available. Boots and clothing frozen on the body should be thawed by immersion in warm water before removal. Vigorous manipulation of frozen parts or attempts at range of motion or massage should be avoided. If the hands are affected, rings should be removed from the fingers early after presentation.

4. If the injured parts are still frozen when first seen, they should be rewarmed rapidly by immersion in water at 100° to 104°F (37.5° to 40°C) with added antiseptic soap, such as pHisoHex, and with agitation of the bath water to hasten the warming. A whirlpool apparatus is most satisfactory for this.

5. General body warmth must be maintained. Sleep and rest should be encouraged.

6. A booster dose of tetanus toxoid should be given to those previously immunized. No evidence exists that prophylactic use

of antibiotics is valuable either in promoting healing or in preventing superficial or deep infection. In fact, the use of prophylactic antibiotics may result in the emergence of a resistant strain of organisms.

7. Large vesicles or bullae should be protected and kept intact if possible. Once ruptured, it is usually desirable to debride the vesicle. Ointment dressings have no place in the usual management of cold injury. Protective dry dressings are desirable during transportation, and sterile cotton should be used between the toes to prevent maceration.

8. Smoking is prohibited.

LATER MANAGEMENT

When the casualty reaches a definitive care facility, the following treatment should be employed:

1. Continued diligence to avoid injury of already compromised tissue should be maintained. In general, for lower extremity injuries, this is accomplished by keeping the patient at bed rest, with the part elevated on surgically clean sheets under a foot cradle and with sterile pledgets of cotton separating the toes. Bearing-weight on injured feet should not be allowed until mature epithelial tissue has developed over the affected areas. In upper extremity injuries, elevation is also desirable on sterile towels, with special care to avoid injury to bullae.

2. In an effort to reduce superficial bacterial contamination, the affected part is treated by whirlpool bath at 98.6°F (37°C), with povidone iodine or hexachlorophine added, on a twice-daily basis, encouraging active motion on the part of the patient during the whirlpool treatment. Whirlpool baths assist in superficial debridement and make active range of motion exercises more tolerable to the patient and less traumatic to the tissues.

3. Analgesics may be required in the early post-thaw days, but a continued requirement for analgesics in uncomplicated injuries is uncommon.

4. The patient should be encouraged to take a nutritious diet with adequate fluids to maintain hydration.

5. Patients should be placed on surgically clean sheets and all lesions should be exposed to the air at the normal room temperature.

6. Superficial debridement of ruptured blebs should be per-

formed, and suppurative eschars and partially detached nails should be removed. Close attention should be paid to circumferential eschars or eschars where vascular compromise could be a problem. Such eschars at least should be bivalved, although complete debridement is occasionally necessary. Early amputation has no place in the management of cold injury. Surgical intervention should be deferred until a distinct line of demarcation has developed. There is usually healthy granulation tissue under an eschar at the line of demarcation. Delay of surgical procedures, especially in upper extremity injuries, will enhance the potential for a functional result. Rarely, generalized sepsis from large areas of necrotic and infected tissue will necessitate amputation. Skin grafting, while not a function of forward facilities, is occasionally indicated to protect denuded areas over vital structures.

7. Active physiotherapy should be instituted during daily whirlpool as soon as possible.

8. Newly epithelialized areas are susceptible to minor trauma, as in walking, and are especially sensitive to cold. Therefore, continued protection must be offered until normal keratinization has occurred. Subsequently, special skin care may be required to deal with residual hyperhydrotic states.

PROPHYLAXIS

The successful prevention and control of cold injuries depend, first of all, upon vigorous command interest, the provision of adequate clothing, and a number of individual and group measures. These measures include:

1. A thorough appreciation and comprehension by command, staff, technical personnel, and all combat components regarding the potential losses that may occur from cold injury, both in winter combat and in other circumstances in which cold injury has been known to occur.

2. There should be full command support, by echelon, of a comprehensive and practical cold injury prevention and control program. It should be emphasized again that this is a command, not a medical, responsibility.

3. Indoctrination of all personnel in the prevention of cold injuries individually and by units.

4. The provision of adequate supplies of clothing and footgear and their correct utilization to avoid exposure to cold. The pro-

gram of supply must provide adequate dry clothing for the daily needs of the soldier who is farthest forward in combat; it must also provide for the correct fitting of clothing and boots. All articles of clothing must be sized and fitted to avoid constriction of the extremities and tightness over the back, buttocks, and thighs.

Clothing for cold weather, based on the layering principle, is now designed as an assembly for protection of the head, torso, and extremities. The clothing is worn in loose layers, with air spaces between the layers, under an outer wind-resistant and water-resistant garment. Body heat is thus conserved. The garment is flexible, and inner layers can be removed for comfort and efficiency in higher ambient temperatures or during strenuous physical exertion. Prevention of loss of body heat by the proper protection of the body is as important as the efficient use of appropriate dry footgear and warm dry gloves. Finally, the most efficient clothing is of no value unless a high level of individual and unit clothing discipline are maintained through training.

5. Special protection for certain groups who may be especially susceptible to cold injury, together with the regular rotation of all troops. It should be remembered that casualties with exposed wounds and injuries are particularly liable to cold injury because blood and transudate from their wounds will freeze from the clothing inward.

6. Effective policies of sorting in forward areas, with provision for early evacuation and treatment of casualties actually suffering from cold trauma.

7. The identification of factors responsible for cold injury in special situations, which is a command responsibility. Significant numbers of cases occur as a result of barehanded contact with cold metal or gasoline; as a result of rapid deployment of troops seated in unheated vehicles, without interruptions for short rewarming marches every few hours; as a result of airdrops of troops into cold areas without adequate protective equipment and training; or as a result of several hours' confinement of artic-equipped airborne troops in heated aircraft, followed by a drop into a subzero environment after their insulating clothing has been saturated with perspiration. Only by the evaluation of these factors can the specific measures necessary in particular units or groups be put into effect.

HYPOTHERMIA

Hypothermia victims, depending on their core temperatures and the durations of their exposure, present with different degrees of physiologic depression. Cold suppresses metabolic function and decreases oxygen demand, thereby enhancing survival. Recognition of this survival potential is critical to successful resuscitation. Everyone involved in the treatment and evacuation of these casualties must be cognizant of the phrase "No one is cold and dead, only warm and dead." Failure to respond to rewarming is the only criterion for death in hypothermia.

Two major defenses against hypothermia are peripheral vasoconstriction and shivering. Peripheral vasoconstriction reduces ·cutaneous blood flow, which conserves core heat by decreasing both radiant and convective heat losses to the environment. Shivering is an involuntary muscle activity that increased heat production. The end result of peripheral vasoconstriction, which decreases circulating volume, is cold diuresis. Shivering produces significant metabolite production, including lactic acid. The longer one is exposed to cold, the greater will be one's metabolic derangement. Dry land hypothermics shiver violently and diurese for long periods of time. This experience diuresis results in more severe metabolic abnormalities. On the other hand, water-immersion hypothermics who cool rapidly do not shiver quite as long and often present with a normal electrolyte and pH profile. As cells drop below 30°C in an acid medium the sodium pump fails and potassium leaks out of cells into the general circulation. As the core temperature drops in the presence of acidosis and hyperkalemia, severe cardiac arrhythmias occur. Hemorrhage from wounds in a cold environment leads to rapid hypothermia.

Hypothermics have decreased cerebral metabolic activity. They show a stumbling gait, incoordination, slurred speech, and a psychological inward retreat. Their senses are dull; they are apathetic, drowsy, and more exhausted than their activity would warrant. This state progresses to unconsciousness. The disorientation, confusion, irrational judgment, and poor decision-making ability pose a significant threat in leadership roles since the small-unit leader is usually exposed to the same physical and cold stresses as his troops. The leader may, in fact, not be able to recognize the signs and symptoms of hypothermia in those he leads if he is experiencing the same symptoms himself. This scenario can result in disaster.

FIELD MANAGEMENT OF HYPOTHERMICS

Individuals must be stripped of their wet clothing; insulated; given warm, sweet drinks; and encouraged to do large-muscle activities that will warm them up. Warming the core with external heat is an extremely difficult physiologic problem. Conscious individuals will shiver and initiate rewarming. If other muscle activity is added, they will warm up quickly. Replacement of fluids is essential to improve peripheral circulation, cutaneous perfusion, and cardiac output. Comatose individuals must be handled carefully, as rough handling can produce ventricular fibrillation arrest. The airway should be patent. Wet clothes should be carefully stripped. They should be well covered and insulated. They should then be transported as rapidly as possible to definitive medical care. Positive pressure ventilation is advised but chest compression is not. Such compressions may convert sinus bradycardia to ventricular fibrillation.

Field rewarming procedures for the comatose individual are time consuming. If possible, it is better to move the casualty to a nearby medical facility. A heated, humidified oxygen rewarming device, if available, may be effective, but is certainly not a major method of heat input for the comatose hypothermic victim. Management throughout the evacuation chain involves improving cardiac output, decreasing blood viscosity, adding heat to the core, improving acid-base balance, and the hyperkalemia. Treatment of imbalances in these parameters depends on the level of sophistication at each treatment site. Hospital management should include active core rewarming utilizing peritoneal dialysis, arterio-venous shunts, or peripheral rewarming involving torso water immersion. Rewarming blankets are slow but may be the only rewarming devices available. Volume replacement is essential to decrease viscosity and increase cardiac output. Low central venous pressures are advisable early and are increased slowly as there is an indication of the ability to hold fluid in the vascular space. Lactate-free and potassium-free fluids are advisable, as lactate conversion to pyruvate by the liver does not occur below 32°C and hyperkalemia probably already exists. Hyperkalemia is improved by fluid replacement and glucose and insulin infusions. Sodium bicarbonate is indicated early to begin correction of acidosis. However, overzealous correction is ill advised. The patient should be kept mildly acidotic throughout the treatment process. Improved ventilation during the resuscitation can improve pH significantly. Antiarrthymic drugs are contraindicated. Excessive early manipulation can result in cardiac arrest. This complication is managed by continuing the rewarming process, along with half-rate, closed-chest cardiac massage until the temperature reaches 31° or 32°C, at which point electrical conversion is more likely to be successful. The patient with severe acidosis and hyperkalemia should not be rewarmed past 30°C. Post rewarming complications include pneumonia, pancreatitis, intravascular thromboses, gastric erosions, and acute tubular necrosis. Pneumonitis is by far the most common problem. It is managed by pulmonary toilet and appropriate antibiotics.

CHAPTER V

Blast Injuries

Explosions inflict injury in a number of ways. *Primary blast injury* is due solely to the direct effect of the pressure wave on the body. *Secondary blast injury* results from penetrating or nonpenetrating damage caused by ordinance projectiles or secondary missiles, which are energized by the explosion and strike the victim. *Tertiary blast injury* results from whole body displacement and subsequent traumatic impact with environmental objects. Tertiary effects generally result from the bulk flow of gases away from an explosion and occur when the individual is in very close proximity to the explosion. Displacement may take place relatively far from the point of detonation if an individual is positioned in the path that gases must take to vent from a structure, such as in a hatch, in a doorway, or by a window. Thermal injury from radiation, hot gases, or fires started by the explosion are considered to be miscellaneous blast effects. Other indirect effects include crush injury from the collapse of structures and toxic effects from the inhalation of combustion gases.

The pressure wave close to the explosion moves outward at supersonic speed. As the wave spherically propagates, it decelerates and loses energy. In water, because of its incompressibility, the speed of wave propagation is much greater and the wave loses energy less quickly with distance. The lethal radius around an explosion in water is about three times the lethal radius of a similar explosion in air.

A typical pressure wave from an explosion in air is shown in Figure 17. Pressure rises almost instantaneously in the ambient environment and then decays exponentially. The peak pressure and duration of the initial positive phase are a function of the size of the explosion and the distance from the detonation. In air, the peak pressure is proportional to the cube root of explosive weight and the inverse of the cube of the distance from detonation. If the pressure wave is in close apposition to a solid barrier, the pressure exerted at the reflecting surface may be many times that of the incident wave.

A blast wave that causes only modest primary injury in the open can be lethal if the casualty was caught near a reflecting surface, such as a solid wall. The bulk flow of gases away from the explosion (blast wind) travels much slower than the shock wave, but may be of importance in causing displacement close to the point of explosion, especially with very large explosions.

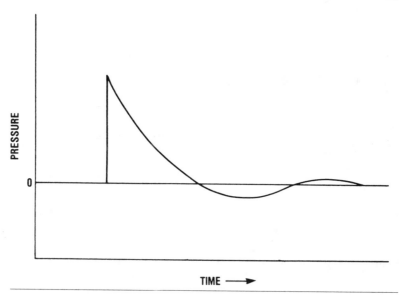

Figure 17.—Idealized representation of pressure · time history of an explosion in air.

For a sharp rising blast wave, damage to both inanimate and biological structures has been shown to be a function of the peak pressure and the duration of the initial positive phase (Figure 18). This figure illustrates the estimated blast levels necessary to cause a range of primary effects in man.

PATHOLOGY OF PRIMARY BLAST INJURY

Primary blast injury is seen almost exclusively in gas containing organs: the ear and the respiratory and gastrointestinal tracts. Of the three organ systems, the ear is the most sensitive. The pinna and the external canal collect and in some cases, amplify pressure signals so that the tympanic membrane, converting acoustic energy to mechanical displacement, is displaced into the middle

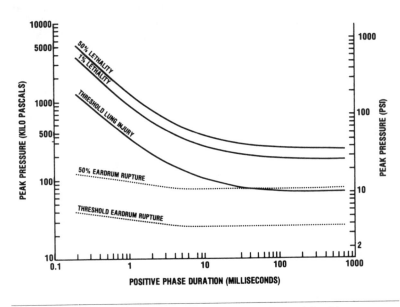

Figure 18.—Estimated human tolerances for single, sharp, rising blast waves.

ear. At pressures of approximately 35 kiloPascals (kPa, with 7 kPa equalling 1 pound per square inch), the human eardrum may rupture (Figure 18). Above 100 kPa, almost all eardrums will be ruptured. The eardrum generally perforates inferiorly in the *pars tensa* but there may be hemorrhage into the membrane without rupture. At higher pressures, the drum may be almost obliterated and the ossicles can be dislocated or fractured. Vestibular function is usually not affected.

Injury to the lung is the cause of the greatest morbidity and mortality. Grossly, one sees diffuse, pleurally-based pulmonary contusions with a stiffened, heavy lung. The costal surface may show transverse stripes called "rib markings" which, in fact, are more closely associated with intercostal spaces. Lung weights may be two or three times normal. Pleural rents or blebs may result in pneumothorax, hemothorax, or mediastinal extravasation of air. Rib fractures or evidence of significant chest wall damage are not seen in the absence of other mechanisms of trauma. Microscopically, the hemorrhage is mainly intra-alveolar with some perivascular or peribronchial disruption and bleeding. Alveolar walls are torn, sometimes producing giant blood-filled alveolar spaces. Alveolar-pulmonary venous communications, the source of air emboli within the arterial circulation, are created. These fistulae are responsible for most of the early mortality resulting from primary blast injury. Critical vascular beds in the central nervous or coronary arterial circulations can be occluded by entrained air emboli with subsequent disastrous results.

The gastrointestinal tract may be damaged wherever there are collections of gas. Injury to the gut is particularly severe in under-water blasts. While hollow visceral injury is also present in airblast, it is generally overshadowed by the more dramatic presentation of air emboli or acute respiratory insufficiency. The colon is the hollow viscus most commonly disrupted. Gastric injuries are usually less common and less severe. Rarely, one encounters rupture of the spleen or liver in the absence of superimposed blunt abdominal trauma. Pathologically, injuries to the bowel range from subserosal or intramural hemorrhage to frank rupture. The natural history of such bowel wall hemotomas is not known, but it is clear that some can progress to perforation during the post-injury course.

MECHANISMS OF INJURY

The blast wave exerts a force (pressure times exposed area) on the body surface. That force is transmitted to internal structures by bulk movement of tissue. Inertial effects may play a role in the injuries seen around the relatively massive airways and vessels suspended in the lighter tissue of the lungs. Mass differences, the compressibility of isolated gas pockets, and the material proper-ties of the foam-like lung tissue are probably critical factors in blast injury. Pressure waves propagate in the lung parenchyma as a result of blast exposure. At some point, the lung is unable to pass on the local stresses generated at the pleural surface as fast as the chest wall moves and delivers energy. In such a case, the local com-pressions, shears, or tensile stresses exceed the physical limits of the lung substance and injury occurs.

For the gut and tympanic membrane, the physical events leading to injury are probably much simpler. Isolated collections of gas within the bowel lumen are compressed by the pressure wave within the abdomen. At some point, the bowel wall is stressed to the point of failure, manifested as either intramural hemorrhage or frank rupture. The eardrum is a relatively simple membrane which completely closes one end of a tube, the other end of which is open to the air. The middle ear airspace behind the drum is unable to equilibrate pressures rapidly enough through the Eustachian tube. When the stress on the drum exceeds the limits of the tissue, the tympanic membrane ruptures.

CLINICAL PRESENTATION OF PRIMARY BLAST INJURY

Primary blast injury effects may be only a part of the problem in a casualty suffering from multiple trauma. In the setting of injury associated with a large blast, the basic principles of trauma care still apply, and resuscitation and evaluation should proceed by the usual numbers. The key to recognizing that primary blast injury is present is a history or setting suggestive of a powerful explosion. One should then search for corroborative findings with a careful examination of the tympanic membranes, retinal arteries, chest, and abdomen. Specialized military ordinance such as a fuel air explosive or underwater blast may cause a relatively pure form of primary blast injury. Fuel air explosive ordinance is a particularly powerful air blast designed to clear mine fields by detonating the land mines in place.

The ear and the upper respiratory tract are the structures most sensitive to primary blast injury. Rupture of the tympanic membrane may cause tinnitus, pain, and hearing loss. Physical examination will reveal blood in the external canal and otoscopic evidence of perforation. In severe injury, there can be vestibular damage with disordered equilibrium. Pressure levels high enough to cause serious injury to the lungs or gut almost invariably rupture the eardrums. This may not be the case when ears were protected by ear muffs or ear plugs. Often the tympanic membranes are not ruptured by high-grade underwater explosions if the head is above water and the tympanic membranes are not exposed to the underwater pressure wave. Petechial hemorrhage in the hypopharynx and larynx is also observed at relatively low pressure levels and, like tympanic rupture, its absence speaks against exposure to high levels of blast. Upper airway petechial hemorrahge such as this is unlikely to cause airway compromise or other symptoms.

Arterial air emboli represent an immediate threat to life. Clinical evaluation in the presence of air emboli will reveal evidence of cerebral dysfunction such as altered affect, confusion, disorientation, or focal neurologic signs. When such findings are noted after an explosion, one must first consider a skull fracture or other closed head injury. Direct trauma to the skull from secondary or tertiary blast effects is more likely than air emboli in most settings. It may be possible to directly visualize air bubbles in the retinal vessels or to observe patchy blanching of the tongue. Emboli to the coronary arteries will be evidenced by arrhythmias or ischemic electrocardiograph changes. Emboli to other vascular beds might be expected to give a clinical picture similar to the "bends" or decompression illness.

Primary blast injury of the lung presents a clinical picture similar to that of pulmonary contusion from blunt chest trauma, but without rib fractures or chest wall injury. Chest tightness, pain, and hemoptysis are common complaints. One observes tachypnea, the employment of accessory muscles of respiration, and other signs of respiratory distress. Evidence of pulmonary consolidation may indicate either contusion or a hemothorax. A pneumothorax may present as unilateral hyper-resonance with decreased breath sounds and a contralateral shift of the trachea and mediastinum. A precordial systolic crunch on auscultation indicates extravasation of air into the mediastinum. Roentgenographic examination of the chest is mandatory. A simple, frontal view will be diagnostic in most instances of significant barotrauma. Pneumothorax, hemothorax, pneumomediastinum, pleural blebs, subcutaneous emphysema and pulmonary interstitial emphysema can be confirmed by the chest X-ray. The manifestations of contusion may develop over the course of hours and may have the appearance of a local or diffuse infiltrate. The clinical picture of "blast lung" may develop over 24—48 hours. In a complex trauma setting, it is very difficult to differentiate the respiratory insufficiency of the adult respiratory distress syndrome with its varied etiologies from that due solely to primary blast injury to the lungs. Aside from arterial blood gas determinations, laboratory studies have little to offer early on.

Gastrointestinal injury usually presents a less dramatic clinical picture and its diagnosis may be suppressed by the more life-threatening effects of air emboli or respiratory insufficiency. Signs of peritoneal irritation such as involuntary guarding, rebound tenderness, and absent bowel sounds may indicate visceral rupture. Bright red rectal bleeding has occurred with low sigmoid injury. Contused bowel may necrose and perforate several days after the initial trauma. Abdominal X-rays may reveal free peritoneal air or air within the lumen of the bowel wall. Although multiple organ injury is the usual case in underwater blast injury, visceral injury may predominate and may represent the sole major injury.

TREATMENT OF PRIMARY BLAST INJURY

The individual with primary blast injury usually presents with associated injuries. The basic principles of triage and trauma care management still pertain. Airway establishment, control of hemorrhage, and reversal of shock should proceed without consideration of the presence of blast injury. Since an overly generous administration of fluids during the resuscitation may complicate pulmonary injury, pulmonary artery catheterization and pressure monitoring may be necessary to guide fluid therapy in complex cases. When possible, blast victims should be kept sedentary, as exercise may increase mortality by increasing air emboli or by worsening lung hemorrhage.

Tympanic rupture is treated conservatively. After examination, any debris should be cleared from the external canal; however, no irrigation should be attempted. The majority of tympanic tears will heal spontaneously. About one fourth will require surgical closure which can be delayed for weeks.

Air emboli from a severe blast may be lethal within minutes. The incidence of severe air embolism can be lessened by placing the individual in the prone position with the left side down, the back at a 45° angle to the ground, and the head lower than the feet. This position is thought to distribute emboli to the lower extremities rather than to the head vessels, and is also thought to trap air in the right heart. If seen early enough, prompt use of a compression chamber may be lifesaving. Hyperbaric therapy works both by physically reducing the size of the bubbles and by speeding their absorption. The addition of oxygen to the hyperbaric environment probably adds little to the effect of the increased pressure. In the absence of hyperbaric capability, empiric therapy for CNS injury or cardiac ischemia should be instituted.

Respiratory distress should be immediately treated with supplemental oxygen, and the individual should be evaluated to establish whether the etiology is pneumothorax or pulmonary parenchymal failure from blast or other causes (e.g., inhalation of toxic gases). Progressive respiratory failure poses a particular problem since positive pressure ventilation may increase the incidence and severity of both air emboli and pulmonary barotrauma. If oxygen delivery via conventional binasal prongs or a face mask is insufficient to produce adequate tissue oxygenation, constant positive airway pressure (CPAP), either by face mask or endotracheal tube, should be employed to keep small airways open and to improve oxygenation. Positive pressure ventilation assistance should not be withheld if the clinical situation deteriorates.

Inhalation anesthesia carries a very high morbidity in blast injury. This is probably due to the unmonitored use of positive pressure ventilation intraoperatively and to the difficulty of neurologically assessing the patient. Every effort should be made to perform surgical procedures under regional or spinal anesthesia. Airway pressures during inhalation anesthesia should be kept as low as possible since intraoperative pneumothorax can be produced. Consideration should be given to the prophylactic use of chest tubes. One should anticipate the very possible occurrence of pleural complications by performing frequent physical examinations and chest roentgenograms.

Blast injury of the gastrointestinal tract should be managed in the same way as blunt trauma. Hypovolemic shock in the absence of other obvious etiology should suggest visceral rupture, and warrants diagnostic peritoneal lavage and consideration of laparotomy. Decompression via a nasogastric tube should be undertaken with any peritoneal signs and whenever ventilatory assistance is instituted. The patient should be observed for several days because of the risk of delayed perforation. The role of antibiotics and anti-inflammatory medication is unclear, although both have their advocates.

CONCLUSION

Primary blast injury may present in individuals exposed to powerful explosions in military operations. It is likely to coexist with missile injuries, blunt trauma, burns, and other injuries.

Diagnosis is suspected in the presence of tympanic rupture or hypopharyngeal petechial hemorrhage. Treatment is similar to that for blunt trauma to the chest or abdomen. An important feature is the recognition of pneumothorax and arterial air emboli, both of which may be made worse by positive pressure ventilation.

CHAPTER VI

Chemical Injury

INTRODUCTION

This chapter provides updated guidance for initial care of chemical casualties so as to save life and limb and to aid in the soldier's early return to duty. The recommendations include current research views and should be considered as an adjunct to, not a substitute for, doctrinal management as outlined in Army TM 8-285, *Treatment of Chemical Agent Casualties and Conventional Military Chemical Injuries*, dated May 1974 (Change #2, November 1985).

BACKGROUND

Since some of our potential adversaries maintain large stocks of chemical agents, train under realistic conditions, and aim for tactical surprise, the threat from chemical warfare (CW) agents on the battlefield is very real. It should also be borne in mind that CW agents are easily synthesized from readily available chemicals and could therefore be employed to advantage by third-world nations. The operational scenario may well be one of initial chemical attack compelling defending troops to "button up," followed by assault with conventional weapons. Thus, the high likelihood of having to deal with combined chemical and traumatic injuries must always be kept in mind.

CLASSIFICATION

The operational classification of CW agents is shown in Table 3. Riot control agents (e.g., tear gas) are not considered CW agents since symptoms are transient and self-limiting. Conversely certain extremely potent chemicals, such as mycotoxins and neurotoxins, are classified with the biological warfare (BW) agents.

TABLE 3.—*Chemical Warfare Agent Classification*

Category	US Code	Common Name
Nerve Agents	GA	Tabun
	GB	Sarin
	GD	Soman
	VX	——
Blister Agents	HD	Distilled Mustard
	L	Lewisite
	CX	Phosgene oxime
Blood Agents	AC	Hydrogen cyanide
	CK	Cyanogen chloride
Choking Agents	CG	Phosgene
	CL	Chlorine
Incapacitation Agents	BZ, QNB	Quinuclidinyl benzilate

IDENTIFICATION AND DIAGNOSIS

Table 4 provides rough initial identification guidance based on the time lag between CW agent exposure and onset of symptoms and signs. Table 5 then aids in diagnostic differentiation once the early signs and symptoms of chemical exposure are established.

TABLE 4.—*Time of Onset*

Precipitous Onset	Rapid Onset	Delayed Onset
Choking Agent: CL	Inhaled Nerve Agent	Absorbed Nerve Agent
Blister Agent: L	Blood Agent	Inhaled Blister Agent
Incap Agent	Liquid in Eye: HD	Choking Agent: CX

TABLE 5.—*Early Signs and Symptoms of Chemical Exposure*

	Signs/Symptoms	Causative Chemical Agent
CNS	convulsions	nerve; blood
	confusion, odd behavior	incap
	stupor	any agent
Respiration	copious oro-nasal secretions	nerve
	chest pain, wheezing	nerve; choking; blister
	frothy sputum	blister; choking
	hyperpnea, dyspnea	choking; blister; blood
	apnea	nerve; blood
	cyanosis	blood; nerve; choking
Circulation	bradycardia	nerve; blood
	tachycardia	blood; nerve; incap
	shock	any agent
Skin	hot, dry, flushed	incap
	vesication	blister
	pain on contact	lewisite
	muscle tremors	nerve
	erythema	unknown liquid
GI/GU	involuntary evacuation	nerve
	vomiting	any agent

DELAYED EFFECTS

While several CW agents produce immediate signs and symptoms, the effects of others may be delayed, depending on the agent concentration and duration of exposure (Table 4). For instance, mustards can seriously damage the skin without immediately producing pain; likewise, pulmonary edema from phosgene may take hours to become manifest. Mixtures of CW agents or newly introduced chemicals further complicate the diagnostice picture. Hence, a holding period following unidentified CW agent(s) exposure, and careful re-examination prior to discharge, may be prudent, circumstances permitting.

General Principles of Management

Personal Hazards. First, do not become a casualty yourself: protect yourself and instruct your personnel to do likewise. Next, prevent further injury of the casualty: apply his protective mask and cover him, administer treatment, remove clothing, and decontaminate exposed body surfaces. Casualty decontamination may not always be as complete as desired because of the urgency of the situation or resource constraints. Thus, the potential for vapor exposure from an off-gassing residual agent or inadvertent contact with unsuspended, undetected liquid is an ever-present hazard for medical personnel.

Route of Entry. The nerve agents and blood agents are liquids, the vapors of which gain systemic access mainly via the respiratory tract. Their onset of action is precipitous and lethality can be swift. Other nerve agents, VX and thickened GD for instance, are absorbed percutaneously so that the onset of first effect may be delayed. Once in the blood stream, however, they act as quickly as the inhaled nerve agents.

Although agents such as mustard rapidly fix in the skin, the visible dermal injury takes time to develop. One observes both the early irritant effect of a mustard gas on the eyes and respiratory tract, and the delayed systemic effects of leukocytopenia with mustard and hemolysis with lewisite.

Persistent (non-volatile) agents also can contaminate uncovered food or water supplies. Ingestion of blister agent, for instance, may cause necrotic changes in the gastrointestinal tract.

Initial Priorities

Casualties may present with combined injuries on the integrated battlefield—that is, chemical/nuclear exposure combined with trauma or illness. Body heat build-up inside the protective ensemble, with resultant dehydration or hyperthermia, further complicates the picture. The initial issue facing the medical officer, then is determination of treatment priorities for such combined injuries.

There is no single "best" way to prioritize emergency treatment for chemical or mixed casualties. In general, respiratory insufficiency and circulatory shock, whatever the cause, present the more immediate life-threatening problems. One possible approach is suggested below:

1. Treat respiratory failure and control massive hemorrhage.
2. Administer chemical agent antidote(s).
3. Decontaminate the face (and protective mask if donned).

4. Remove contaminated clothing and decontaminate exposed skin.

5. Render emergency care for shock, wounds, and open fractures.

6. Administer supportive medical care as resources permit.

7. Transport the stabilized patient to a chemically clean area.

The following five sections group CW agents according to the categories of Table 3.

Nerve Agents

Nerve agents inhibit the ability of choline esterase to hydrolyz acetylcholine (ACh) which in turn stimulates muscarinic and nicotinic receptors as well as the central nervous system (CNS) directly. As a result, the casualty will manifest a classic cholinergic syndrome that, depending on exposure and treatment, can span the range from simple miosis and "red eye" to a fulminanting cholinergic crisis progressing within minutes to respiratory arrest and death.

Diagnosis: The diagnosis of nerve agent exposure is readily made from physical signs: fasciculation of skeletal muscle (perhaps progressing to depolarization paralysis), smooth muscle contraction of airways, bladder, and bowel; intense miosis and cycloplegia; marked bradycardia (may be masked by excitement or atropine); copious secretions; convulsions; rapidly weakening respiratory effort; pale cyanosis; and terminal apnea.

Treatment: Immediate IM or IV injection with atropine to block muscarinic cholinergic receptors, and with 2-PAM (if given soon after exposure) to reactivate cholinesterase, is effective. Each U.S. soldier has in a pocket of his protective mask carrier three MARK I kits for intramuscular self-injection, each kit delivering 2 mg injections of atropine sulfate and 600 mg pralidoxime chloride (3-PAMC1). Additional 2 mg injections of atropine may need to be given by medical personnel until clear clinical evidence of atropinization is obtained (dry red skin, easier breathing, decreased wheezing, dry mouth and, less consistently, dilating pupils).

Airway obstruction requires the clearing of secretions (by suction, if possible, or else by prone turning for postural drainage), the placement of an oropharyngeal or nasopharyngeal airway, and supplementary oxygen, if available. Endotracheal intubation or cricothyrotomy may be required in conjunction with manual or mechanical ventilation. If the environment is chemically contaminated, a closed system or charcoal-filtered air must be used for ventilation.

Experimental evidence suggests that benzodiazepine anticonvulsants reduce the morbidity associated with organophosphate-induced convulsions. Suggested doses are 5 mg Valium (IM) repeated as needed, or 2.5 mg increments of (IV) Valium.

Blister Agents

The blister (vesicant) agents are cytotoxic alkylating compounds exemplified by the mixture of compounds collectively known as "mustard" or "mustard gas" (H). Other blister agents are sulfur mustard (HD), nitrogen mustard (HN), phosgene oxime (CX), and Lewisite (L), an arsenical vesicant. Mustard vapor injury is a particular threat in hot climates. High humidity in a hot environment further enhances contact damage to the skin.

Diagnosis: The diagnosis of chemical skin injury is straightforward once blisters have appeared, but early and correct recognition of blister agent exposure can be difficult because:

a. Eye inflammation and upper respiratory tract irritation, often the first effects noted, present a picture similar to that produced by choking agents.

b. Although dermal damage occurs within minutes of contact, it cannot always be seen immediately and is commonly painless until subdermal layers become involved and blisters form several hours later.

After a 1-12 hour (or more) latent period, during which burning and itching may occur, erythema appears on exposed skin. In dark-skinned casualties, sulfur mustard lesions may turn coal-black in such areas as the face, neck, axilla, groin, and genitalia. Erythema is followed by coalescing, translucent, yellowish blisters on a red base. Healing and resorption of non-infected blisters occur in 1-3 weeks. Broken blisters must be protected to minimize chances for infection and subsequent scarring of denuded skin.

Lewisite is differentiated from the mustards by pain immediately upon skin contact. Nasal irritation, sneezing, and pungent odor provide early warning of the presence of Lewisite vapor. Only those without, or incapable of donning the mask will suffer serious respiratory effects.

Treatment: Forward treatment of vesicant injuries is mainly preventive and supportive. Immediate decontamination of the casualty has top priority. Agent droplets should be removed as expeditiously as possible by blotting or flushing. The M-258A1 decon kit is extremely effective in inactivating mustard, but it is also quite caustic. A surgical soap and cool water wash suffices, particularly for widely contaminated skin. Neither scrubbing nor hot water is recommended since both accelerate absorption and increased vapor formation. Army TM 8-285 provides further details regarding proper decontamination procedures.

Eye. Immediately flush the contaminated eye with water. Antibiotic ointment, with or without steroid, helps minimize infection. In more severe cases, blepharospasm and pain are extreme, requiring local anesthetic drops or ointment (e.g., tetracaine). Irrigation with sterile saline will remove crusted exudate.

Respiratory Tract. Inhalation of mustard vapor produces severe irritation of the upper respiratory tract, with painful cough, bloody sputum, chest pain, and dyspnea. Treatment is symptomatic at first, since the severity of the broncho-pulmonary lesion may not become evident for some time. Even asymptomatic patients should be observed for at least 4-6 hours, and not released until after re-examination of the chest. Lewisite vapor produces similar effects, except for more pronounced nasal irritation and sneezing.

Tracheitis and bronchitis are prominent; however, fulminant pulmonary edema is much less common with the blister agents than with the choking agents. Bronchopneumonia is a common complication; a change in the appearance of the sputum (culture if possible) is a clear indication for antibiotic therapy.

Prophylactic antibiotic administration is neither necessary nor recommended.

Skin. Doctrinal (TM 8-285) treatment recommends the opening and draining of blisters with removal of the blister fluid. Syringe aspiration of bullous fluid from large blisters might be as effective. Supportive therapy for mustard burns is essentially similar to that for thermal burns: aggressive fluid replacement, pain relief, and vigilance against bacterial infection. From the standpoint of personnel, facilities, and re-supply, forward-positioned medical resources would be severely stressed in the event of widespread utilization of mustard gas by the enemy.

Systemic. Bone marrow depression with severe leukopenia and thrombocytopenia follows extensive mustard absorption. Resistance to infection is diminished, with correspondingly high mortality from pneumonitis or other bacterial infections. Mustard ingested with water or food may damage gastrointestinal epithelium, resulting in blood and fluid losses.

Arsenical vesicants, such as Lewisite, increase capillary permeability, causing extensive third-space fluid shifts. Intravascular hemolysis of erythrocytes, and subsequent hemolytic anemia, complicate the clinical picture and may lead to renal failure. Intramuscular BAL (1ml per 50 pounds, not to exceed 4 ml) is given at 4-hour intervals for a total of 4 doses. In severe cases, follow-up treatment for 3-4 days with the daily deep IM injections of 1 ml per 100 pounds is recommended.

Choking Agents

This group, so called because of the pronounced irritation of the upper as well as the lower respiratory tract, consists of phosgene (CG), diphosgene (DP), and chlorine (CL). Phosgene gas, approximately three times heavier than air, hugs the ground as a white cloud that spills into bunkers and fighting pits.

The choking agents are treacherous in that the onset of fulminating pulmonary edema is delayed several hours following exposure. Thus, a soldier with dyspnea and mild substernal discomfort may have normal auscultatory and radiographic signs and be returned to duty, only to progress to extremis a few hours later.

It is imperative that any casualty with known phosgene exposure, no matter how minor his dyspnea or upper respiratory irritation, be observed for 4-6 hours at the very least, then carefully checked for impending pulmonary edema before being returned to duty (see below).

Diagnosis: Phosgene has the characteristic odor of freshly mown grass. The threshold for detecting phosgene's characteristic odor is so close to the irritant threshold as to be useless as a warning. The individual's sense of dyspnea as the lung stiffens still serves as the best indicator of impending pulmonary edema.

Irritant effects on the eyes and tracheo-bronchial tree—accompanied by tearing, cough, or chest discomfort—and dyspnea or tachypnea are the first effects noted. These symptoms may appear to be rather minor at first, resembling the symptoms of a common cold or anxiety reaction. From one-half hour to four or six (rarely twelve) hours following exposure, cough, chest pain, cyanosis, and progressive dyspnea herald impending overt pulmonary edema. Painful cough, frothy sputum, cyanosis, rales, dullness to percussion, and radiographic evidence support the diagnosis.

Uncomplicated cases recover without permanent after-effects. However, the possibility of secondary bacterial pulmonary infection is considerable. Circulatory failure or the patient appearing "mouse-grey cyanotic" are ominous signs. The "plum-blue cyanotic" patient, conversely, has a good chance to survive. These gross observations may be helpful in mass casualty triage.

Treatment: Recall the treacherous "silent period" that follows the inhalation of a pulmonary irritant. Observe the symptom-free patient with known exposure to a choking agent for at least 4-6 hours and the casualty with known exposure and minimal symptoms (itching eyes, runny nose, mild cough, vague chest discomfort) for at least 12 hours. In either case, do not release these personnel to duty without a careful re-examination of the chest.

Treatment of non-cardiac pulmonary edema in the field is mostly supportive, with enforced rest to minimize exertion. Oxygen with air admixed to 40% is sufficient and will help conserve limited supplies. Intravenous fluids (as in any case of pulmonary edema) should be administered sparingly. The risk of bronchopneumonia is greatest when pulmonary edema begins to subside. The clinician must be alert for changes in sputum color or a sudden rise in body temperature.

According to current thinking, (a) prophylactic antibiotics are of no proven benefit, (b) steroids, whether given intravenously or by inhalation, appear to offer no advantage, (c) early positive end-expiratorypressure (PEEP) breathing may well reduce the severity of the subsequent pulmonary edema, and (d) patients in severe distress will require endotracheal intubation or tracheostomy and positive pressure mechanical ventilation.

Phosphorus pentoxide, the dense white smoke associated with white phosphorus munitions, presents the same clinical picture as phosgene exposure. Experience has shown that the chemical burn of the alveolus produced by phosphorus pentoxide is irreversible and fatal in those who progress to pulmonary edema. It is a sobering and frustrating experience to observe a totally asymptomatic soldier, exposed to phosphorus pentoxide inhalation, progress from the asymptomatic state to intractable pulmonary edema and death over the span of eight hours in spite of every supportive effort.

Blood Agents

Hydrogen cyanide (AC) and certain of its congeners form highly stable complexes with metalloporphyrins such as cytochrome oxidase. Aerobic cellular metabolism comes to a virtual halt. Venous blood remains as oxygen rich as arterial blood, accounting for the "cherry red" postmortem appearance of cyanide victims. Death is due to cytotoxic hypoxia.

High volatility and relatively low toxicity (50-100 times less than those of nerve agents) limits its operational utility in open spaces. Potassium cyanide poisoning of water and food supplies is an old terrorist tactic that one should be aware of.

Diagnosis: The diagnosis of hydrogen cyanide inhalation is difficult to make without a history. Cyanogen chloride (CK) is more readily recognized because its irritant properties cause tearing and coughing in sublethal does.

Treatment: Immediate removal of casualties from the contaminated atmosphere prevents further inhalation. Nitrites are effective antidotes. They form methemoglobin, to which the cyanide ion binds preferentially; however, overly enthusiastic methemoglobin conversion reduces available hemoglobin, imperiling intravascular oxygen transport. Sodium nitrite for intravenous use (10 ml of 3% solution) is stocked in forward field medical facilities. (The amyl nitrite "pearl" for inhalation has been removed from issue.) Sodium thiosulfate (50 ml of 25% solution, IV) provides free sulfur to convert toxic cyanide to a far less toxic thiocyanate ion.

Manual or mechanical ventilation is central to resuscitation of apneic casualties. Those in respiratory distress will be aided by oxygen inhalation.

Incapacitation (INCAP) Agents

Incapacitation agents (incaps) are a heterogenous group of chemical agents with potent CNS effects that seriously impair normal function but do not endanger life or cause permanent tissue damage in operationally effective doses. Atropine and scopolamine were early forerunners; other cholinolytics such as benactyzine followed. Quinuclidinyl benzilate (BZ or QND) is a potent glycolate representative of this class. The diagnosis of incap exposure may be extremely difficult to make in isolated instances due to the paucity of distinct diagnostic signs and criteria.

An essential precaution with these confused, perhaps disturbed, casualties is immediate removal of firearms and other weapons to insure the safety of themselves, other patients, and nearby personnel. Be aware that interaction between incaps and pharmacologic agents such as analgesics, antidotes, and anesthetics is probable, but little specific information is available. Caution in their use is advisable.

Belladonna-type drugs: These cholinolytics cause widely dilated pupils, tachycardia, dry mouth, hot dry skin, and decreased intestinal motility and bladder tone. The CNS symptoms and signs run the gamut from inattention, confusion, anxiety, restlessness, and hallucinations on up to delirium.

Recommended treatment is physostigmine, given IM in 2-3 mg doses every 45 minutes. Since the CNS effects of BZ may persist for days, close observation and continued treatment with 3-4 mg physostigmine orally every 1-2 hours are essential elements in managing toxic delirium. Titrate therapeutic dosage against clearing of mental status, should heart rate fall below 70, in which case dosage may be decreased, but physostigmine should not be discontinued. The ability of the body to thermoregulate is damaged by cholinolytics. This is of concern, particularly with personnel in protective clothing. Administering fluids, recording body temperature and urine output, and catherizing the bladder to relieve distention are key supportive measures.

CNS Depressants. In this group are cannabinols, barbiturates, and morphine-like compounds that destroy motivation and produce tranquillity and sedation. If treatment of severe indolence is required, CNS stimulants such as the amphetamines have been effective.

CNS Excitants. These agents incapacitate by raising the level of neurotransmitters, causing cerebral hyperstimulation. Indoles such as lysergic acid diethylamide (LSD) produce inappropriate behavior, restlessness, fear, perceptual aberrations, and a general schizoid psychosis-like syndrome. In hyperexcitable casualties, sedative barbiturate or chlorpromazine administration has been proposed. Benzodiazepines may be useful, with Valium having the advantage of ready oral absorption.

CHAPTER VII

Mass Casualties in Thermonuclear Warfare

GENERAL

Nuclear weapons range in size from very small (not many times larger in total energy yield than the largest conventional bombs), to immensely large (the so-called thermonuclear or hydrogen devices), with yields in the megaton range. Total energy yield of nuclear weapons are rated in terms of equivalent amounts of TNT. Therefore, a weapon with a 20-kiloton yield has the same total energy output as 20,000 tons of TNT. A 1.0-megaton weapon has the energy output of 1,000,000 tons of TNT. Energy is released by nuclear detonations in three forms: thermal radiation, blast, and ionizing radiation. The relative-casualty causing potential of each depends primarily upon three factors: the yield of the weapon, the environmental conditions in which the detonation occurs, and the distribution of troops in the target area. The thermal output may be the most significant casualty producer, particularly for the larger weapons; however, blast will produce nearly as many casualties, and blast and thermal injuries together will account for most of the casualties under almost all circumstances. Radiation, either at the time of detonation or later from fallout, will be responsible for significant numbers of delayed casualties.

Radiation-associated injuries pose many new challenges to medical management. Many organ systems are affected by radiation, often compounding problems produced by conventional injuries. These challenges are magnified by the very real potential of nuclear weapons to produce very large numbers of casualties instantaneously. Thus, new concepts of mass-casualty medicine that utilize simplified and standardized regimens will be required to accomplish what is now done by labor and resource-intensive means.

LOGISTICS OF CASUALTY MANAGEMENT

If nuclear weapons are employed within the theater, the entire medical evacuation and treatment system will be severely overburdened and some system of classification and sorting of casualties must be added to the normal procedures of evacuation and hospitalization. In addition, a system must be established to hold casualties who are too seriously injured to remain with their units, but who do not need to or cannot be hospitalized. These two requirements, the sorting of casualties and the holding of the excess numbers, must be planned for as part of the normal organization and operation of the medical support system in a theater of operations.

In applying the principle of providing the greatest good for the greatest number to the management of mass casualties, a field medical system must face and solve several problems. The location and number of casualties must be determined. This requires intact communications, since isolated units on a dispersed battlefield could suffer severe casualties and be unable to notify higher headquarters. Subsequent delay in initiating treatment and hospitalization will result in greatly increased morbidity and mortality.

The casualties must be evacuated. In frontline areas, follow-up enemy action exploiting the use of nuclear weapons could greatly hinder or prevent evacuation. In rear areas, adequate evacuation means may not be available to handle the massive number of casualties produced by an attack. The availability of helicopters would help since they can be diverted from one area to another much more readily than ground transportation. The use of nonmedical transportation systems may be required but cannot be planned on.

TRIAGE

If nuclear weapons casualties are encountered, the basic principles of mass casualty management (triage, evacuation, and the use of standardized care interventions) will have to be followed. Our relative inexperience in dealing with these types of patients will make matters worse. Life-threatening doses of acute total body radiation are so infrequently encountered that management policies must be derived in part from different but analogous clinical situations and from studies in experimental animals.

Conventional injuries should be treated first and initial triage should be based on these injuries, since no immediate life-threatening hazard exists for radiation casualties who can ultimately survive. The patient with multiple injuries should be resuscitated and stabilized. During this process, standard preoperative preparation for surgery will accomplish much radioactive decontamination. More definitive evaluation of the radiation injury can be initiated postoperatively.

Three groups of conventional injury patients will have to be considered:

1. Those with minimal injuries that do not incapacitate them completely and are not a significant threat to life. These casualties could continue as at least partially effective soldiers and would not qualify for immediate or early evacuation.

2. Those with severe multiple injuries who obviously are going to require extensive, time-consuming care. These also would be delayed.

3. Finally, those with relatively simple injuries which require immediate surgical treatment. These would get first priority for evacuation.

Further classification of patients will not be required prior to evacuation. The presence or absence of radiation injury, in general, will be ignored in this preliminary sorting, since there are no reliable guidelines to aid in the early diagnosis of extent of radiation injury. Eventually, however, all casualties unable to continue as effective soldiers will have to be evacuated.

As noted, there is a requirement for appropriate holding facilities to which patients who cannot be treated immediately or who require only minimal treatment can be evacuated. These facilities should be set up with limited equipment and staffed with small numbers of medical personnel, and should be part of the expansion plans of all field hospitals regardless of size or location. Holding facilities should be as close to hospitals as possible so as to optimize the availability of appropriate additional care and to allow the transfer of patients as the overall situation and balance between medical resources and patient load change. A great variety of patients, including those not fit for field duty but not requiring full-care-type hospitalization, as well as the very severely injured, should be kept there. These should include patients in the following categories:

1. Minimal burns.
2. Mild trauma cases.
3. Mild chemical injury cases.
4. Severely injured patients who are not expected to survive and for whom treatment is not immediately available, but for whom supportive measures may be enough to keep them alive until treatment does become available.

Radiation injury introduces many complications into the patient's course. Hematologic injuries cause anemia, infection, bleeding, and delayed wound healing. Performance decrements due largely to neuromediator release can also impact the patient. At higher doses of radiation, dehydration due to severe fluid and electrolyte losses through the intestinal wall will be encountered.

After conventional injuries have been managed, the physician is faced with the problem of triaging the patients according to the severity of their radiation injuries so that appropriate treatment can begin. This problem is difficult since the response of any given individual may vary greatly, and a nonhomogenous exposure of radiation (especially if bone marrow and gut are spared) may result in a markedly decreased effect. U.S. forces do not carry individual personal dosimeters that measure neutron and photon exposures. Finally, dose rate effects can be very profound, especially in a fallout environment. In this situation, tactical dosimeters (two per platoon) may be useful to a commander deciding whether to commit exposed troops to battle, but they are less useful to the health care provider. Other problems will also exist. Casualties will be numerous and resources certainly will be strained. Complicating this will be the occurrence of blast and thermal injuries (in addition to radiation injuries). Improved dosimetry is needed for triage since the goal of military medical personnel should be the appropriate allocation of precious resources to salvage the maximum number of casualties. Improved dosimetry is currently unavailable, but its desirability is currently undergoing evaluation by the U.S. Army Academy of Health Sciences.

Based on recent recommendations, the following guidelines apply to medical personnel operating in austere field conditions. The lymphocyte level can be used as a biological dosimeter to confirm the presence of pure radiation injury, but not in combined injuries. If the physician has the resources of a clinical laboratory, additional information can be obtained to support the original working diagnosis suggested by the presence of prodromal symptoms. An initial blood sample for concentrations of circulating lymphocytes should be obtained as soon as possible from any patient classified as "radiation injury possible" or "radiation injury probable." After the initial assessment, or at least no later than 24 hours after the event in question, additional comparative blood samples should be taken. The samples may be interpreted as follows:

(1) Lymphocyte levels in excess of $1500/mm^3$: There is minimal likelihood of significant dose that would require treatment.

(2) Lymphocyte levels between 500 and $1000/mm^3$: These indicate treatment for severe radiation injury. These patients should be hospitalized to minimize the complications from hemorrhage and infection that will present within 2-3 weeks postexposure.

(3) Lymphocyte levels of less than $500/mm^3$: These patients have received a radiation dose that may prove fatal. All of these patients need to be hospitalized for the inevitable pancytopenic complications.

(4) Lymphocytes not detectable: These patients have received a supralethal radiation dose. Survival is very unlikely. Most have received severe injuries to their gastrointestinal and cardiovascular systems and will not survive for more than two weeks.

A useful rule of thumb is: If lymphocytes have decreased by 50% or are less than $1000/mm^3$, the individual has received a significant radiation exposure. In the event of combined injuries, the diagnostic use of lymphocytes may be unreliable. It should be borne in mind that those with severe burns or multisystem trauma often develop lymphopenia.

It is difficult to establish an early definitive diagnosis. Therefore, it is best to utilize a simple, tentative classification system based on three possible categories of patients as discussed below.

1. Radiation Injury Unlikely. If there are no symptoms associated with radiation injury, patients are judged to be at minimal risk for radiation complications. These patients should be triaged according to the severity of their conventional injuries. If the patients are free of conventional injuries or disease states that require treatment, they should be released and returned to duty.

2. Radiation Injury Probable. Anorexia, nausea, and vomiting are the primary prodromal symptoms associated with radiation injury. Priority for further evaluation will be assigned after all life-threatening injuries have been stabilized. Casualties in this category will not require any medical treatment within the first few days for their radiation injuries. Evidence to support the diagnosis of significant radiation injury in the absence of burns and trauma may be obtained from serial lymphocyte assays taken over the next two days. If the evidence indicates that a significant radiation injury was received, these casualties should be monitored for pancytopenic complications.

3. Radiation Injury Severe. These casualties are judged to have received a potentially fatal radiation dose. Nausea and vomiting will be almost universal for persons in this group. The prodromal phase may also include prompt, explosive bloody diarrhea, significant hypotension, and signs of neurologic injury. These patients should be sorted according to the availability of resources. Patients should receive symptomatic care. Lymphocyte analysis is necessary to support this classification.

Categorization of these patients into one of these three irradiation categories will be facilitated by an appreciation for the characteristic symptoms induced by radiation. These are:

a. Nausea and Vomiting. Nausea and vomiting occur with increasing frequency as the radiation exceeds 100-200 centiGrays (cGy). Their onset may be as late as 6-12 hours postexposure. They usually subside within the first day. The occurrence of vomiting within the first two hours is associated with a severe radiation dose. Vomiting within the first hour, especially if accompanied by explosive diarrhea, is associated with doses that frequently prove fatal. Due to the transient nature of these symptoms, it is possible that the patient will have already passed through this initial phase of gastrointestinal distress before being seen by a physician. It will be necessary to inquire about these symptoms at the initial examination.

b. Hyperthermia. Casualties who have received a potentially lethal radiation injury show a significant rise in body temperature within the first few hours postexposure. Although our experience is limited, this appears to be a consistent finding. The occurrence of fever and chills within the first day postexposure is associated with a severe and life-threatening radiation dose. Hyperthermia may occur in patients who receive lower (200 cGy or more) but still serious radiation doses. Present evidence indicates that hyperthermia is frequently overlooked. Individuals wearing a chemical ensemble will normally be hyperthermic; consequently, this may not be a useful sign.

c. Erythema. A person who receives whole-body radiation in excess of 1000-2000 cGy will experience erythema within the first day postexposure. This is also true for those who receive a comparable dose to a local body region in which case the erythema will be restricted to the affected area. With lower but still potentially fatal doses (200 cGy or more), erythema is less frequently seen.

d. Hypotension. A noticeable and sometimes clinically significant decline in systemic blood pressure has been recorded in victims who received a supralethal whole-body radiation dose. A severe hypotensive episode has been observed in one person who had received several thousand rads. In persons who received several hundred rads, a drop in systemic blood pressure of more than 10% has been noted. Severe hypotension after irradiation is associated with a poor prognosis.

e. Neurologic Dysfunction. Experience indicates that almost all persons who demonstrate obvious signs of CNS injury within the first hour postexposure have received a supralethal dose. Symptoms include mental confusion, convulsions, and coma. Intractable hypotension will probably accompany these symptoms. Despite vascular support, these patients succumb within 48 hours.

Casualties receiving a potentially fatal dose of radiation will most likely experience a pattern of prodromal symptoms that is associated with the radiation exposure itself. Unfortunately, these symptoms are nonspecific and may be seen with other forms of illness or injury, thereby seriously complicating the radiation exposure diagnosis. Therefore, the triage officer must determine if the symptoms occurred within the first day postexposure, evaluate the possibility that they are indeed related to radiation exposure, and then assign the patient to one of the three categories:

"Radiation Injury Unlikely," "Radiation Injury Probable," or "Radiation Injury Severe." In the last two categories, the observation of changes in circulating lymphocyte counts may either support or rule out the original working diagnosis. All individuals with multiple injuries should be treated initially as if no significant radiation injury is present. Triage and care of any life-threatening injuries should be rendered without regard to the probability of radiation injury. The medical officer should make a preliminary diagnosis of radiation injury only in those patients for whom radiation is the sole source of the problem. This is based on the appearance of nausea, vomiting, diarrhea, erythema, hyperthermia, hypotension, and neurologic dysfunction.

Decontamination of the Patient. Radiation injury per se does not imply that the patient is a health hazard to the medical staff. Studies indicate that the levels of intrinsic radiation present within the patient from activation (after exposure to neutron and high-energy photon sources) are not life-threatening to the medical staff.

Patients entering a medical treatment facility should be routinely decontaminated if monitoring for radiation is not available. Removal of the patient's clothing will usually reduce most of the contamination. Washing exposed body surfaces will further reduce this problem. Both of these procedures can be performed in the field or on the way to the treatment facility. Once the patient has entered the treatment facility, care should be based on the obvious injuries. Care for life-threatening injuries should not be delayed until the decontamination procedures are completed.

When radiation safety personnel are available, decontamination procedures will be established to assist in rendering care and to minimize the hazard from radioactive contaminants. A more extensive decontamination procedure is to scrub the areas of persistent contamination with a mild detergent or a diluted strong detergent. Caution should be taken to not disrupt the integrity of the skin while scrubbing, because disruption can lead to incorporation of the radioisotopes into deeper layers of the skin. Contaminated wounds should be treated first, since they will rapidly incorporate the contaminant. Washing, gentle scrubbing, or even debridement may be necessary to reduce the level of contaminants.

Wearing surgical attire will reduce the possible contamination of health personnel. If additional precautions are warranted, rotation of the attending personnel will further reduce the possibility of significant contamination or exposure. The prevention of incorporation is of paramount importance. The inhalation or ingestion of radioactive particles is a much more difficult problem, and resources to deal with it will not be available in a field situation.

SPECIFIC MEDICAL EFFECTS OF NUCLEAR WEAPONS

Proper management of radiation casualties of nuclear war requires an understanding of the medical problems to be expected. Nuclear weapons are sufficiently different in their casualty-producing potential from conventional weapons that the types of injuries will be different. It is important to understand these differences if triage and medical treatment are to be accomplished effectively and quickly. As has been said, the biologic effects of nuclear weapons are due to thermal burns, blast, and radiation injuries.

Thermal Burns. The extremely high temperatures produced by a nuclear explosion cause release of a large part of the energy in the form of thermal radiation. This radiation travels at the speed of light and is capable of producing severe burns at great distances. In nuclear warfare, burn casualties will constitute a large fraction of the patient load. All echelons of medical care must plan for this increased burden of thousands of burn cases.

A major problem will occur during the initial evacuation of burn patients if massive numbers of casualties must be handled. Sorting will be essential to conserve medical resources and should be done in accordance with the following criteria:

1. Cases involving 20% or less of the body surface should be treated on a outpatient basis or at minimal care facilities. These patients can care for themselves with minimal supervision. They will not be fit for duty and should not remain with their units if those units are actively engaged in combat.

2. Patients whose burns involve certain critical areas, such as the head and neck, hands, or feet will require hospitalization even if the total body surface involvement is less than 20%.

3. Patients with more than 20% body surface involvement, or

with associated blast injuries, will require hospitalization for resuscitative treatment and surgical care.

4. Cases with more than 50% involvement have a decreasing chance of survival with increasing degree of involvement and should be given a low priority for needed surgical care. They should be retained in a delayed status in the minimal care section of a medical facility where they will be available for more extensive treatment if resources and time allow. It must be realized that young healthy adults, without other injury or disease, may be more likely to survive such burns with adequate treatment; thus, a rigid classification system denying them available treatment is not desirable.

All patients should receive as much treatment as possible and the above criteria must be flexible. However, any treatment must be accomplished as efficiently and quickly as possible, and long, time-consuming procedures may have to be delayed, or not performed. The greatest good for the greatest number is best achieved by treating each patient as quickly and simply as possible by doing first what is essential to save his life, then what may be possible to save limbs, and last what might be required to save and restore function.

Depending on the weapon yield, some burn patients will have associated radiation injury and will develop bone marrow depression during the course of their illness. These patients cannot be recognized upon admission, since the bone marrow depression does not become clinically evident until after a latent period of 2-6 weeks after the radiation exposure. A blood count in such cases during the first few days after exposure will show a variable leukopenia, particularly of lymphocytes. These patients will have high morbidity and mortality rates due primarily to infection. Unless a procedure is required to save life, these patients should not be subjected to surgery during the phase of bone marrow depression. If there is no evidence of bone marrow recovery, the patient will not survive with the treatment modalities presently available in the field.

Blast Injuries. Blast injuries caused by nuclear detonations are of two types: direct (due to overpressure effects) or indirect (due to drag forces of the winds accompanying the blast wave). This latter category includes a wide variety of missile and translational injuries.

Direct blast injuries will be rare, since persons close enough to the point of detonation to sustain significant direct overpressures will almost invariably sustain lethal thermal and indirect-blast injuries. However, those few patients who survive the direct blast should be managed the same as any other direct blast injury. Their injuries will be complicated by other trauma and they will suffer a high incidence of radiation-induced bone marrow depression during their post-injury phase, resulting in increased morbidity and mortality. Direct blast-induced internal injuries can easily be overlooked in a mass casualty situation.

The blast wave of a nuclear detonation is unlike conventional blast waves in that its formation is associated with the production of severe, transient winds from the violent movement of large masses of air to form the wave itself. These blast winds, perpendicular to the plane of the wave, have velocities reaching several hundred kilometers per hour. They last only a few seconds but can produce considerable damage through drag forces and by the production of large numbers of low-velocity secondary missiles, the size and nature of which depend on the environment. A high percentage of blast trauma will be caused by such missiles, and a large number of patients will have multiple missile injuries. Many Japanese at Hiroshima and Nagasaki had dozens of superficial wounds caused by flying glass and debris. These types of injuries will vary greatly in severity, but in general, there will be a relatively low incidence of deeply penetrating injuries. However, when massive numbers of casualties must be quickly sorted and prepared for evacuation and treatment, a significant number will have penetrating wounds which might be overlooked until clinical signs become obvious. Otherwise, the nonpenetrating missile injuries will not be severely disabling unless critical parts of the body are involved, such as the head, face, neck, or hands.

Radiation Injuries. The detonation of a nuclear weapon produces large amounts of ionizing radiation in two basic forms: electromagnetic (gamma) radiation, which travels at the speed of light and is highly penetrating, and particulate (alpha, beta, and neutron) radiation. Of the particulate radiations, only the neutron is highly penetrating, whereas the alpha and beta are not. All four types are present at the time of the detonation, but the gamma and neutron are by far the most important clinically. All but the neutron radiation are present in fallout and, in this instance, the gamma is the most important.

Ionizing radiation is emitted both at the time of the nuclear detonation and for a considerable time afterward. That which is emitted at the time of the detonation is termed "prompt radiation", and is produced by the nuclear reactions of fission and fusion. The significant part of prompt radiation consists of a mixture of gamma and neutron radiation, most of which is emitted within a few seconds of the onset of the detonation. However, the duration of significant emission may be longer, particularly with larger weapons. One minute has been established as a reasonable time parameter, after which there is no significant amount of prompt radiation, regardless of the type of weapon or circumstances of the detonation.

Residual radiation is that which persists beyond the first minute after detonation. Its source is the variable amount of residual radioactive material produced by a nuclear detonation. A nuclear fission reaction transforms uranium or plutonium into a large number (about 150) of radioactive isotopes, termed fission products, which constitute by far the most important source of residual radiation. In addition, small amounts of unfissioned bomb material, and material in which neutron radiation has induced radioactivity, are present. All of these residually radioactive materials will be found in fallout.

Fission products are the major radiation hazard in fallout, since a large number of them emit penetrating gamma radiation and, as a result, can be hazardous even at great distances. They have half-lives varying from fractions of seconds to several years, but most have half-lives in the range of days to weeks. As a result, the total amount of radiation emitted by a typical mixture of fission products is quite intense early and remains hazardous until the activity decays to negligible levels. This takes several days to several weeks, depending on the original level of activity; however, some isotopes with very long half-lives will be present and detectable for many years.

Figure 19 shows that fallout activity decays down to 1/10 of its initial level within seven hours post detonation. At H plus one hour a significant part of the early fallout will have deposited itself close to the point of detonation. Deviation from this decay curve will be common, depending on the interplay between the various factors controlling the rate of deposition of fallout and the distance involved. At greater distances from the point of detonation, it may take several hours before fallout will be deposited and become detectable. A significant amount of radioactive decay will have already occurred while the radioactive material has been airborne and, as a result, the rate of decay, once all the fallout is on the ground, will be similar to the later part of the curve shown in Figure 19. If fallout in a given area is a mixture from several detonations at different times, the observed rate of decay may be quite different from this ideal example. Under these circumstances, the rule of thumb that fallout will have decayed to negligible values by two weeks may not be applicable. It should be obvious that instruments designed to measure fallout activity must be available and used to evaluate the true hazard.

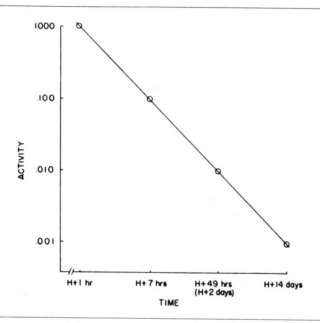

FIGURE 19.—Fallout decay with time after detonation. Fallout activity decreases by a factor of 10 for every sevenfold increase in time after burst. Fallout activity is referenced to 1 hour after burst (H + 1 hour) , which is used as the base value in fallout calculations.

Not all the uranium or plutonium in a weapon is fissioned, and fallout, which contains residual weapon material, will contain small amounts of these elements. They add little to the hazards of fallout since they are alpha emitters and are not an external hazard unless ingested or inhaled. They must be incorporated into body tissue to do damage and their relative insolubility greatly minimizes this hazard. Obviously, ingestion or inhalation of contaminated material should be avoided.

Because of the exceedingly high temperatures generated in a nuclear detonation, all the fission products and the weapon residues are vaporized. As they cool and recondense, they solidify as extremely small particles. In an airburst, these particles will remain suspended in the upper atmosphere (stratosphere) for long periods of time, descending slowly over a period of years and over large parts of the earth's surface. This occurred during the atmospheric testing of weapons. Under such circumstances, there is no significant early or local fallout. When a detonation occurs within a certain critical distance of the surface, however, severe updrafts cause large amounts of terrain debris to be sucked up into the fireball. As a result, as the radioactive materials cool and condense, they become affixed to relatively large particles of dirt and debris. These large particles, with their radioactive contamination attached, tend to fall back to earth rapidly and locally, resulting in high levels of radioactivity downwind from the point of detonation. On occasion, this type of fallout is visible while it descends.

The major hazard in this type of fallout will be external whole-body irradiation from gamma-emitting isotopes, since they do not actually have to be on a person's skin to cause damage. Gamma radiation has a very long range in air, and large amounts of gamma-emitting material scattered uniformly over many square kilometers can produce a high level of penetrating radiation, which is a hazard to anyone occupying or passing through the area, even though he avoids direct contact with the fallout material. Even personnel traveling through in vehicles will be exposed, although vehicles can provide significant reduction of exposure because of the ability of most metals at least partially to scatter or absorb gamma radiation. The dose rate inside a tank, for example, may be only 4-10% of that outside.

The potential injury incurred from gamma radiation is a function of the amount of time spent in the fallout field as well as the dose rate present, since these factors together determine the total dose absorbed.

The beta-emitting isotopes in fallout are not a significant hazard, unless a person is directly contaminated with or ingests them. External contamination can result in a moderate degree of skin damage somewhat similar to a thermal burn, and incorpora-tion into body tissues can result in organ damage of long-term significance. These later effects—that is, interferences with specific organ functions, carcinogenesis, and accelerated aging changes—are not manifested for months or years, and acute whole body irradiation, with resulting radiation sickness, will not occur. Therefore, in combat situations, the beta-emitting components of fallout are not considered to be a serious hazard.

RADIATION SYNDROMES

Radiation sickness caused by whole body irradiation may be lethal within a few days to several weeks, depending upon the dose sustained. Clinically, radiation sickness occurs in a dose-dependent pattern of three syndromes, determined by the organ system most seriously involved. These are (1) the neurovascular syndrome, caused by very high doses and uniformly fatal within 2-4 days; (2) the gastrointestinal syndrome, due to somewhat lower doses but also uniformly fatal; and (3) the hematopoietic syn-drome, caused by still lower doses and associated with the possibili-ty of recovery and survival.

The neurovascular syndrome will be extremely rare in combat. The gastrointestinal syndrome will be relatively uncommon but may be seen. The hematopoietic syndrome will be the most com-monly seen.

All three syndromes have certain characteristics in common. These include:

1. An initial nonspecific response.
2. A latent period.
3. A clinical phase

1. Initial Response. Within a few hours after a prompt exposure, all patients, regardless of which syndrome later develops, pass through a nonspecific, transient period of malaise, weakness, anorexia, vomiting, and diarrhea. This response is probably tox-ic in nature due to tissue, breakdown products associated with radiation-induced cellular damage. The exact mechanism respon-sible or the cell mass involved is not known. The initial response to irradiation lasts up to a few hours and then subsides. It is followed by a latent period during which there are no significant symptoms or obvious physical signs of radiation injury. At present,

no diagnostic clues are available to establish firmly the presence or extent of radiation injury during the initial response phase. Its severity and duration are not reliable indexes of the degree of radiation exposure and it may be absent following low dose-rate fallout exposures, despite their magnitude.

2. Latent Phase. All three syndromes have latent periods between the initial response and the onset of the clinical phase. This latent period is shortest for the neurovascular syndrome, from an almost negligible period to three days, and longest for the hematopoietic syndrome, lasting 2-6 weeks, with an occasional patient demonstrating an even longer latent period. The gastrointestinal syndrome has an intermediate latent period of a few days. This phase is characterized by a feeling of relative well-being.

3. Clinical Phase. The clinical phase follows the latent period and many patients will not be hospitalized until this time, unless they have had other injuries for which they require treatment. As noted previously, there are three distinct syndromes (Figure 20), depending upon the dose of radiation sustained, as follows:

(a) Neurovascular Syndrome. The dose of radiation required to cause each type of clinical response varies considerably. The neurovascular syndrome requires very high doses (3,000 cGy or more). Such doses are rare in a battlefield situation, except for unprotected personnel exposed to extremely intense fallout very close to the point of surface detonation of a large weapon or in an armored vehicle near the detonation of a small device. Therefore, these patients will be rare and in most cases will usually not survive to be seen in medical facilities because of other lethal injuries.

The clinical course of the neurovascular syndrome is one of progressive depression leading to coma and finally death. In its early stage, patients will be ataxic; convulsions are frequent as the clinical condition deteriorates. This syndrome progresses too rapidly for significant hematologic changes to occur; therefore, diagnosis will not be easy, particularly if patients have sustained head injuries.

(b) Gastrointestinal syndrome. The gastrointestinal syndrome is caused by doses in the range of about 1,000 cGy and higher.

These doses will not be common, but exposure to prompt radiation from small weapons or to intense levels of fallout will result in a small number of such patients. Small numbers of patients with this type of radiation sickness were seen among the victims at Hiroshima and Nagasaki.

A typical patient with this syndrome will have to be hospitalized for other injuries and will, within four to 4-5 days of injury, develop severe, bloody diarrhea. A peripheral blood count will show a depression of lymphocytes and beginning depressions of other leukocytes and platelets. Differentiating between this syndrome and an infectious, nonradiaton-induced diarrhea, superimposed upon radiation-induced bone marrow depression, could well be difficult because of the widespread occurrence of various dysenteries in combat. As the bone marrow depression becomes more severe, a point will be reached from which recovery will be impossible. Such patients eventually will succumb to the effects of overwhelming infection and hemorrhage, despite antibiotic therapy and massive fluid, electrolyte, and blood replacement. If patients with gastrointestinal damage are not treated, they will die early due to their massive fluid and blood losses. Replacement therapy can prevent this type of death, but then such patients will progress to the clinical phase of irreparable bone marrow injury. The survival time of such patients will vary, but may be a few weeks. They could constitute a severe burden on all echelons of medical care.

(c) Hematopoietic syndrome. Patients with exposures below levels causing the gastrointestinal syndrome will have longer latent periods before the clinical picture of bone marrow depression becomes evident. This may take from less than two weeks to more than six weeks to develop, but, in most cases, the latent period will be from 2-3 weeks.

The degree of bone marrow depression will vary with the dose of radiation sustained, and the probability of survival is directly related to the probability of recovery of the bone marrow.

The clinical picture presented by patients with bone marrow depression will vary, depending upon the presence and nature of other injuries. In uncomplicated radiation sickness, the clinical picture will reflect the increased bleeding tendencies which develop. These patients will develop extensive hemorrhages throughout their bodies. Subcutaneous petechiae and ecchymoses and extensive gastrointestinal bleeding will be common. Decreased resistance to infection will accompany the hemorrhagic diathesis, and infection will be the primary cause of death. Treatment will be limited to supportive measures, such as fluids and antibiotics. Bone marrow transplantation is obviously not practical therapy in the field. Transfusion of blood or blood components will become impractical if the number of casualties is too high.

This syndrome is associated with a chance for survival, depending upon the ability of the bone marrow to recover. Bone marrow recovery and an associated favorable prognosis can be determined by serial peripheral blood counts.

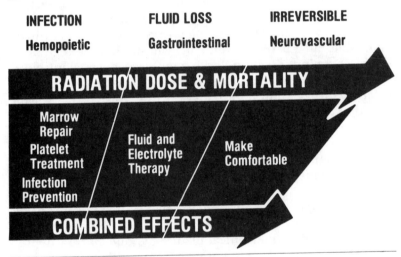

FIGURE 20.—Postradiation syndrome dose and time relationships.

INITIAL TREATMENT FOR PATIENTS WITH WHOLE-BODY RADIATION INJURY

The primary determinants of survival among most patients receiving intermediate (serious but not uniformly fatal if treated) radiation doses are the management of microbial infections and the arrest of bleeding. If high intermediate doses have been received, fluid and electrolyte loss may cause early deaths. If properly resuscitated, however, these patients can survive until the consequences of hematologic failure become apparent.

For those casualties who have received sublethal whole-body

radiation doses, gastrointestinal distress will predominate in the first two days. Antiemetics (metoclopramide, dazopride) may be effective in reducing the symptoms, but currently available drugs have significant side effects. Unless severe radiation injury has oc-curred, these symptoms will usually subside within the first day. For those patients who continue to experience gastrointestinal distress, parenteral fluids should be considered. If explosive diar-rhea occurs within the first hour postexposure, fluids and elec-trolytes should be administered, if available. For triage purposes, the presence of explosive diarrhea (especially bloody) is likely to be related to a fatal radiation dose.

Cardiovascular support for patients with clinically significant hypotension and neurologic dysfunction should be undertaken only when medical resources permit. These patients are not like-ly to survive injury to the vascular and gastrointestinal systems combined with bone marrow aplasia.

New means of radioprotection and repair of radiation damage are presently on the horizon. Furthermore, immunomodulators are now under study which may not only facilitate marrow regeneration, but also help reduce the profound immunosuppres-sion responsible for infections associated with severe injury. These agents may be used in combination with radioprotectors and an-tibiotics to further enhance survival. Leukopenia is a significant problem in irradiated casualties, but hazards exist with leukocyte transfusion into patients. Induction of stem cell regeneration agents into selected populations probably offers the best oppor-tunity to correct this deficiency. Although platelet transfusions are certainly desirable for radiation victims, they are presently not practical for mass casualty scenarios. Enormous progress is being made in autologous bone marrow transplants, but this procedure is not practical in forward facilities. Again, repair by stimulation of surviving stem cells is probably the best near-term hope of solv-ing this problem. Problems of effective wound management and fluid and electrolyte replacement remain to be overcome in the neutropenic patient. Pharmacologic means to regulate perfor-mance decrements, such as emesis and early transient incapacita-tion are still not available for use by military personnel.

DIAGNOSIS AND TREATMENT OF THE PATIENT WITH COMBINED INJURIES

As already noted, radiation injury will be associated with other injuries in a large number of patients, in which event the clinical phase of radiation sickness will come sometime during the course of recovery from the other injuries. With supralethal doses of radiation resulting in the gastrointestinal syndrome, the primary clinical picture of the syndrome will predominate and any lesser effects from radiation on other injuries will be secondary. Following lower doses, however, the bone marrow depression will have significant effects upon the clinical course of certain types of wounds and injuries.

In the event of a nuclear detonation, those patients with burns and traumatic injuries in addition to radiation should be managed on the basis of their conventional injuries. Further reclassification may be warranted on the basis of prodromal symptoms associated with radiation injury. The prognosis for all combined injuries is worse than for radiation injury alone. Animal studies indicate that, when other injuries are accompanied by sublethal doses of radiation, their effects are synergistic: infections are much more difficult to control, and wounds and fractures heal more slowly. Thus, potentially survivable burns and trauma will be fatal in a large percentage of persons who have also received significant injury from sublethal doses of radiation. Because of the delays in wound healing and the subsequent granulocytopenia and thrombocytopenia with injuries from nuclear weapons, most lifesaving and reconstructive surgery must be performed within 36 hours after the exposure. Then, if possible, no surgery should be performed for the next 6-8 weeks postexposure.

Closed wounds will not be affected greatly, but open wounds, particularly burns, will demonstrate delays in healing. Granulation tissue will disappear and the wounds will become pale. In addition, they will bleed quite easily. Wound infection, caused by both exogenous and endogenous organisms, can become a severe problem. Closed simple fractures will not be markedly affected, although some delay in union may occur. Open fractures, or severe fractures in which infection is a probable complication, are dangerous.

MANAGEMENT OF INFECTION

In spite of antibiotics, infections with opportunistic pathogens are still a major problem. The majority of these organisms today are gram-negative bacteria such as Escherichia coli and Pseudomonas aeruginosa. These infections occur as a consequence of profound immunosuppression, abnormal colonization of body surfaces, and invasive medical devices. Susceptible body surfaces include the oropharyngeal-respiratory tree and the intestine. Wound sites and artificial invasive devices, such as catheters, are also important sources of infection. Infections may be more prevalent and severe if patients are maintained for long periods in environments containing antibiotic-resistant pathogens.

Wound debridement, appropriate wound dressings, and antibiotics are key elements in infection control. Since infections will be extremely difficult to control in neutropenic subjects, every effort at preventive measures should be made. Antibiotics, preferably in combination therapy, should be used promptly to treat any new fever. When signs or symptoms of infection do appear in the granulocytopenic patient, treatment should be started without waiting for culture and sensitivity studies. Initial coverage should be directed against gram-negative organisms and Staphylococcus aureus. Prevalent organisms and antimicrobial susceptibility patterns in the particular medical facility should also be considered. The drugs most often used now for the initial treatment are the synthetic penicillins, such as ticarcillin, combined with an aminoglycoside such as tobramycin. It is recommended either that the treatment continue until the granulocytes return to more than 500, or that the treatment continue for only two weeks and then stop, even if the white cell count is still depressed, as long as all signs of infection have cleared.

Decontamination and Decorporation After External Contamination by Radioactive Materials

The tremendously increased use of radionuclides in medicine, research, Navy nuclear power, and space, in addition to the increased transport of these materials, has increased the likelihood of exposure to military personnel. A nuclear weapon may have its high-explosive detonate, scattering plutonium debris. In addition, a weapon may be detonated by a terrorist, a third-world country, or by a major power in a single strike. All of these scenarios may result in radionuclide contamination and traumatic injury one or many casualties. Because of the increased probability of exposure, it is important for military physicians to be trained in decontamination procedures and in the decorporation of radionuclides.

SKIN DECONTAMINATION

Skin contamination with radionuclides is almost never immediately life threatening. As in every other aspect of radiation accident management, the serious medical problems have priority over decontamination. The primary objectives of skin decontamination should be to remove as much radionuclide as possible to reduce the surface dose rate and minimize entry into the body. Decontamination also increases the accuracy of determining incorporated radionuclide burdens by whole-body counting. Zealous decontamination to decrease the percutaneous absorption is to be discouraged. Simple removal of the victim's clothing can remove as much as 70-80% of the contamination. No human exposure to date has represented a significant risk to the personnel giving assistance. Additionally, the principles of time, distance, and shielding can reduce any potential radiation exposure to the attending personnel. Personnel participating in decontamination should wear protective clothing, including surgical gowns, gloves, shoe and head covers, and aprons. Health physics monitoring may suggest the need for additional protective gear. Clothing, personal effects, and biological samples from swabs of the nares, aural canal, and mouth should be placed in plastic bags and glass-stopped tubes with proper identification for later analysis.

The first priority of surface decontamination should be open wounds. Since these areas may allow the rapid incorporation of radionuclides, they should be copiously irrigated with physiological saline for several minutes. If contamination persists, gentle surgical debridement may be necessary. Experiments with plutonium oxides have shown translocation to regional lymph nodes within a few minutes to several hours. After one month, the concentration absorbed is 60% of the implanted dose. For this reason, contaminated wounds must receive first decontamination priority. If the radionuclide is plutonium or other alpha emitters for which DTPA is an effective chelating agent, treatment should begin immediately. An effective irrigating solution for americium or plutonium contamination is 1 gram calcium DTPA and 10 ml of 2% lidocaine in 100 cc of normal saline. If an extremity is so severely contaminated that it is not possible to decontaminate it adequately, a decision may be required of whether or not to amputate. Amputation should be seriously contemplated only when the extremity injury is so severe that it precludes functional recovery or when the contamination burden is so great that severe radionecrosis will occur. The best conservative advice is still "decontaminate, but do not mutilate."

After contaminated wounds have been treated, other areas can be decontaminated. The eyes, ears, nose, mouth, areas adjacent to uncontaminated wounds, and remaining skin surface should be decontaminated. Gentle, frequent irrigation and suction of the eyes and ears should be sufficient to decontaminate them. Decontamination of the mouth is important because of possible incorporation. The mouth should be irrigated. A nasogastric tube should be inserted and aspirated for analysis. If radionuclides have been ingested, lavage and decorporation therapy should be begun. Decontamination of the skin usually requires only soap and warm water with gentle scrubbing. The use of hot water is contraindicated because of the subsequent vasodilation. If more aggressive decontamination is necessary, a mixture of half cornmeal and Tide (detergent) has been shown to be very effective. Hair can usually be decontaminated with soap and water. If this is inadequate, the scalp should be clipped rather than shaved, to avoid disruption of the skin barrier.

MANAGEMENT OF INTERNAL CONTAMINATION WITH RADIOACTIVE MATERIAL

Radionuclides within the body represent a state of either internal contamination or incorporation. In internal contamination, radionuclides reside in the respiratory and gastrointestinal tracts, and have not crossed the mucous membranes. In incorporation the radionuclide has been transported across mucous membranes, or the radionuclide has been injected or absorbed through the skin or a wound. Once radionuclides are incorporated, they are significantly more difficult to remove; consequently, internal contamination must be removed before it is incorporated. The treatment involves reducing the absorption and internal deposition, and enhancing the excretion of the absorbed radionuclides. A number of important factors must be understood in assessing the hazards and therapy of incorporated radionuclides. These include absorption, excretion, concentration, biologic half-life, and effective half-life. A definitive review of these factors and incorporated radionuclides is provided in Report No. 65 of the National Council on Radiation Protection and Measurements (NCRP). Blocking agents can enhance elimination of the radionuclide or decrease the quantity incorporated. After incorporation, chelating agents or agents that mobilize the radionuclides are much less effective. It should be obvious that the least incorporation will occur with early administration of the proper drug. Chelating agents bind metals into complexes, thus preventing tissue uptake and allowing urinary excretion. These agents were previously referred to with regard to CaDTPA and transuranic incorporation through a skin wound. A handy checklist is provided in the front of NCRP Report No. 65 for guidance in rapidly treating and preventing transuranic incorporation.

Blocking agents are chemicals that saturate a tissue with a nonradioactive element, thereby reducing the uptake of the radionuclide. Dilution of an isotope involves administering large amounts of a stable isotope so that the hazardous radioisotope is diluted. Incorporated radioiodine can be treated by either approach. Radioiodine is an especially important radionuclide because of the increasing number of potential sources of exposure in medicine, nuclear weapons, and nuclear reactors. A power reactor may contain 10-100 million curies of iodine-131. A loss-of-coolant accident releasing 1% of the radionuclide under the most adverse weather conditions could give an iodine-131 exposure of 500 cGy (R) to a child's thyroid at 75 km. Since most of a dose of radioiodine is taken up by the thyroid within several hours, rapid administration is necessary. Early administration is not the only requirement, however, since exposure from a reactor accident will continue for a period of time. Many recommendations have recently been made to prevent the uptake of radioiodine. A recommended protective dose of stable potassium iodide (KI) for a person over 1 year of age is 130 mg per day, while a dose of 65 mg per day is recommended for children under 1 year of age.

A multitude of other radionuclides of potential importance should be encountered only rarely. Extensive guidance for these can be obtained from NCRP Reports No. 65 and 55 and the *Manual on Early Medical Treatment of Possible Radiation Injury*.

To reiterate, the first several hours after exposure to radionuclides is the best time to prevent uptake, whether by local removal, chelation, physiologic treatment, or limitation of absorption.

CHAPTER VIII

Multiple Injuries

Casualties with multiple injuries are more difficult to treat because of synergistic effects of the pathophysiological disturbances on more than one organ system, the increased frequency and severity of shock, and the competing priorities for immediate care of the various injuries. Wounds involving more than one organ are characteristically more frequently lethal.

ETIOLOGICAL CONSIDERATIONS

The patients in this group most often have sustained multiple missile wounds involving a number of organs or anatomical areas. In addition to missile wounds, these casualties frequently present with associated traumata of other kinds, as follows:

1. Thermal traumata (burns or cold injuries)

2. Physical traumata, including blast injuries, underwater compression as seen in submarine or ship crews, injuries following decompression (aviation or diving crews), crush injury, electrical injury, and rapid deceleration injuries as commonly seen in aircraft and vehicular accidents.

3. Chemical traumata such as phosphorus burns; exposure to organic fuels or propellants; injuries resulting from other chemical agents causing either cutaneous, respiratory or other systemic irritation, or depression of the nervous system.

4. Ionizing radiation injuries with either local or systemic effects.

These special injuries are seen with increasing frequency either in combination with the usual battle wounds or in combination with each other. Personnel working in various military specialties are subject to combinations of injuries which may be unique to their specialty or environment. Physiological disturbances secondary to multiple factors, such as climatic or environmental temperature extremes, dietary inadequacies, superimposed acute or chronic infectious diseases, and systemic poisoning, must also be considered and dealt with.

MANAGEMENT

Diagnosis, Triage, and Evacuation at the Division Level

A thorough examination is carried out at the battalion or division medical facility that initially receives the casualty. Additional problems to be countered are those imposed by the tactical situation and often the generally unfavorable condition of the combatant (dehydrated, grimy clothed, burdened with equipment, and frequently confused after blood loss or sedation given in the field). Under these circumstances, an accurate medical history is difficult to obtain. Unless great care is taken, it is easy to overlook injuries.

The best way to avoid a serious oversight is to remove the patient's clothing completely and consider systematically all the injuries that may have resulted either from a particular missile type and its trajectory, or from other trauma. In addition to obvious lower extremity trauma, a thoracoabdominal blast injury should be considered following a mine explosion. Carbon monoxide poisoning and burns of the respiratory tract must be considered in casualties with burns about the face and those involved in a fire in a closed environment, such as tank or armored personnel carrier. Shock, frequently present, is often severe. It is usually proportionate to the number and magnitude of injuries sustained.

After examination and identification of injuries, the degree of urgency and priorities of treatment must be established. Immediately, life-threatening problems must be corrected; general first aid measures, establishment of the airway, control of hemorrhage, and initiation of resuscitation are carried out according to usual routines. The patient with multiple injuries presents special problems for consideration during evacuation. If these casualties are to survive, essential care must continue en route to the definitive treatment center. Skilled medical attendants are needed to maintain the airway, support the respiration, control hemorrhage, and insure the adequacy of blood or fluid volume replacement. Rapid helicopter evacuation alone is not a substitute for adherence to the above principles, nor does it permit one to ignore the need for adequate fracture immobilization. Concise, accurate records of the injury, of the types of wounds, and of the treatments administered are mandatory to facilitate subsequent medical care.

Preparation for Initial Surgery

Casualties who are seen by medical personnel for the first time at a hospital are evaluated carefully in the manner already described. The accuracy of findings and the response to previous treatment are reassessed with each admission along the evacuation chain. Priorities for care of various wounds in the same patient must be established. While many patients with multiple, extensive wounds can be treated successfully, the potential lethality of certain wounds, such as a massive central nervous system injury or a 90% third-degree burn, must be realistically assessed as the lowest priority for treatment.

Although an oral airway may be adequate in some patients, an endotracheal tube is mandatory in others to assure an adequate airway. Where indicated, chest tubes are inserted and connected to closed drainage. Major bleeding must be controlled and blood volume replenished. Intravenous routes are established with due regard for the site of major injury; for example, a major abdominal injury is best managed with large-gauge cannulae placed in the upper extremities or neck. Other measures important in a patient with multiple injuries are evacuation of the stomach by nasogastric suction and the insertion of an indwelling catheter to measure the urinary output and determine the presence or absence of hematuria. Unstable fractures must be splinted either by conventional means or with the radiolucent inflatable splint before further transport. These splints are ill-suited for fractures of the femur or humerus. While inflatable splints may reduce blood loss, they can present a threat to the circulation if inflated other than by mouth, due to the expansion of air in the splint during evacuation at flight altitude.

Appropriate roentgenograms must be obtained and should include special studies when indicated, such as intravenous pyelograms or cystograms in abdominal and pelvic wounds. Intraperitoneal injuries, produced by missiles entering through the thigh, buttock, or back, are easily overlooked. Abdominal radiographic studies in such wounds is particularly indicated.

The lack of response to vigorous resuscitation may necessitate immediate surgical intervention to control major internal blood loss. However, other causes, which produce or simulate shock must be considered (for example, drug overdose or other poisoning, cardiac tamponade, cerebral malaria, and other infectious diseases).

The complication of cardiac arrest usually is treated by closed cardiac compression; however, open cardiac compression may be required.

Operative Management

The order of priority of wound care is often difficult to establish. In general, those injuries most life threatening are treated initially; thereafter, good judgment must prevail. For example, a patient with both thoracic and abdominal injuries should have definitive operative correction of a lacerated bronchus before a repair of multiple intestinal injuries. Definitive care of intracranial, facial, ocular, and hand injuries frequently must be delayed until other more immediately threatening injuries have been dealt with. Usually, initial operative management of major chest, abdominal, and extremity wounds is performed at a forward hospital. After stabilization, the patient can be transferred to a larger supporting hospital for the appropriate care of remaining injuries. This staged approach, even though it requires a second anesthetic, is much safer than the evacuation of an unstable casualty.

Surgical staffing should provide sufficient personnel to insure appropriate care and to keep operating room and anesthesia time to a minimum. When the situation permits, this may best be accomplished by having separate teams operating on different regional injuries simultaneously. If the wounds are unrelated, it may be necessary to operate on various anatomical areas in successive procedures. Where possible, for example, a buttock wound should be debrided and bleeding controlled before exploring the abdomen. Patients in shock with continued blood loss are extremely unstable after lengthy operative procedures, and cardiac arrest is likely to occur if the procedures are performed in reverse order.

The simplest lifesaving surgical procedure consistent with established principles of combat surgery is all that should be attempted at this time. Unnecessary or meddlesome procedures, such as resection of an undiseased appendix or a Meckel's diverticulum during laparotomy and bowel repair, impose an unacceptable added risk to the patient.

Special Considerations

Despite optimal medical treatment by personnel at all echelons of care, the patients in the multiple injury category are at an extremely high risk. Respiratory support with mechanical ventilators is frequently the only way to counteract the pulmonary insufficiency and fatigue factor common to this group. This is particularly true in casualties with major blast injuries, hepatic wounds with concomitant pulmonary contusion, thoracoabdominal wounds or severe sepsis, and in patients who have required cardiorespiratory resuscitation.

A policy of restraint in intravenous crystalloid fluid administration during resuscitation and operations should be considered in cases where the development of postraumatic pulmonary insufficiency is likely. This policy does not preclude the administration of large volumes of blood or colloid where indicated.

Experience has repetitively demonstrated that constant vigilance and an inquiring attitude will help to define confusing problems and provide practical solutions to what at first may have seemed an impossible problem.

TRAINING

Resuscitation and operations are performed by teams of medical officers, corpsmen, nurses, and other support personnel rather than by individuals. Each medical officer or surgeon has the responsibility of continually training his supporting personnel. The Advanced Trauma Life Support (ATLS) course of the American College of Surgeons provides a good starting point for training applicable to the evaluation and resuscitation of the casualty with multiple injuries. However, medical officers should not forget that ATLS was developed by civilian physicians for use by civilians in dealing with typically civilian trauma. It has not been tested in war and may not be entirely appropriate for combat casualty care. Certainly, a more problem-oriented approach may be necessary, especially during mass casualty situations in exposed field medical units.

ADVANCED TRAUMA LIFE SUPPORT

Primary Survey.   During the primary survey, life-threatening conditions are identified and their simultaneous management is
begun.
  (1)   A — Airway maintenance with cervical spine (C-spine)
          control.
  (2)   B — Breathing.
  (3)   C — Circulation with hemorrhage control.
  (4)   D — Disability; neurologic status.
  (5)   E — Expose; completely undress the patient.

Resuscitation Phase.   During this phase, the oxygenation and
ventilation are reassessed. Shock management is initiated and
hemorrhage control is reevaluated. A urinary catheter and
nasogastric tube may also be inserted during this phase if their
use is not contraindicated.

Secondary Survey.   The secondary survey does not begin until
the primary survey (ABCDE) has been completed and the
resuscitation phase (management of other life-threatening conditions) has begun. The secondary survey is a head-to-toe evaluation of the casualty. Each section of the body is examined in an
organized fashion, utilizing look, listen, and feel techniques. Chest
and C-spine X-rays may be obtained during this section, but only
after the patient is stabilized.

Definitive Care Phase.   In this phase, the patient's less-life-
threatening injuries are managed (setting of fractures, stabilization, wound debridement, and transfer).

TREATMENT AND MANAGEMENT

Primary Survey:
  (1) Airway and C-spine. Upper airway problems are not uncommon in the combat casualty arriving for definitive care. Initial attempts to establish a patent airway include the chin-lift, the jaw
thrust maneuver, or simply the removal of foreign debris. Patients
in whom blunt trauma has been a mechanism of injury, such as
from a helicopter crash or blast displacement injury, should have
a consideration for protection of the C-spine. Excessive movement

of the C-spine can result in permanent injury. In any patient in whom a C-spine injury is suspected, a lateral C-spine X-ray should be taken. All seven vertebrae must be visually confirmed as normal. Pain, tenderness, swelling, and neurological exam are all unreliable indicators of C-spine injury.

(2) Breathing. Ventilatory exchange should be assessed by looking at the chest and listening with a stethoscope. Airway patency does not assure adequate ventilation. The three traumatic conditions that most often compromise ventilation are tension pneumothorax, open pneumothorax, and a large flail chest with pulmonary contusion. Ventilation may be accomplished with an oral or nasal airway and a bag valve device. Chemical injuries may create life-threatening breathing problems. Blast injuries can result in acute pulmonary dysfunction.

(3) Circulation. Adequate circulatory volume can be assessed by examining pulse, skin color, capillary refill, and blood pressure. If the radial pulse is palpable, the systolic pressure will be above 80mm of mercury. If the femoral or carotid pulse is palpable, the systolic pressure will be above 70mm of mercury. A quick and easy method of assessing the peripheral perfusion is the capillary blanch test, done on the hypothenar eminence, the thumb, or the toenail bed. In a normal volemic patient, the color returns to normal within two seconds. Extremity hemorrhage should be controlled by direct pressure. Tourniquets may be of value, but the use of clamps directly into the wound should not be employed. Pneumatic splints may be helpful in controlling bleeding as well. Occult bleeding into the major body cavities will result in shock if left unchecked, and bleeding around crush injuries and fractures will also contribute to hypovolemia. Blast injury can result in arrhythmias.

(4) Disability. A brief neurologic examination should be conducted to establish the level of consciousness and the status of the pupils. A more detailed neurologic examination will follow later in the secondary survey. Simply identifying the level of consciousness and the status of the pupils in the primary survey is sufficient.

(5) Expose. The patient should be completely undressed to facilitate thorough examination and assessment.

b. Resuscitation:
(1) Maintenance of airway, establishment of ventilatory

mechanism, and resuscitation of circulating volume should be initiated when the problem is identified rather than after completion of the entire primary survey.

(2)   Supplemental oxygen therapy should be instituted. Nasal cannulae provide the simplest method of providing this; however, rebreathing masks provide a higher level of inspired oxygen.

(3)   Two large-bore IVs should be started and a Ringer's lactate infusion begun. Percutaneous IV sites have the lowest incidents of complications. Cutdowns may be employed in the antecubital fossa or in the lower extremities. Central line placement in the internal jugular or subclavian veins may also be employed and are of value for central venous pressure monitoring. Resuscitation may also include type-specific whole blood or low-titer type O blood. Hypovolemic shock is not treated by vasopressors, steroids, or sodium bicarbonate. Adequate resuscitation is assessed by following pulse blood pressure and urinary output. Careful electrocardiogram (ECG) monitoring may be indicated by clinical circumstances, such as blunt chest trauma.

(4)   Placement of urinary and nasogastric catheters should now be considered. Urinary catheters are contraindicated in the presence of suspected urethral transection, and nasogastric tubes are contraindicated in the presence of cribriform plate fractures.

c.   Secondary Survey:

(1)   Head. The secondary survey begins with an evaluation of the head and proceeds downward. The scalp and bony structures of the head should be checked for evidence of blunt penetrating trauma. The eyes should be examined for chemical irritation, foreign bodies, and pupillary integrity.

(2)   Maxillofacial trauma. Maxillofacial trauma is important because of its relationship to the airway, the central nervous system and the cervical spine. Maxillofacial trauma by itself can usually be managed at some later time. Patients with midface fractures may have fractures of the cribriform, plate and in these patients gastric intubation should be performed by the oral route.

(3)   C-spine/neck. Patients with maxillofacial trauma produced by blunt injury should be presumed to have a C-spine fracture until proven otherwise. The absence of a neurologic deficit, pain, or deformity does not rule out a C-spine injury. A lateral C-spine X-ray is the only way to completely rule out a C-spine injury. Following blunt trauma to the head and neck, the C-spine should be mobilized utilizing sandbags and tape until such time as the injury

has been ruled out. Penetrating wounds of the neck should not be explored in the emergency area with probes or fingers, but should be evaluated in the operating room. Arteriography may be indicated prior to exploration.

(4)   Chest. Visual examination of the chest, both front and back, will identify most penetrating trauma. Sucking chest wounds should be covered with vaseline gauze or treated with chest tube insertion. Evaluation of ventilatory function is best performed utilizing the stethoscope. A check for the status of the neck veins may be helpful in making an assessment of cardiac tamponade.

(5)   Abdomen. All penetrating abdominal traumata should be explored in the operating room. Blunt trauma to the abdomen requires special assessment. Close observation and frequent reevaluation are important in the management of blunt abdominal trauma. Patients with neurologic injury resulting in an impaired sensorium may present special difficulties in evaluating blunt abdominal trauma. Peritoneal lavage may be of assistance in these instances.

(6)   Rectum. A complete rectal exam is important in all trauma patients: look at the perineum, examine sphincter tone, check the integrity of the rectal wall, check the location and mobility of the prostate, and look at the examining finger for the presence of gross blood. This is especially important in blunt trauma.

(7)   Fractures. Extremities should be examined for contusions or deformity. Palpation and examining for tenderness, crepitation, or abnormal movements along with shafts will help identify fractures. A special check for fractures of the pelvis in blunt trauma is particularly important, because the identification of a fractured pelvis usually indicates the need for significant blood volume replacement. Pulses should be examined in each of the extremities in which there is blunt or penetrating trauma.

(8)   Neurologic. An indepth neurological examination should be conducted in which the physician looks for reflexes, evaluates motor and sensory function, and reevaluates the level of consciousness. The Glasgow Coma Scale is important in assessing the patient with head trauma.

d. Definitive Care. The definitive care of each injury will be discussed in subsequent chapters.

Most combat casualties are young, healthy individuals; however, senior personnel and civilian combatants may provide the opportunity to care for individuals with preexisting medical problems and possible medication complications. An "AMPLE" history is important.

A —Allergies
M —Medication
P —Past illnesses
L —Last meal
E —Events preceding the injury

Reevaluation of the patient is an essential part of all patient assessment, whether for blunt or penetrating trauma. Many injuries may not be evident when the patient first presents. As the patient remains in the health care system and is transported from one location to another, injuries and altered physiology may be evident. Continuous monitoring of vital signs is essential.

Meticulous recordkeeping is extremely important since more than one provider will be participating in the care of the patient along the evacuation chain. Precise records are essential in order to keep up with the patient's clinical status. As the patient is transported along the evacuation chain, all records of laboratory tests, treatments, and X-ray evaluations should accompany him.

PART II

Response of the Body to Wounding

CHAPTER IX

Shock and Resuscitation

One encounters multiple classifications of the shock syndromes. The common denominator in all forms of shock is inadequate capillary perfusion. This chapter concerns itself with the diagnosis and treatment of hemorrhagic shock, that clinical state in which the capillary perfusion is inadequate to satisfy tissue requirements as a result of the loss of blood. For the sake of completeness, we will briefly mention the other forms of shock:

(1) Septic Shock — This syndrome results from the absorption of bacterial toxins or toxic products from infected muscle or other tissues in which debridement has not been performed or was performed inadequately. Massive infection of serous cavities especially predisposes to this potentially catastrophic complication.

(2) Neurogenic Shock — Neurogenic shock results from autonomic nervous system stimulation, causing either widespread vasodilatation or the inhibition of vasoconstriction. This can result in vascular collapse. Neurogenic shock may occur after head injury, may be brought on by pain, or may occur on an emotional basis. The pulse is slow, usually around 60/minute. The syndrome is most often encountered in the operating room in association with the use of certain pharmacologic agents.

(3) Oligemic Shock — Oligemic shock, like hemorrhagic shock, results from loss of circulation volume. The volume loss in this situation usually results from severe, unreplaced, nonhemic losses, such as those arising from severe vomiting or diarrhea, ileus, intestinal obstruction, or enteric fistulas. Loss of plasma by seepage, as occurs with burns, intestinal infarction, and crush injury, also results in external or extravascular "third spaces" losses.

The combat surgeon should bear in mind that the most common cause of death on the battlefield and during evacuation to the hospital is exsanguination. Hemorrhagic shock is far and away the most commonly encountered shock syndrome. Experience has also shown that the majority of casualties, presenting in advanced shock will require surgical intervention to achieve hemostasis before stabilization and hemodynamic improvement can be achieved and maintained.

ORGANIZATION OF A TRIAGE AND RESUSCITATION FACILITY

Prompt, preoperative resuscitation saves lives. Careful preliminary preparations must be made and resuscitative measures instituted with the least possible delay once a casualty has been received in the resuscitation facility. The triage and resuscitation of casualties in shock require considerable clinical experience and acumen. An experienced medical officer, assisted by an experienced and well-trained staff, should be in charge of the triage and resuscitation facility. There must be coordination between the triage officer, the resuscitation personnel, and the operating room personnel. The triage surgeon not only sets individual resuscitation and operative priorities but also must be intimately involved in coordinating and facilitating casualty flow.

PHYSICAL SETTING

1. The facility should be a large, well-lighted expanse of uninterrupted space, allowing free movement of people and an unobstructed view of the entire room. Partitions or unnecessary structures which interfere with communication have no place. To effectively direct activities within the receiving area, the triage officer must be able to see and be seen throughout the area.

2. Such a facility should be capable of handling a large number of casualties. Its location is important in relation to the transportation which delivers the casualties, to the other supporting services, and to the overall internal patient flow. It should be immediately adjacent to the ambulance unloading area or the helicopter pad so that transfer into and out of secondary vehicles is not required. The area should be situated close to the operating room. Portable X-ray apparatus should be close at hand. These arrangements reduce the necessity of moving the patient, which is always deleterious in shock.

3. Supplies and equipment should be immediately visible and accessible without obstructing floorspace. A large number of open shelves lining the walls circumferentially about the triage area will be valuable for this purpose.

4. The blood bank and X-ray facility should adjoin the triage area. Laboratory tests other than cross-matching of blood and determination of arterial blood gases are not needed for initial resuscitation and can be set up in a laboratory closer to the wards and intensive care unit.

5. The facility should be arranged so that casualties can be moved easily and rapidly from the triage area or X-ray facility to the preoperative area and the operating rooms. After initial evaluation and treatment, the wounded should be separated according to priorities. Those most critically wounded are moved to an appropriate surgical stabilization area or, in dire circumstances, may require immediate movement into the operating room. Those that require general anesthesia and can be stabilized are managed in a preoperative area while awaiting their turn in the operating room. Those needing only debridement of minor wounds under local anesthesia may be cared for in a separate area.

EQUIPMENT AND SUPPLIES

1. The frames upon which stretchers will be placed should always be in position, carefully arranged to allow enough space between patients for easy movement. A minimum of other furnishing is necessary. Aside from a desk or countertop work space for record keeping, there should be no chairs or furniture about the working area. Stethoscopes, sphygmomanometers, intravenous administration sets, IV fluids, and devices for suspension of IV bottles or bags should be at every stretcher position.

2. Sterile prepacked sets for emergency procedures, such as cutdowns, tracheostomies, insertions of chest tubes, and control of bleeding, should be conveniently located. These sets must include all of the instruments, sutures, and fittings needed for the purpose and should be plainly marked.

3. Suction equipment must be immediately available for airway aspiration.

4. Laryngoscopes and endotracheal tubes with inflatable cuffs should be conveniently located in the resuscitation area. Oropharyngeal airways prevent the tongue from obstructing the oropharynx in the unconscious patient. Insertion of the endotracheal tube is a rapid means of assuring upper airway integrity and facilitates the later performance of a tracheostomy under more controlled circumstances. A ventilating bag with mask

and endotracheal tube fittings for manual ventilation should be available at numerous locations.

5. Large bandage scissors should be in each corpsman's pocket and at numerous other places to allow quick removal of the casualty's clothing.

6. Intravenous fluids, in large quantities, should be immediately available in the triage area. One bottle of Ringer's lactate with tubing inserted should be hung in place over each set of litter frames. A blood filtration set should be at hand for those who require subsequent administration of blood.

7. Percutaneous venous catheters are preferable to needles in administering intravenous fluids. The intravenous pathway should be at least 18 gauge.

8. Large-bore catheters for chest drainage and sterile tubing for insertion of underwater drainage or suction should be available. Heimlich one-way valves attached to chest tubing are acceptable only for temporary purposes.

9. Quantities of prepackaged sterile dressings in various sizes should be in ample supply at every stretcher.

10. Prepackaged sterile syringes in 5, 10, and 20 ml sizes should be within reach. In addition, preheparinized 5 ml syringes should be available for blood gas determination samples.

11. Sterile prepackaged sets of urinary catheters will be needed and should be available. Only large balloon Foley catheters should be used.

PATHOPHYSIOLOGY

Early post-hemorrhage circulatory changes are compensatory, all serving to preserve perfusion of the vital organs. Vasoconstriction, shunting, and fluid shifts all contribute to the attempt to maintain perfusion of vital vascular beds. A more detailed account of these homeostatic mechanisms operative in the shock state is provided in Chapter X, dealing with the physiologic response to trauma. For our purposes here, suffice it to say that the response to hemorrhage is graded and complex. The circulating blood volume represents approximately 7% of body weight, or about 5 liters in the 70 kg man. In the young healthy individual, a significant blood loss can be tolerated without major changes of the blood pressure early on. The foregoing may not apply to the older casualty, to the depleted casualty, or even the younger casualty as the interval between wounding and initiation of therapy lengthens. The following is offered as a guide in assessing the volume of acute blood loss:

(1) Up to 15% blood volume loss (Class I hemorrhage). Mild tachycardia is the only clinical sign in an uncomplicated situation. This represents a blood loss of 500 cc or less in the 70 kg person. The blood pressure, respiratory rate, urine output, and mental status are within normal limits. The capillary blanch test is normal, refilling occurring within two seconds. These casualties should be resuscitated with crystalloid solutions.

(2) 15-30% blood volume loss (Class II hemorrhage). This degree of loss in the 70 kg soldier amounts to 750-1500 cc of blood. Clinical findings include a pulse greater than 100/minute, a slight decrease in the blood pressure, an altered capillary blanch test response, and subtle central nervous system changes including inordinate anxiety or fright. The urine output is only minimally depressed. This class of patients can also be resuscitated with crystalloid alone.

(3) 30-40% blood volume loss (Class III hemorrhage). This represents a 1,500-2,000 cc blood loss in the standard male. Tachycardia (usually at greater than 120), tachypnea, diastolic and systolic hypotension, and scanty urine output are apparent. These casualties will require blood in addition to crystalloid for resuscitation.

(4) Over 40% blood volume loss (Class IV hemorrhage). This degree of hemorrhage is clearly life threatening. It amounts to a hemorrhage in excess of 2,000 cc. All of the classic signs of shock are present. The skin is cold, clammy, and pale, and the mental faculties are clearly depressed. These casualties not only require large-volume blood replacement in addition to crystalloid, but in addition to volume replacement often times require immediate surgical intervention if resuscitation is to be successful. That is to say, they require operation for resuscitation rather than resuscitation for operation.

PREDISPOSING AND AGGRAVATING FACTORS

Circulatory collapse is hastened or aggravated by a number of factors. Preexisting fluid or electrolyte imbalances resulting from excessive sweating, diarrhea, or vomiting all contribute. The same effect occurs when handling of the casualty during evacuation is rough and traumatic, when injured extremities are not splinted, or when there is sudden shifting of the casualty's position.

Relative overdoses of morphine and certain operating room drugs can make matters worse, as can operation with inadequate anesthesia, prolonged operation, excessive mesenteric traction, or massive contamination of the peritoneum.

INITIAL HOSPITAL EVALUATION

The approach to the casualty in the shock state should be directed to the adequacy of the airway, control of bleeding, and the restoration of the blood volume. Simultaneously, with the institution of initial fluid administration, the surgeon ascertains the mechanism of injury, the wounding agent, the time elapsed since wounding, and, if possible, the position of the casualty when wounded, the estimated initial and enroute blood loss, the drugs administered prior to hospital arrival and the presence or absence of known allergies. Since most combat casualties are young and were previously healthy, history of past or preexisting diseases or chronic medication requirements is usually of little value. This may not be the case in older casualties, especially civilian casualties.

On arrival, a rapid but thorough physical examination is performed to determine vital signs and to identify the number, location, and extent of wounds. The casualty should be completely undressed to allow head-to-toe front and back examination. Blood pressure, respiratory rate, mental status, skin color, capillary refill, and temperature are recorded in the abbreviated clinical record. The capillary refill test is performed by depressing the fingernail or tip of the finger. A normal response is refill of the capillary bed as manifested by the return of color within two seconds. Hidden blood loss into the chest, abdomen, fracture sites (pelvis and thigh) or crush injury sites may be present. These fractures can account for 1.5-2 liters of acute blood volume loss. In the presence of shock, with a chest wound or probable chest wound, a closed-tube thoracostomy should be performed without delay.

As the large-bore intravenous infusion lines are placed, blood is aspirated for type and crossmatch. If additional laboratory tests are indicated, blood is drawn at this time. Usually this amounts to a hematocrit determination for future comparison as therapy progresses. It should be emphasized that the hematocrit has no place in the estimation of the volume of acute blood loss.

HEMOSTASIS

Early in the evaluation and resuscitation phase of the unstable casualty, extremity dressings should not be removed, as the ensuing bleeding will only serve to further deplete circulating volume and will impede therapy by diverting attention away from the business at hand. Direct pressure will adequately control most external hemorrhage. Blind clamping in deep wounds is usually time consuming and frustrating, and in general should be avoided. Tourniquets should be used only after other methods of control have failed. If indicated, the properly applied tourniquet can save the life, but endangers the limb. A common mistake with tourniquets is inadequate compression, which occludes the veins but fails to occlude the artery, resulting in an increased rate of blood loss. The tourniquet should be placed as distally as possible on the extremity, just proximal to the wound. Once in place and adequately controlling hemorrhage, it should not be released until the casualty reaches the operating room. When applied in the field or enroute, the time of tourniquet application should be recorded on the field medical card.

Expedient evacuation of the shock casualty to a definitive facility should not be delayed by application of military antishock trouser (MAST). Some controversy still surrounds their use. MAST trousers can produce ischemia and compartment syndromes if improperly used. A recent combat casualty with abdominal wounds and no lower extremity wounds was treated with MAST trousers in addition to fluid resuscitation and operation. Instability was such that the trousers were left inflated for 18 hours. This casualty subsequently required bilateral above knee amputations. The trousers should never be inflated beyond 100 mm Hg. If there has not been a hemodynamic response within 30 minutes, the inflation pressure should be reduced as the resuscitation continues.

Operation in the resuscitation area of the hospital is rarely necessary; however, the casualty that arrives with penetrating or perforating chest wounds and very recent loss of vital signs is an exception. Salvage may be attempted by immediately opening the unprepped chest of the unanesthetized casualty in an attempt to temporarily control hemorrhage, as fluids are pumped in and the casualty is ventilated via endotracheal tube. An occasional young man will be salvaged in this manner. If some degree of stability is achieved, the casualty is moved to the operating room for definitive repair and closure.

Autotransfusion devices may be available in future wars. There are basically two types of such devices. Both add small amounts of anticoagulant to the collected blood. One simply collects the blood, filters it and reinfuses it. The other type collects the shed blood, washes and centrifugally separates out the red blood cells, and then reinfuses them. These devices may be practical in the resuscitation area for casualties with substantial and ongoing hemothorax. In the operating room, these devices may be applicable in extremity wounds or in cases of uncontaminated hemoperitoneum.

VENOUS ACCESS

Multiple sites of venous access, utilizing large-bore, relatively central catheters, provide both rapid infusion and venous pressure monitoring capability. The most commonly employed percutaneous approaches are the internal jugular, the subclavian, and the median basilic veins. If a cutdown is required to achieve large-bore venous access, the median basilic, the greater saphenous in the groin, or the distal saphenous vein at the median malleolus are all easily isolated. Cutdowns performed under emergency conditions are prone to infection and should be discontinued about 24 hours after the emergency. The magnitude and location of the casualty's wounds will influence the site selected for infusion. Except for the most emergent situations, such as cardiac arrest, one should avoid using the common femoral vein for direct access, as the incidence of injury of adjacent structures and deep vein thrombosis can significantly complicate the postoperative course.

REPLACEMENT THERAPY

Lactated Ringer's solution is the resuscitation fluid of choice. It has advantages over solutions such as Dextrone (5% dextrose in lactated Ringer's solution) since the glucose is poorly metabolized in the presence of the catecholamine response. The incremental elevation in blood glucose levels results in an osmotic diuresis, misleading urine output levels, and dehydration. Colloid solutions are expensive and do not equilibrate with the interstitial space as rapidly as Ringer's lactate. Even though smaller volumes of colloid are required for initial resuscitation, the consensus is that colloid-containing fluids have no significant advantage over Ringer's lactate for resuscitation of the shock casualty.

The shock casualty should be given 1,000-2,000 cc of lactated Ringer's solution, infused as rapidly as possible. Another rule of thumb is an initial fluid challenge of 10-25 ml/kg given over a ten minute period. Some will respond promptly and remain stable with only this therapy. If the hemorrhage has been severe or is ongoing, the response will usually be only transient, but nevertheless may allow time for typing and crossmatching of blood. Lactated Ringer's solution, in addition to providing a rapid increase in circulating volume, will begin the correction of the reduced extracellular volume space resulting from compensatory fluid shifts induced by the shock state. Crystalloid solution rapidly equilibrates between the intravascular and interstitial compartments. For this reason, adequate restoration of hemostatic stability may require large volumes of Ringer's lactate. It has been empirically observed that approximately 300 cc of crystalloid is required to compensate for each 100 cc of blood loss. This 3:1 rule is a good beginning point for fluid resuscitation, but obviously is not a hard and fast rule for those with massive hemorrhage. If the 3:1 ratio were adhered to in a casualty requiring 5,000 cc of blood replacement, inundation would result. About 3,000-4,000 cc of Ringer's lactate seems reasonable.

Several clinical parameters are utilized by the medical officer in determining the casualty's response to the therapeutic intervention. Assessment of clinical response can be made on the basis of changes in blood pressure, pulse rate, capillary refill, urine output, and mental status. Where large volumes of fluid and blood are required, the progress of therapy is facilitated by central venous pressure monitoring. The centrally-placed catheter affords an accurate measure of the right heart's volume requirement and its ability to accept additional fluid loading. Serial measurements are clearly of greater value than a single determination. Sophisticated systems that measure cardiac output and the pulmonary artery wedge pressure do not add a great deal to the early treatment or treatment assessment of the combat casualty.

Blood transfusion is an integral part of the resuscitation of casualties presenting with Classes III and IV hemorrhages and in those with continuing hemorrhage. Whole blood is preferred due to its lower viscosity, faster infusibility and potential provision of some of the clotting factors. Prior to hospital arrival, a more forward echelon may have already infused low-titer type O blood. Those casualties that have been started on type O blood should continue to receive type O. Switching to type-specific blood, especially after several units of type O blood have been given, can result in a transfusion reaction secondary to the reaction between anti-A and anti-B introduced into the recipient by donor O blood and the antigens A and B in the patient's blood. As a general rule, if four units or less of low-titer O blood have been given, a change to type-specific blood is possible without producing ill effects. It is recommended that type-specific blood be withheld for 2-3 weeks or longer if more than four units of type O was initially administered. Female casualties who require the immediate use of type O blood should be given Rh-negative, if available, to avoid the potential of future problems associated with sensitization. Ideally, the casualty is given type-specific, cross-matched blood. This was the practice of American forces in Vietnam, where 80% of the blood administered was type-specific. In the Korean conflict, the practice was to use type O, low-Rh titer blood.

Whole blood should be filtered during administration to remove small clots and other aggregations. A 160 micron macropore filter accomplishes this objective. Blood infusions should be warmed to prevent not only cardiac arrhythmias but also hypothermia. The incidence of cardiac arrhythmia is highest when almost-outdated, old blood with high potassium levels is infused, when the blood is not warmed prior to infusion, and when the infusion catheter rests in a cardiac chamber. When using packed cells, it is recommended that every fourth unit be followed by a unit of fresh frozen plasma. Banked blood in the combat zone, not uncommonly, is close to its expiration date. After an infusion of about ten units of this product, coagulation defects and bleeding diatheses often arise. They should be anticipated and may be avoided by interspersed transfusions of fresh frozen plasma and platelet packs, or by intermittently infusing freshly-drawn local donor blood. The majority of those requiring blood transfusions do not require calcium supplementation; however, when infusion rates exceed 100 cc/minute, 250-500 mg of calcium chloride should be given as a slow bolus through a separate infusion line.

Adequate volume replacement is reflected by a normal central venous pressure and a urine output of 0.5-1 cc/kg/hour. This level of urinary output should be substantially increase, in cases of crush injury.

The tachypnea of trauma tends to produce a state of respiratory alkalosis; however, this effect is more than overcome by the metabolic acidosis resulting from the perfusion deficit. Persistance of the shock state results in shifts to anaerobic metabolism, and further worsens the acidosis. Bicarbonate should be administered in those whose pH approaches 7.2. Serum potassium levels may rise to dangerously high levels as a result of acidosis-triggered potassium shifts. Hyperkalemia can in turn evoke cardiac arrest.

In situations in which infusion therapy fails to initiate a favorable response, conditions other than hypovolemia should be suspected. Cardiac tamponade, tension pneumothorax, myocardial injury, nerogenic shock, and acute gastric dilation may be responsible or contributory. Continued and unrecognized hemorrhage into the chest or abdomen is the most common cause of poor response to fluid therapy. In this sort of situation, the surgeon must operate to resuscitate rather than resiscitate to operate.

The following chart outlines the classes of shock, their presenting signs and symptoms, and the guidelines for resuscitation. These are guidelines only. The amount of blood lost is estimated only as a starting point for resuscitation. Clinical parameters must guide the response to therapy.

TABLE 6.—*Estimated Fluid and Blood Requirements in Shock*

(Based on Patient's Initial Presentation)

	Class I	Class II	Class III	Class IV
Blood Loss (ml)	up to 750	750-1500	1500-2000	2000 or more
Blood Loss (%BV)	up to 15%	15-30%	30-40%	40% or more
Pulse Rate	100	100	120	140 or higher
Blood Pressure	Normal	Normal	Decreased	Decreased
Pulse Pressure (mm Hg)	Normal or increased	Decreased	Decreased	Decreased
Capillary Blanch Test	Normal	Positive	Positive	Positive
Respiratory Rate	14-20	20-30	30-40	> 35
Urine Output (Ml/hr)	30 or more	20-30	5-15	Negligible
CNS-Mental Status	Slightly anxious	Mildly anxious	Anxious & confused	Confused-lethargic
FluidReplacement (3:1 Rule)	Crystalloid	Crystalloid	Crystalloid & blood	Crystalloid & blood

Adequate volume replacement can be guided by urinary output. Fifty cc per hour is a minimum objective of resuscitation for an adult. This figure should be doubled in cases of crush injury.

PROCEDURES
(Adopted with permission from the ATLS Providers Manual, ACS, 1984)

Internal Jugular Venipuncture

1. Place the patient in a supine position, at least 15° with the head-down to distend the neck veins and to prevent an air embolism. Turn the patient's head away from the venipuncture site.

2. Cleanse and prep the skin around the venipuncture site and drape the area. Sterile gloves should be worn when performing this procedure.

3. Introduce a large-caliber needle, attached to a 6 ml syringe, into the center of the triangle formed by the two lower heads of the sternomastoid and the clavicle.

4. After the skin has been punctured, turn the bevel of the needle upward, and expel the skin plug that may occlude the needle.

5. Direct the needle caudally, parallel to the sagittal plane, at a 30° posterior angle with the frontal plane.

6. Slowly advance the needle while gently withdrawing the plunger of the syringe.

7. When a free flow of blood appears in the syringe, remove the syringe and occlude the needle with a finger to prevent an air embolism. If the vein is not entered on the first attempt, the needle generally is too medial. Withdraw the needle and direct it 5-10° more laterally.

8. Quickly insert the catheter to a predetermined depth (such that the catheter is above rather than within the right atrium).

9. Remove the needle and connect the catheter to the IV tubing.

10. Suture the catheter in place, apply antibiotic ointment, dress the area, and tape the tubing in place. Label the adhesive with the date of the procedure.

11. Obtain a chest film to check the position of the IV line and to rule out pneumothorax.

Infraclavicular Subclavian Catheterization

1. Place the patient in a supine position, at least 15° head down

to distend the neck veins and to prevent an air embolism. Turn the patient's head away from the venipuncture site.

2. Cleanse and prep the skin around the venipuncture site and drape the area. Sterile gloves should be worn when performing this procedure.

3. Introduce a large-caliber needle, attached to a 5 ml syringe, 1 cm inferior to the junction of the middle and medial thirds of the clavicle.

4. After the skin has been punctured, with the bevel of the needle upward, expel the skin plug that may occlude the needle.

5. Direct the needle medially, slightly cephalad, and posteriorly behind the clavicle towards the posterior, superior angle of the sternal end of the clavicle (toward a finger placed in the suprasternal notch).

6. Slowly advance the needle while gently withdrawing the plunger of the syringe.

7. When a free flow of blood appears in the syringe, remove the syringe and occlude the needle with a finger to prevent an air embolism.

8. Quickly insert the catheter to a predetermined depth such that the catheter does not rest within a cardiac chamber.

9. Remove the needle and connect the catheter to the IV tubing.

10. Suture the catheter in place, apply antibiotic ointment, dress the area, tape the tubing in place, and label the adhesive with the date of insertion.

11. Obtain a chest film to check the position of the IV line and to rule out pneumothorax.

Saphenous Vein Cutdown at the Ankle

1. One site for a peripheral venous cutdown is the greater saphenous vein at the ankle, just anterior to the medial malleolus. Another secondary site is the antecubital median basilic vein, 2 cm lateral to the medial epicondyle of the humerus at the flexion crease of the elbow. Another site is the proximal greater saphenous vein caudad to the fossa ovalis.

2. Cleanse and prep the skin of the ankle, and drape the area.

3. Infiltrate the skin over the saphenous vein with local anesthetic.

4. A full-thickness transverse skin incision is made through the area of anesthesia to a length of about 2 cm.

5. By blunt dissection, using a curved hemostat, the saphenous vein is indentified and dissected free from the saphenous nerve, which is attached to the anterior wall of the vein.

6. Dissect the vein from its bed and elevate the vein for a distance of approximately 2 cm.

7. Ligate the distal mobilized vein leaving the suture in place for traction.

8. Pass a tie about the vein, proximally.

9. Make a small transverse venotomy and gently dilate the venotomy with the tip of a closed hemostat.

10. Introduce a plastic cannula through the venotomy and secure it in place with the upper ligature about the vein and cannula. The cannula should be inserted an adequate distance to prevent dislodging.

11. Attach the IV tubing to the cannula and close the incision with interrupted sutures.

12. Apply a sterile dressing with a topical antibiotic ointment. Label the adhesive with the date of the insertion.

Needle Thoracentesis

NOTE: This procedure is applicable to the rapidly deteriorating casualty with a life-threatening tension pneumothorax.

1. Identify the second intercostal space, in the midclavicular line on the side of the pneumothorax.

2. Insert a 14 or 16 gauge needle into the skin and direct the needle just over (i.e., superior to) the top of the rib into the intercostal space.

3. Puncture the parietal pleura. If the patient has a tension pneumothorax, a rush of air will exit from the hub of the needle.

4. Prepare for a chest-tube insertion. The chest tube should be inserted at the nipple level anterior to the midaxillary line of the affected side.

5. Connect the chest tube to an underwater seal device or a flutter-type valve apparatus.

6. Obtain a chest X-ray.

Chest Tube Insertion

1. Fluid resuscitation via a large-caliber IV, and monitoring of vital signs should be in process.

2. Determine the insertion site, usually the nipple level (5th intercostal space) anterior to the midaxillary line on the affected side. A second chest tube may be required for a hemothorax.

3. Prep and drape the chest at the predetermined site of the tube insertion.

4. Locally anesthetize the skin and rib periosteum.

5. Make a 2-3 cm transverse (horizontal) incision at the predetermined site and bluntly dissect through the subcutaneous tissues, just over the top of the rib.

6. Puncture the parietal pleura with the tip of a clamp and put a gloved finger into the incision to insure that the pleural space has been entered and the area is free of adhesions.

7. Clamp the end of the thoracostomy tube and advance the thoracostomy tube into the pleural space to the desired length.

8. Look for "fogging" of the chest tube with expiration, or listen for air movement.

9. Connect the end of the thoracostomy tube to an underwater-seal apparatus or flutter valve.

10. Suture the tube in place.

11. Apply a dressing and tape the tube to the chest.

12. Obtain a chest X-ray.

Pericardiocentesis

1. Monitor the patient's vital signs, central nervous pressure (CVP), and ECG before, during, and after the procedure.

2. Prep the xiphoid and subxiphoid areas, if time allows.

3. Using a #16-18 gauge, 6-inch or longer over-the-needle catheter, attach a 35 ml empty syringe with a three-way stopcock.

4. Assess the patient for any mediastinal shift that may have caused the heart to shift significantly. This is best determined by noting the position of the palpable trachea and the point of maximal intensity of the apical heart beat.

5. Puncture the skin 1-2 cm inferior to the left of the xiphichondral junction, at a 45° angle to the skin.

6. Carefully advance the needle cephalad and aim toward the tip of the left scapula.

7. If the needle is advanced too far (into the ventricular muscle) an injury pattern (e.g., extreme ST-T wave changes, or widened and enlarged QRS complex) will appear on the ECG monitor. This

pattern indicates that the pericardiocentesis needle should be withdrawn until the previous baseline ECG tracing reappears. Premature ventricular contractions may also occur, indicating undesired needle contact with the ventricular myocardium.

8. When the needle tip enters the blood-filled pericardial sac, withdraw as much unclotted blood as possible.

9. In a simple tamponade, the aspiration of pericardial blood will cause a rapid drop in the CVP and a slower improvement in the blood pressure.

10. As aspiration progresses and blood is withdrawn, the surface of the heart will reapproach the pericardial surface and the tip of the needle. An ECG injury pattern may reappear. This indicates that the pericardiocentesis needle should be withdrawn slightly. Should this injury pattern persist, withdraw the needle completely.

11. After aspiration is completed, leave the pericardiocentesis catheter in place with the stopcock closed. Secure the catheter in place.

12. Reassess all vital signs and the CVP. A full 12-lead ECG should also be done upon completion of this procedure.

13. Should cardiac tamponade persist, the stopcock may be reopened and the pericardial sac reaspirated. The plastic pericardiocentesis needle can be sutured or taped in place, and covered with a small dressing to allow for continued decompression en route to the hospital or the operating room.

CHAPTER X

Compensatory and Pathophysiological Responses to Trauma

Major combat wounds initiate sudden and intense physiological and metabolic responses. The magnitude and duration of the response are directly proportional to the extent of injury and the interval between wounding and treatment. The development of post-traumatic complications also influences the duration and magnitude of the response. The combat surgeon who has an understanding of the pathophysiological responses to trauma is better able to provide both acute and chronic care to these casualties.

SYSTEMIC PATHOPHYSIOLOGIC RESPONSE

The magnitude of the systemic response to trauma is proportional to the extent of the injury and the local changes at the site of injury. The response is biphasic, with early post-injury hypofunction followed by later hyperfunction in most organ systems. The acute phase is characterized by progressive circulatory insufficiency, decreasing cardiac output, decreasing oxygen consumption, developing acidosis, and discharge of the adrenergic nervous system. If adequate resuscitation is provided, a chronic hyperdynamic, hypermetabolic state persists until resolution of the traumatic injury and any post-traumatic complications. This phase is characterized by an increase in cardiac output and oxygen consumption, tachycardia, and negative nitrogen balance with depletion of lean body mass. This response occurs following a variety of injuries and is modified by any pre-existing metabolic disorder or post-traumatic complications that may arise.

CARDIOVASCULAR RESPONSE

Loss of blood triggers a compensatory vasoconstriction and tachycardia, which permit a reduction of blood volume of 20-30% while maintaining the blood pressure at nearly normal levels. If hypovolemia persists or rapidly progresses below these levels, hypotension results, and, if not corrected promptly, may cause death. Changes that are characteristic of the hypovolemic shock state are decreased cardiac filling pressures, decreased systemic arterial pressure, tachycardia, and increased systemic vascular resistance secondary to catecholamine release.

Liberation of histamine, serotonin, and prostaglandins, leukocytosis; the activation products of complement and coagulation systems; and neutrophils liberated from injured tissue all contribute to a local state of increased vascular permeability. This response can aggravate the intravascular volume deficit. The acute discharge of catecholamines from the sympathetic nervous system and the adrenal glands serves to maintain tissue perfusion in the face of acute intravascular volume loss.

The catecholamines exert an inotropic influence on the heart tending to increase cardiac output which is falling secondary to decreasing preload. Peripherally, there is a redistribution of blood flow, which is in part secondary to a graded autonomic innervation in the vascular beds of various organ systems. Blood flow to vital organs, such as the brain and heart, is maintained at the expense of decreasing flow to skin, muscle, renal, and enteric beds in a prioritized fashion. This response is regulated by the density of alpha receptors responding to the vasoconstrictive influence of circulating catecholamines and by that tissue's inherent local sympathetic nervous system innervation. Hence, we see a casualty with rapid, thready pulse, and pale cool skin, before development of hypotension. If this casualty is administered anesthetic agents that depress these compensatory autonomic responses in the hypovolemic patient, hypotension and shock may result.

Following these acute reflexes, which tend to maintain perfusion, a series of endocrine responses occurs, which serves to replenish the intravascular volume. As an initial response, vasopressin (ADH) is released from the posterior pituitary. ADH exerts a direct action on the renal collecting tubule to increase passive diffusion of water across the cell and back into the peritubular vessels. Under normal conditions, ADH is primarily regulated by hypothalamic osmoreceptors; however, in the response to acute blood loss, volume stretch receptors, hypotholamic osmoreceptors, and a neural pain/stress response appear to play an important role. Subsequently, the release of aldosterone, mediated through the renin-angiotensin system, following stimulation of the juxtaglomerular apparatus of the kidney, acts to maintain extra-cellular fluid volume. Aldosterone, acting at the proximal renal tubular level, causes the reabsorption of sodium and the conservation of water.

RESPONSE TO THERAPY

The hemodynamic response to the initial fluid infusion falls into one of three categories. A small number of patients will respond to the initial fluid bolus with a prompt normalization of blood pressure and will maintain hemodynamic stability. Further therapy is directed at replacing ongoing losses. This response is usually seen in patients with volume deficits of less than 20%. The majority of patients will show a transient response to the fluid bolus. Over time, the initial improvement dissipates, requiring further administration of volume to restore and maintain hemodynamic stability. Most of these patients have experienced a 20–40% volume loss, and may have ongoing bleeding necessitating surgical intervention for control. The third category consists of that small number of patients who show minimal or no response to fluid boluses and usually have an exsanguinating hemorrhage, requiring immediate surgical control. The clinical picture of this subset of patients may be compounded by myocardial dysfunction, necessitating invasive assessment of volume status and myocardial function.

The use of blood transfusions should be limited to cases of severe and ongoing hemorrhage where blood loss exceeds 30% of the total blood volume (i.e. 1500–2000 cc). Red blood cell concentration (hematocrit) determines the blood's viscosity and oxygen-carrying capacity. The goal in blood transfusion is to optimize oxygen delivery to the cells. While an increasing hematocrit allows for a greater oxygen-carrying capacity, the concomitant elevation in viscosity can cause a decreased cardiac output secondary to increased vascular resistance, which impedes the delivery of oxygen to the cell. Viscosity varies little between hematocrits of 20-35%, however, it rapidly increases above this level. In patients who are hypermetabolic and able to elevate their cardiac output, a hematocrit of 30–35% is adequate to ensure sufficient oxygen transport in the systemic circulation. However, in the maximally stressed patient, there may be no further reserve to increase cardiac output to meet the fixed elevated peripheral oxygen needs. Under these circumstances, an infusion of red cells will increase the hematocrit and may increase delivery of oxygen to the tissues.

Transfusions may be associated with complications, including transfusion reactions, transmission of disease (donor pool dependent), and coagulopathy (in patients receiving massive transfusions) secondary to either dilution or a disseminated intravascular coagulation (DIC)-like state. Transfusion related transmission of an immunosuppressing virus is but one of many transfusion-related infectious complications. Transfusion of massive quantities of blood may result in hypothermia, which may be partially avoided through the use of a blood-warming apparatus.

METABOLIC/ENDOCRINE RESPONSE

Trauma produces a sympatheticoadrenal response which partially initiates a hypermetabolic state. Following resuscitation, oxygen consumption increases to supranormal levels. The extent of hypermetabolism is proportional to the severity of injury. The hyperdynamic response is mediated by elevated levels of the counter regulatory hormones: catecholamines, glucagon, and cortisol, which acutely maintain blood glucose levels and later maintain an accelerated body catabolism while opposing the anabolic functions of insulin. In the early post-injury period, insulin levels are low, contributing to hyperglycemia. With time, insulin levels rise toward normal, even in the presence of persistent hyperglycemia. There appears to be an altered tissue receptor sensitivity to insulin in peripheral tissues. Additionally, hepatic glucose production from peripheral precursors is elevated proportionately to the extent of injury. Epinephrine promotes glycogenolysis, also contributing to the hyperglycemia; high concentrations of epinephrine may even inhibit the production of insulin.

Anaerobic glucose utilization at the injury site represents up to 80% of the consumed glucose. The byproducts produced by the wound, lactate and pyruvate, are recycled to the liver where gluconeogenesis occurs. Accelerated peripheral proteolysis occurs during the hypermetabolic state, resulting in an erosion of lean body mass and an increased nitrogen excretion. Amino acids from skeletal muscle are mobilized and serve as additional substrates for hepatic gluconeogenesis. In order to prevent the depletion of lean body mass in the hypermetabolic injured patient, nutritional support should be initiated following resuscitation. Nutritional support must provide sufficient protein and carbohydrate to match the elevated energy demands of the patient. The hypermetabolic response is exaggerated by post-traumatic complications such as sepsis, and is especially detrimental in casualties who are already at the limits of their metabolic reserves.

PULMONARY SUBSYSTEM

Pulmonary vascular changes parallel the systemic circulatory response to trauma. The increase in pulmonary vascular resistance is proportionately greater and more persistent than that seen in systemic vascular beds. Although the etiology of the increase in pulmonary vascular resistance is not fully understood, studies of burn patients suggest that release of vasoactive agents, primarily thromboxane, may play an important role. There appears to be little, if any, change in pulmonary capillary permeability. As a component of the hypermetabolic response to injury, minute ventilation increases significantly as a result of increases in both tidal volume and the respiratory rate. This increase in minute ventilation results in a respiratory alkalosis. Post-injury respiratory alkalosis is appropriate under these circumstances and attempts should not be made to correct it pharmacologically or to suppress the respiratory drive. Hyperventilation can be further aggravated by post-traumatic fever, anemia, or sepsis.

Post-traumatic pulmonary insufficiency can result from penetrating or perforating pulmonary injury, pulmonary contusion secondary to blunt or blast trauma, and smoke inhalation. Aspiration of gastric content is another common cause, especially in the unconscious casualty. Aspiration can result in chemical and/or bacterial pneumonitis. Respiratory insufficiency may also result from the pulmonary edema of excessive fluid resuscitation. Massive blood transfusion, usually greater that ten units over 24 hours, also predisposes to pulmonary insufficiency. The common end result of these divergent pulmonary insults can be the adult respiratory distress syndrome (ARDS). Although the specific pathogenesis of ARDS remains undefined, it has been postulated that activation of the complement system via an alternative pathway causes aggregation and activation of neutrophils, which in turn damage the pulmonary microvasculature resulting in increased vascular permeability.

Clinically relevant ARDS manifests itself by tachypnea and an increased respiratory effort. Pulmonary secretions may be minimal and the breath sounds dry. Pulmonary compliance decreases and pulmonary arteriovenous shunting increases, with a resultant decrease in the PaO_2. Characteristically, the decreased PaO_2 is relatively unresponsive to increases in the inspired oxygen content (FIO_2).

Chest X-ray changes may lag 12-24 hours behind pathophysiological changes. When they appear, one sees diffuse alveolar infiltrates, which commonly progress to complete consolidation.

ARDS therapy usually requires endotracheal intubation, mechanical ventilation, and the maintenance of positive end expiratory pressure (PEEP). Failure to respond to treatment is often related to pulmonary or remote infection. In those cases where treatment fails and the process progresses, the lungs become less compliant and more difficult to ventilate, even with inordinately high inspiratory pressures. In these casualties, the PaO_2 progressively falls and the $PaCO_2$ progressively rises, in spite of maximal FIO_2, maximal levels of PEEP and maximal inspiratory pressures and rates. Ultimately, the hypoxemia, hypercarbia, and acidosis can result in death; however, the majority of these patients die of sepsis.

Because of the lethal problems associated with ARDS, efforts should be directed at preventing the development of the full-blown syndrome. Prophylactic pulmonary care should include avoidance of overly zealous fluid resuscitation, prevention of aspiration, and frequent pulmonary toilet. In the presence of progressively worsening ARDS requiring very high ventilatory pressures, the surgeon should consider the placement of prophylactic chest tubes. Prompt identification and treatment of both local and remote infections decreases the likelihood of sepsis-related ARDS. It may be appropriate to choose a more appropriate or effective antibiotic in some cases. Humidification of inspired oxygen and, if possible, the avoidance of prolonged utilization of high inspired oxygen concentrations are also major considerations.

The early use of diuretics and parenteral albumin, may reduce pulmonary fluid.

GASTROINTESTINAL SUBSYSTEM

Preferential redistribution of blood flow in the shock state results in splanchnic ischemia. The ischemic mucosal insult can subsequently result in gastric stress ulceration, especially in the presence of associated sepsis. Gastrointestinal hemorrhage of significant degree is usually the presenting symptom. The onset of bleeding usually presents about ten days post injury. These gastric ulcerations are frequently multiple. Perforation can occur. Prophylactic therapy consists of antacid buffering of the gastric content, and administration of a histamine hydrogen receptor antagonist, such as cimetidine. Enteral alimentation is also thought to provide gastric mucosal protection and should be instituted when feasible.

Intractable upper gastrointestinal hemorrhage from stress ulceration may require gastric resection or vagotomy and pyloroplasty. Perforation is another indication for operative intervention.

Acalculous cholecystitis may occur in trauma victims at a time when it is most difficult to diagnose. Presumably, it develops under the conditions of dehydration or lack of stimulation by oral intake, or from the effects of drugs. All of the foregoing occur in trauma casualties, oftentimes in association with abdominal wounds. It may mimic other more common conditions following trauma, and may progresses to gangrenous cholecystitis and rupture before it is suspected.

The generalized ileus usually seen in the shock state necessitates nasogastric decompression to prevent emesis and possible aspiration.

HEMATOLOGIC AND CLOTTING SUBSYSTEMS

Certain casualties, such as those with heart or liver wounds and those with pelvic crush injuries, require very substantial infusions of whole blood. Very often, ten units of blood will have been infused before operative control of the source of hemorrhage is controlled. In the combat zone, it is not uncommon for bank blood to be nearing its expiration date. This combination of circumstances set the stage for catastrophic cardiac arrhythmia. The elevated potassium concentration of old bank blood, when infused directly into a cardiac chamber, can precipitate fatal arrhythmias. The same complication can result from infusion of large quantities of cold blood. The blood should be warmed, and infusion directly into the right atrium should be avoided.

Another common and very serious complication in this sort of circumstance is the development of a diffuse bleeding diathesis. Some degree of coagulopathy occurs routinely after about ten units of infusion and worsens as the blood requirement increases. The diathesis can be avoided, lessened, or corrected with infusions of fresh frozen plasma and platelet packs. If these components are not available, freshly drawn blood, less than 24 hours old and procured within the facility from the walking donor pool, should be employed. If the hemorrhage or diathesis persists, requiring massive transfusion, about every fourth unit should be freshly drawn. Bank blood becomes progressively platelet- and clotting-factor-deficient from the third day on. Citrate in banked blood aggravates the situation. When available to the surgeon, therapy is based on the results of the platelet count, partial thromboplastin time, prothrombin time, and the fibrinogen level. With lesser laboratory capability, the surgeon must anticipate the diathesis and resort to empiricism.

Anemia will develop in those casualties where large volumes of asanguineous fluids were utilized to treat hemorrhagic shock. Reticuloendothelial system removal of damaged bank red cells and the excessive drawing off of blood for laboratory tests will contribute to the anemia.

Disseminated intravascular coagulation (DIC) may develop in association with shock, tissue injury, or sepsis. Consumption of clotting factors by disseminated intravascular microthrombi give rise to the consumptive coagulopathy. The casualty with DIC may present a clinical spectrum ranging from a simple hypercoagulability state to fulminant consumptive coagulopathy resulting in massive diffuse bleeding. Therapy includes correction of the shock state, appropriate wound debridement, and treatment of sepsis. In the presence of laboratory evidence of DIC and elevated levels of circulating fibrin degradation products, patients with a bleeding diathesis may be treated with repeated small doses of heparin.

RENAL SUBSYSTEM

Urinary output: The decrease in urinary output that occurs as a physiological response to wounding is the result of both metabolic and vascular changes. Normally, the urinary output is in excess of 500 ml per 24 hours when the blood pressure is within the normal range and the urinary flow is not mechanically obstructed. As the systolic blood pressure is lowered by hemorrhage to a level of 60–80 mm Hg or even lower, the urinary flow decreases and may progress to oliguria; that is, to a volume of urine less than 20 ml per hour, or less than 400 ml per 24 hours.

Obstruction of a urinary catheter is a particularly likely cause of absence of detectable urinary output. Most patients, even those with acute renal failure, excrete 50 ml or more of urine per day. When anuria develops, a mechanical reason for it should be suspected. Frequent causes are obstruction or actual destruction of the urethra or ureters by wounds in the pelvic region, spasm of the urethral sphincter, and atony of the bladder. Careful physical examination; catheterization of the urinary bladder; and intravenous pyelography, cystoscopy, or exploration, as indicated, will establish the presence or absence of adequate urinary flow from the kidneys. If a urethral catheter has been inserted, it may be obstructed by mucous plugs or blood clots. These are such obvious causes of oliguria and anuria that, paradoxically, they are sometimes overlooked.

Acute renal insufficiency: Acute renal insufficiency or acute renal failure indicates sudden and essentially complete failure of the excretory function of the kidneys. This complication, in which the pathological process is acute tubular necrosis (lower nephron nephrosis), must be suspected if less than 400 ml of urine is excreted in a 24 hour period. It is important to recognize, however, that some casualties who develop the syndrome of acute renal failure do not have oliguria but may become uremic nonetheless (high-output renal failure). Although urine volumes may be normal to high, a lack of concentration indicates failure to clear solutes. Failure to recognize this fact and to monitor the patient's fluid administration may result in overhydration and fatal circulatory embarrassment of the nonoliguric as well as the oliguric patient with acute renal failure. Failure to recognize high-output nonoliguric renal failure can result in worsening the hypovolemic state, further compounding the renal insult. Paradoxical polyuria should be replaced at 0.5 cc per cc of urine output, but care should be taken to avoid "chasing" the urine output and causing overhydration. Excessive urine output may be associated with significant urinary potassium losses, requiring frequent monitoring of the serum potassium level and replacement as indicated.

Factors which frequently cause acute renal insufficiency are long periods of hypotension, crushing injuries, burns, hemolytic reactions (most frequently from blood transfusions); drug nephrotoxicity, sepsis, and hypersensitivity phenomena.

At first, the urine is pale and dilute unless blood or hemoglobin is present. If hemolysis has occurred, it is characteristically dark brownish red. Proteinuria may be conspicuous for a day or two. Granular and heme-pigment casts soon appear. The specific gravity falls rapidly, and by the third day it may be as low as 1.010 and fixed.

The BUN (blood urea nitrogen) level rises rapidly. The rate of increase is closely related to the extent of trauma or to factors which influence the catabolic rate. In a massively wounded and catabolic patient with renal failure, the BUN may rise as much as 120 mg percent per day. Hyponatremia is a frequent finding and is usually attributed to an excessive administration of water rather than to an actual sodium deficit. With the development of metabolic acidosis, the serum bicarbonate falls. Hypocalcemia is frequently present. Anemia and leukocytosis are usually present, even in the absence of infection. Because infection is a leading contributory cause of death in acute renal failure, search for foci of infection is mandatory. Diarrhea, sometimes with bloody stools, may develop if uremia persists. Abdominal distention may be marked. Drowsiness, disorientation, muscular twitchings, and even convulsions may occur. Diastolic hypertension of considerable degree is not unusual. Acute pulmonary edema and congestive heart failure are more likely to develop when hypertension is marked, especially if an excess of fluid has been given. Weight loss and hypoproteinemia, progressing to emaciation, reflect the catabolic state, and dependent edema may occur even when the fluid allowances are less than conventional. The clinical course may be complicated by extensive and progressive infection, impairment of wound healing, and a distinct tendency to bleed.

Many of the abnormalities observed in acute renal insufficiency are the result of potassium intoxication. Because of catabolism, the potassium ion shifts from its normal intracellular location to the extracellular fluid compartments. The process may be more rapid in the presence of necrotic tissue or hematoma formation and should be suspected whenever major injury to muscles is present. In the presence of acidosis and uremia, the plasma potassium levels are abnormally high, and potassium intoxication can occur on the first day after wounding in casualties who are oliguric. Frequently, physical signs or symptoms do not reflect the gravity of the situation until death is imminent. Neuromuscular and cardiac changes are manifestations of potassium intoxication. Tendon reflexes are diminished to absent, and complete paralysis may follow. Potassium intoxication causes certain electrocardiographic changes, such as high-peaked T waves in the precordial leads, a widening of the QRS complex, a depression of the P waves, and a sloping ST segment in the limb leads. Conduction disturbances can lead to ventricular arrhythmia and death. Fatalities from cardiac arrest secondary to potassium intoxication have been observed as early as the fourth day after wounding.

The earliest sign of acute renal failure is usually the appearance of oliguria with no other obvious cause for a decreased urinary output. Volume expansion, monitored by the CVP, will help in identifying and treating cases of prerenal oliguria. This is accomplished by rapidly administering a test load (500–1,000 ml) of intravenous fluid, rapidly followed by a single dose of diuretic agent. The urine specific gravity is usually 1.010 in the syndrome of acute tubular necrosis, and the urine sodium concentration is relatively high (60 to 100 meq/l). The UUN/BUN (urine to serum urea ratio) is usually less than 10:1. Electrocardiographic and chemical determinations may confirm the presence of hyperkalemia.

The clinical manifestations of sepsis, shock, and necrosis of undebrided tissue are quite similar to those of uremia, but the differential diagnosis is seldom difficult because these manifestations appear considerably earlier than those of uremia. Even though both oliguria and azotemia may be present in the first few days after wounding, the nausea, vomiting, disorientation, and convulsions which occur at this time are not likely to be of uremic origin.

Since renal insufficiency usually is not diagnosed in its incipiency, treatment during this phase, when the only manifestation is oliguria, is vascular volume expansion using blood and other suitable electrolyte solutions, with monitoring of the central venous pressure, adequate debridement of any wounds, a trial of mannitol intravenously injected in a 12.5–25gm bolus, and the administration of antibiotics as indicated. The concern of the medical officer in a forward unit should be the correction of potentially reversible renal failure by prompt restoration and preservation of adequate blood volume and urinary flow.

In a temperate climate, the total fluid intake for 24 hours, exclusive of blood, plasma, or plasma expanders, should be 500 ml to cover insensible loss, plus the measured output. The measured output is the total of urinary excretion, vomitus, diarrhea, fluid removed by gastric suction, and fluid lost from burned surfaces. Allowance must also be made for increased insensible fluid losses. These vary accordingly to climatic conditions and body temperature. In humid tropical regions and febrile states, these losses may be 2,000 ml per day or more.

Maintenance of the proper relationship of fluid intake to fluid output is important, for increasing the fluid intake will not increase the urinary output in acute renal insufficiency. An excessive intake, in fact, will endanger the patient's life. The responsible medical officer must give his personal attention to the calculations. A careful record must be kept, and nurses and aidmen must be instructed specifically about how to keep it. A warning notice to keep the fluid intake-output chart must be displayed prominently on the patient's bed.

The patient's thirst must not be allowed to influence the volume of intake, and close supervision is necessary to insure that he does not overhydrate himself. A daily weight record should be maintained if practical. An increase in weight implies water retention and, therefore, overhydration. A useful general rule is the maintenance of 0.5 pound daily weight loss under usual catabolic conditions.

Administration of fluids should be oral if tolerated and feasible. When parenteral administration is required, as it often is, it should be a continuous intravenous infusion at a constant rate. It is technically simple to pass a polyethylene catheter into the superior vena cava via a peripheral vein, and little trouble need be expected if the tube is allowed to remain in situ for no longer than five days. This technique minimizes the risk of thrombosis, which would be associated with infusion by a needle or cannula in a peripheral vein for this period of time. It also makes movement of the patient simpler and allows CVP monitoring through the same catheter. Although wound management is essentially the same as in patients without renal failure, early debridement is even more critical in that damaged tissue aggravates the effects of renal failure. Hypoxia and respiratory acidosis during anesthesia should be particularly avoided, since they may promote the release of intracellular potassium into the plasma.

Caloric intake should be maintained by the use of carbohydrates and fats, with the complete elimination of protein-containing foods. Hypertonic glucose can be given effectively through a central venous catheter. Potassium should not be administered to the oliguric patient unless the concentration of the ion is deficient.

The early use of mannitol as an osmotic diuretic has been mentioned. If diuresis results from a 12.5–25g bolus, a sustained infusion of 20% mannitol may be used to titrate an adequate urine volume. Furosemide and ethacrynic acid should be used as an initial diuretic. Caution is required in their use, however; serious adverse reactions have been reported, including deafness and death. The treatment of hyperkalemia with cation exchange resins, such as Kayexalate, has decreased the requirement of dialysis for the sole purpose of treating hyperkalemia. Usual doses are 10–50 gm by mouth or enema every two to six hours. Sorbitol, as an osmotic cathartic (5–10 ml) by mouth or by enema, also promotes diarrhea and intestinal potassium losses. Since many drugs are excreted through the kidneys, decreased renal function requires decreased doses of most antibiotics and other drugs such as digitalis. Magnesium-containing compounds, such as antacids, should be used sparingly in the oliguric patient because of the possibility of magnesium toxicity.

An oliguric patient should not be kept in the forward area any longer than necessary. Instead, he should be evacuated as expeditiously as possible to a center that possesses an artificial kidney and that is otherwise specially equipped to treat acute renal insufficiency. If he cannot be evacuated, a patient who remains oliguric for 72 hours should be treated by the following emergency measures, designed to reduce or counterbalance an excess of serum potassium:

1. Intravenous glucose is given in 10% concentration through the superior vena cava. This measure will cause potassium to be reincorporated into intracellular glycogen and will lower the

serum concentration. The concomitant use of insulin may facilitate this process.

2. Since calcium is a specific antagonist of potassium, a continuous infusion of 10% calcium gluconate will counterbalance excess potassium if it is not extreme. Although sodium is also an antagonist of potassium, large amounts of this ion should not be used during the first days of acute renal insufficiency. Sodium, in this setting, is used sparingly and only to replace that lost by urinary excretion, gastric suction, or diarrhea. Generally, one-third normal saline is used to replace urine output, and normal saline to replace gastric fluid loss.

3. Fluid balance is maintained by the use of carefully calculated amounts of the required fluids. Consider, for example, a patient who has excreted 50 ml of urine and who has lost 150 ml of fluid in vomitus or by gastric suction within 24 hours. His measured output is thus 200 ml. This amount should be added to the basic allowance of 500 ml to give a total intake for 24 hours of 700 ml. Of this, 100 ml may be 10% calcium gluconate, 400 ml should be 10% glucose in water with 10 units of regular insulin, and 200 ml should be isotonic saline. Sodium bicarbonate in 7.5% solution may replace saline if the pH determination reveals metabolic acidosis. Since some wounded patients develop respiratory alkalosis, monitoring of serum pH is necessary to determine appropriate fluid replacement. Peritoneal and extracorporeal dialyses are effective techniques of treatment but are not usually feasible outside a special center staffed by personnel trained in these techniques.

CHAPTER XI

Infection

GENERAL PRINCIPLES

War wounds are characterized by lacerated, contused, and devitalized tissue; extravasated blood; disruption of the local blood supply; presence of foreign bodies; and contamination with various microorganisms, all of which predispose to the development of subsequent infection. The devitalized tissue and extravasated blood provide an excellent culture medium to support the growth of microorganisms and thus are conducive to the development of wound infections. Injury-related edema may produce tension within a fascial compartment that compromises the capillary circulation of the tissues within the compartment, resulting in local tissue anoxia. Additionally, the anaerobic character of hypoxic tissue may inhibit leukocyte phagocytosis or limit the function of leukocytes. The time lag between wounding and treatment represents an incubation period during which bacteria may proliferate and initiate infection. Early adequate surgery is therefore the most important step in prophylaxis against wound infection. A wound, debrided of nonviable contaminated tissue and left with an excellent blood supply, is best able to resist infection.

Although early antibiotic therapy plays an important role in the prevention and treatment of wound infections, antibiotics do not take the place of early surgical therapy. Antibiotic therapy should be based upon a knowledge of the likely causative organism and the antibiotic or antibiotics most suitable for controlling the organism.

Prophylaxis and early treatment are of the greatest importance. Once infection is established, it may be lethal and it is always costly in terms of further destruction of tissue, persistance of disturbed body physiology, delayed wound healing, and prolonged morbidity. Underlying medical problems, such as malignant disease, diabetes, malnutrition, and metabolic disease, may reduce an individual's resistance to microorganisms. These factors, however, are uncommon in the typical active duty military casualty.

ETIOLOGIC FACTORS

The development of a wound infection is generally associated with one or more of the following factors:

(1) Delay in surgical treatment.

(2) Inadequate wound debridement.

(3) Associated vascular injury resulting in regional tissue ischemia.

(4) Inadequate hemostasis at the initial wound operation, resulting in subsequent hematoma formation.

(5) Retention of foreign bodies within the wound.

(6) Failure to provide adequate drainage.

(7) Tight packing of the wound or the use of tight circular dressings or casts.

(8) Primary closure of war wounds.

(9) Failure to recognize and treat a perforated hollow viscus.

(10) Wound contamination with bacteria that are resistant to antibiotics.

(11) Secondary contamination from fomites, or exposure to personnel who are carriers of pyogenic bacteria.

(12) Presence of metabolic diseases, such as diabetes, which predispose to the development and spread of infection.

DIAGNOSIS OF INFECTION

The classic signs and symptoms of infection are redness, swelling, heat, and pain. Redness of the skin is due to intense hyperemia and is seen in infections which involve the skin or subcutaneous tissue and, in some patients, in the skin overlying foci of suppurative thrombophlebitis. The hyperemia is responsible for the local increase in temperature. Fever and tachycardia are additional but nonspecific signs of infection. Rigors and chills are suggestive of septicemia.

Leukocytosis commonly accompanies acute bacterial infection. Generally, the more severe the infection, the greater the leukocytosis. The leukocytosis is characteristically accompanied by an increase in the proportion of immature granulocytes, the so-called "left shift."

Exudate from the area of infection should be examined for color, odor, and consistency. A Gram stain of the exudate should be performed immediately to facilitate prompt institution of appropriate antimicrobial therapy. For each bacterial cell observed under microscopic oil immersion lens examination, there are approximately 10^5 similar organisms in each milliliter of exudate from which the smear was prepared.

A wound biopsy is a useful method of confirming the presence of infection in a wound, particularly in a burn wound or wounds of the subcutaneous and soft tissues. Areas of the wound that appear purulent or reveal new focal areas of discoloration should be biopsied. If the technical capability exists, a portion of the specimen should be sent to the microbiology laboratory for quantitative culture. The recovery of 10^5 or more organisms per gram of tissue from a quantitative culture is suggestive but not necessarily diagnostic of infection. This finding is highly sensitive but not specific for infection, since proliferation of colonizing organisms may account for such bacterial densities. The remaining portion of the specimen is forwarded to the pathologist for histologic examination. The histologic finding of microorganisms in viable tissue is highly specific and is diagnostic of infection. Consequently, the examination of histologic sections prepared from a biopsy specimen is the most reliable means of differentiating contamination or colonization of nonviable tissue from infection of viable tissue.

BACTERIOLOGY

Bacterial contamination of a war wound is certain. The wounds are contaminated at the time of injury and secondary contamination may occur at any time during the course of treatment. Clostridium species are commonly introduced at the time of injury. Hemolytic Staphylococci and Streptococci may also be introduced at the time of wounding or by later contamination with such organisms in the hospital. Animal studies have shown heavy growth of Gram-positive cocci and Clostridium species in experimental missile wounds after delayed debridement. Gram-negative bacilli are typically encountered later and are often hospital acquired. Patients with abdominal injuries are also at risk of developing Gram-negative infection, particularly those with an injury to a hollow viscus. Many of these bacteria produce toxins and enzymes to facilitate their spread through tissues within wounds. Coagulase, fibrinolysin, proteinase, collagenase, and hyaluronidase favor the development and spread of wound infection.

The results of cultures taken from wound walls after debridement in animal studies indicate that, even though the degree of contamination or colonization can be significantly reduced by prompt debridement, the wound is not sterilized. Persistance of microorganisms in the wound following mechanical cleansing and removal of damaged tissue justifies the use of prophylactic antibiotics.

SURGICAL THERAPY

Prompt, adequate surgical debridement is the cornerstone of therapy of war wounds, particularly with respect to prevention of infection. In addition to adequate debridement and excision of crushed and lacerated tissue, the removal of foreign bodies and reduction of microbial density are important considerations. The current recommendation is that war wounds be debrided within six hours of injury.

Although such classic signs as impaired contractility, altered consistency, and lack of capillary bleeding have been shown to correlate poorly with tissue viability, they have a useful function. If there is any question about the adequacy of debridement, the wound is dressed and reexplored three to five days later. If there is no residual nonviable tissue and no evidence of infection, the delayed primary closure is performed. Delayed primary closure effects timely closure of an initially heavily-contaminated wound while minimizing the risk of infection. An even longer delay in wound closure may be indicated in some wounds, as was supported by the recent-albeit limited-experience with septic complications in limb wounds during the Falkland's campaign. This study showed that no septic complications developed in those patients undergoing delayed closure eight days or later from time of injury (none of five patients). Fifteen percent developed septic complications when closed at 5-7 days (six of 40), and 75% (three of four) when closed within four days. If at the time of inspection, 3-5 days post injury, nonviable tissue remains or infection is present, further debridement is performed and the infection is treated before closure is attempted.

ANTIBIOTIC THERAPY

The primary emphasis of antibiotic treatment of wounds is early administration before an infection becomes established. During the Yom Kippur War, medical personnel were instructed to administer antibiotics routinely to all wounded. A recent review of infections following soft-tissue limb wounds in soldiers injured during the Falkland Campaign indicated that a delay in surgery and a delay in antibiotic administration were the most important factors related to the subsequent development of infection. When surgical delay was unavoidable, the delay in antibiotic administration assumed an even greater importance. That study showed a greater incidence of septic complications when debridement was delayed more than six hours, as well as an increased incidence of infectious complications when the time from wounding to antibiotic administration exceeded six hours.

An animal study of .223-caliber high-velocity projectiles in a porcine model demonstrated that bacterial proliferation could be prevented with early institution of intravenous penicillin therapy. Another study in wounded pigs suggested that the growth of mixed flora in a contaminated missile wound predisposed the wound to infection with other more pathogenic strains and impaired the ability of reversibly-injured tissue to recover. The mixed flora in that study consisted of bacterial strains usually sensitive to penicillin. Yet another study in wounded pigs demonstrated a decrease in the amount of devitalized tissue during debridement at 12 hours in penicillin-treated animals as opposed to animals not treated with penicillin.

Selection of antibiotic therapy is based upon a knowledge of likely causative organisms, examination of the Gram stain of the wound exudate, and culture and sensitivity studies of the wound. The characteristics of antibiotics useful against various organisms commonly encountered in surgical infections are described in the table at the end of this chapter (Table 7).

HYPERBARIC THERAPY

In 1963, Brummelkamp and associates in Amsterdam reported the first use of hyperbaric oxygen in the treatment of infections caused by gas-producing microorganisms. The patients were placed in a room-sized chamber in which the air pressure was raised to three atmospheres. During the course of three days, the patient inhaled 100% oxygen from a face mask for one-and-a-half hours on seven occasions. This increased the oxygen tension in plasma, lymph, and tissue fluids by 15-20 fold. Dramatic clinical improvement was described for most patients within the first day. Large pressure chambers are available at only a few medical centers in the world and at special military and marine industrial facilities. Much less expensive single patient chambers are now available. Therapy with hyperbaric oxygen, antibiotic administration, and surgical debridement has been reported as effective in patients with clostridial myonecrosis who evidenced toxicity. Hyperbaric oxygen appears to reduce toxemia and diminish the amount of tissue requiring excision. However, patients with gas-producing infections due to anaerobic Streptococci, *Escherichi coli*, and Klebsiella species showed no improvement after exposure to high-pressure oxygen. All of the foregoing notwithstanding, the use of hyperbaric oxygen is not feasible in the theater of operations. Even in referral centers, it is advocated only as an adjunct to the surgical treatment of clostridial infections, and not as a substitute for conventional modes of therapy, including early surgical debridement and the administration of antibiotics.

CLOSTRIDIAL INFECTIONS

Three types of clostridial infections of ascending severity have been described: simple contamination, clostridial cellulitis, and clostridial myonecrosis. Simple contamination of a wound by clostridia is common. It causes no discomfort to the patient and should be of little concern to the surgeon. A thin seropurulent exudate may be present. If the necrotic tissue harboring the microorganisms is debrided, there will be no subsequent invasion of surrounding tissue. The frequent contamination of war wounds with clostridia is due to the ubiquitous nature of this organism. A high oxygen tension in the surrounding healthy tissues prevents invasions in these areas.

Clostridial cellulitis is characterized by the presence of gas in necrotic and viable subcutaneous tissue that produces crepitus on palpation. Intact healthy muscle is not invaded. The cellulitis produces a foul-smelling seropurulent discharge from the depths and crevices of a wound. There are often local extensions along fascial planes, but involvement of healthy muscle and marked toxemia are absent. The predominant organisms are proteolytic and nontoxigenic clostridia, such as *Clostridium sporogenes* and *Clostridium tertium*. Clostridial cellulitis generally has a gradual onset. The incubation period is from 3-5 days; systemic effects are usually mild; there is no toxemia; the skin is rarely discolored;, and there is little or no edema. These characteristics distinguish the infection from gas gangrene.

Clostridial myonecrosis, or gas gangrene, is the most serious of the clostridial infections. This infection occurs most often in association with severe wounds involving large masses of muscle that have been contaminated with pathogenic clostridia, especially *Clostridium perfringens*. Such wounds are commonly caused by the high-velocity missiles of modern warfare and by crush injuries in which the skin is broken. Clostridial myonecrosis principally (although not exclusively) occurs in the lower limbs, buttocks, and upper limbs. In association with the muscle injury, the arterial supply to the limb may be impaired and the damaged tissues may be contaminated by soil, clothing, and other foreign bodies. Glycolysis continues in the anoxic wound with a drop in the oxygen tension, accumulation of lactate, and fall in pH providing an ideal environmental for the growth of clostridia. Once bacterial growth is established and toxins and other products of bacterial metabolism accumulate, invasion of uninjured tissues is promoted and the anaerobic infection is established. Resistance to the infection and its spread is compromised by the avascularity of the necrotic tissue that prevents entry of phagocytes, antibodies, or systemically-administered antibiotics into that tissue.

Culture of sites of clostridial myositis usually yields several species of toxigenic clostridia, particularly *Clostridium perfringens, Clostridium novyi*, and *Clostridium septicum*. The common habitat of these species is the soil, but they also are found in the intestines of many animals, including man. The toxic metabolites elaborated by the anaerobes, together with other substances produced by their actions on the muscle, are responsible for the local pathological changes in the muscle and the associated toxemia and anemia.

The diagnosis of gas gangrene can often be made on the basis of clinical findings alone. The usual onset occurs one to four days after injury; however, onset can vary from 8-10 hours at one extreme to five or six days at the other. The most striking feature is a rapid deterioration of a casualty who had previously been progressing satisfactorily. Pain is frequently the earliest symptom of clostridial myonecrosis and is frequently disproportionate to the apparent severity of the wound. Fever is common and blood pressure falls as the infection advances. Anemia and dehydration are common late findings. Examination of the wound may reveal profuse serous or serosanguineous discharge sufficient to soak through massive dressings. The discharge may contain gas bubbles, and it occasionally yields large Gram-positive rods evident on microscopic examination.

Although clostridial myonecrosis often is described as emitting a characteristic rotten meat odor, this is not always the case. The odor emitted from the wound is variable, ranging from sweet and pungent to foul and fetid, depending upon the species of bacterial present. Gas production is more marked with *Clostridium perfringens* infections than with other types of clostridia. Gas bubbles may be seen dissecting along fascial planes on roentgenograms; however, the absence of tissue gas does not exclude clostridial infection.

Several other conditions must be differentiated from clostridial myonecrosis. Anaerobic cellulitis is characteristically limited to the subcutaneous tissue and fascia, and does not involve muscle. Gas formation is far greater than in gas gangrene. The brownish and purulent discharge is profuse. Pain and toxemia are not prominent. Local changes include cutaneous erythema and swelling. This redness distinguishes it from clostridial myonecrosis. Anoxic gangrene results from ligation or failure to repair a damaged major extremity artery. It is often differentiated from clostridial myonecrosis by the history and absence of toxemia and other evidence of infection.

Although animal experimental data exist showing that penicillin alone will prevent gas gangrene, there are no data from humans to confirm this. Early adequate surgical debridement of war wounds remains the primary means of preventing gas gangrene, its threat to life, and the mutilating effects of the management required when it becomes established.

Preoperative antibiotic therapy consists of penicillin G, three million units IV followed by a total of 10-24 million units over the 24-hour preoperative period. Appropriate volume restoration measures should also be used. Antibiotic and fluid therapy should not significantly delay surgical intervention. In vitro studies have shown that both clindamycin and metronidazole, utilized as single agent therapy, are equally effective if penicillin cannot be used.

Ample exposure of the wound is necessary and rapid removal of the affected tissue is essential. When the infection is confined to a single fascial compartment, surgical excision of the affected muscle or muscle groups may be sufficient. Excision, however, must be as radical as is necessary to remove all discolored muscle and any muscle that does not bleed or contract when it is incised. This may mean removal of an entire muscle from origin to insertion, complete removal of a whole muscle group, or (if the whole limb is involved) amputation of the limb. When infection has extended beyond the practical limits of amputation or disarticulation, the fascial planes and muscle sheaths are incised to relieve tension and promote drainage. If septic shock develops, placement of a Swan-Ganz catheter will permit monitoring of cardiac function and the patient's intravascular volume status. Postoperatively, intravenous fluids should be infused to maintain an adequate hourly urine output between 30-50 cc. Intravenous penicillin is also administered in the postoperative phase.

In World War I, 5% of wounded patients developed gas gangrene with a fatality rate of 28%. In World War II, 0.7% developed gas gangrene with a 31% fatality rate. In Korea, 0.08% developed gas gangrene with no mortality recorded. Its incidence in Vietnam was even lower. This may be attributed to prompt adequate debridement and vascular repairs, attention to casts, and good surgical technique rather than lack of organisms.

STREPTOCOCCAL MYONECROSIS

Anaerobic streptococci may cause necrosis of tissue in association with gas formation. Streptococcal myonecrosis, originally described in the 1940s, resembles subacute clostridial gas gangrene. After an incubation period of 3-4 days, there is swelling, edema, and a purulent exudation from the wound. The infected muscle initially appears pale and soft but as the infection progresses, it becomes bright red and then finally purple and gangrenous. These signs are followed by pain, which rapidly becomes severe. Gas is present in the infected tissue and the involved muscle becomes gangrenous. The seropurulent discharge has a sour odor. The management of streptococcal myonecrosis includes surgery, combined with the antibiotic regimen outlined for gas gangrene. Surgery consists of relaxing incisions, extending through the deep fascia and into muscle, that will provide adequate drainage and relieve tension. Care must be taken to extend the excision beyond the area of obvious infection into the neighboring or adjacent viable tissue.

TETANUS

Tetanus is a severe infection caused by *Clostridium tetani* and its toxin's effects on the nervous system. It carries a mortality rate of approximately 50%. In an analysis of Vietnam War wound infections, no cases of tetanus were reported. The infection is characterized by local and general convulsive spasms of the voluntary muscles. *Clostridium tetani* is a strict anaerobe which exists in spore form in the soil and in the intestines of animals and man. Local necrosis and ischemia provide the conditions necessary for contaminating spores to evolve into their vegetative form and multiply rapidly at the site of infection. Once the vegetative forms have begun to multiply, large amounts of tetanus toxin are produced.

The incubation period is usually 6-12 days but may vary from 4-21 days or longer. In any event, the incubation period is sufficiently long to prevent the development of tetanus in war wounds if proper prophylaxis is employed within a day or two of injury.

Small, deep puncture wounds that often appear trivial are important sources of this infection and must be considered prone to tetanus. Early clinical manifestations may be of a general nature, such as irritability, insomnia, muscular tremors, local spasm, or rigidity in the muscle near the wound. Trismus is usually the first symptom. Sore throat, painful dysphagia, stiff neck, and difficulty in beginning micturition may be early evidence of muscular irritability. The dental officer may be the first to see the patient if trismus has been mistaken for some oral condition.

Trismus and risus sardonicus resulting from spasm of the masseters and muscles of the face are signs of established tetanus. Arching of the spine (opisthotonos) and respiratory difficulty from laryngeal and intercostal muscle spasm may also be present. The contractions are aggravated by additional spasms whenever any sensory excitation occurs. Usually reflex spasms are brought on by external stimuli, such as moving the patient or striking the bed, but later they occur spontaneously at regular and increasingly frequent intervals until the height of disease is reached. Spasms often begin with a sudden jerk. Every muscle in the body is thrown into intense tonic contraction; the jaws are tightly clenched, the head is retracted, the back is arched, the chest and abdomen are fixed, and the limbs are usually extended. A severe spasm may result in respiratory arrest. Spasms may last a few seconds or several minutes. When spasms occur frequently, they lead to rapid exhaustion and sometimes to death from asphyxiation. Without spasms, mortality is low. Few patients with severe spasms survive.

Cephalic tetanus is a form of tetanus in which irritation or paralysis of cranial nerves appears early and dominates the picture. The facial nerve is affected most often. Ophthalmoplegia from involvement of the ocular nerves may develop. Trismus and dysphagia may also follow wounds of the head and face, and the symptoms often appear first on the injured side.

Severe tetanus is often fatal, but those who recover do so completely without sequelae. The patient who has survived tetanus is not immune and, unless immunized, is susceptible to a second attack. Recurrent tetanus in the same patient has been reported. Apparently a sublethal amount of tetanus toxin is not sufficient to provide an adequate antigenic stimulus for production of active immunity.

The diagnosis of tetanus is a clinical one, with bacteriological confirmation sometimes possible. The morphologic appearance of the organism in stained smears (the so-called tennis racket terminal spore in Gram-positive bacillus) usually is not sufficient to differentiate *Clostridium tetani* from other anaerobes with terminal spores. The disease proceeds with fever, sweating, and oliguria while the mind remains clear. Death usually occurs as a result of respiratory arrest during painful generalized convulsions. Toxemia, pneumonia secondary to aspiration, hyperpyrexia, and cardiac failure are other causes of death.

SURGICAL THERAPY

The surgical care of wounds should be immediate. The most important features of surgical wound care are thorough cleansing and debridement. Foreign bodies and necrotic tissue can be contaminated massively with *Clostridium tetani* and establish wound conditions promoting growth and exotoxin production. The wounds should be left open until the patient has recovered from the convulsion stage of disease. Antibiotic therapy with penicillin is effective against the vegetative cells of *Clostridium tetani*. Treatment of patients with severe tetanus involves the use of muscle relaxants and sedation, as well as maintenance of fluid and electrolyte balance. Pulmonary toilet is necessary, as is elimination of visceral stimuli such as distention of the urinary bladder and fecal impaction. Careful nursing care is required. Translaryngeal intubation or even tracheostomy may be useful in maintaining a patent airway in patients who undergo frequent episodes of respiratory failure.

TETANUS IMMUNIZATION

In 1984, the Committee on Trauma of the American College of Surgeons published recommendations concerning prophylaxis against tetanus and the management of wounds. Immunization in adults requires at least three injections of toxoid. A routine booster of absorbed toxoid is indicated every 10 years thereafter. Combined tetanus and diphtheria toxoid is recommended for routine or post-wounding boosters.

In individuals not adequately immunized (that is, the patient who has received only one or no prior injections of toxoid or the immunization history is unknown), 0.5 ml absorbed tetanus toxoid should be given for nontetanus-prone wounds. For tetanus-prone wounds, 0.5 ml absorbed toxoid and 250 units or more of human tetanus immune globulin should be given, using different syringes, needles, and sites of injection. Completion of the series of toxoid immunizations should then follow.

When the medical officer has determined that the casualty has been previously fully immunized and the last dose of toxoid was given within 10 years, no booster of toxoid is indicated for nontetanus-prone wounds. For tetanus-prone wounds and if more than five years have elapsed since the last dose, 0.5 ml absorbed toxoid should be given. When the patient has had three prior injections of toxoid and received the last dose more than 10 years previously, 0.5 ml absorbed toxoid for both tetanus-prone and non-tetanus-prone wounds should be given.

Passive immunization with tetanus immune globulin must be considered individually for each patient. Characteristics of the wound, the conditions under which it was incurred, its treatment, and the patient's age should all be considered. Immunization with human immune globulin is not indicated if the patient has ever received two or more injections of toxoid and the wound is less than 24 hours old. An injection of human immune globulin is indicated if the wound is felt to be a tetanus-prone wound more than 24 hours old and only two prior toxoid injections have been administered. An injection of human immune globulin is also indicated for patients with tetanus-prone wounds who have not received any prior toxoid injections or only one prior injection.

ABDOMINAL WOUNDS

Sepsis is the most common cause of death in patients who sustain penetrating abdominal trauma and survive initial surgical therapy. Prophylactic antibiotic therapy for such patients should be directed toward pathogens encountered in the lower gastrointestinal tract and should be administered perioperatively for 24 hours. A generally accepted regimen of combination antibiotic therapy consists of an agent effective against the anaerobes (clindamycin or metronidazole) and an aminoglycoside (gentamicin) effective against Gram-negative rods. Recent studies of antibiotic therapy following penetrating abdominal trauma suggest, however, that single agent therapy with cefoxitin is equally effective. Given the lack of nephrotoxicity with cefoxitin and considering that the battlefield casualty likely exhibits some degree of dehydration, this regimen represents an attractive alternative. A review of wounded patients in the Vietnam War revealed that abdominal wounds were the wounds that most frequently became infected (6.89%) following initial treatment). Penetrating abdominal wounds accounted for 24% of all wound infections but only 13% of all wounds.

MANAGEMENT OF SEPTIC SHOCK

Shock due to uncontrolled infection in a surgical patient requires prompt identification and treatment of the septic process. Control of infection by surgical debridement or drainage and the use of specific antibiotics represents definitive therapy. An attempt to identify the primary site of infection should be made upon diagnosis of this condition. If the source of infection is amenable to surgical control, this should be carried out expeditiously as soon as the patient's condition is sufficiently stable. Broad spectrum antibiotic therapy is initiated and based upon likely infectious organisms. A typical treatment regimen consists of triple antibiotics, such as ampicillin, gentamicin, and clindamycin. Repletion of the intravascular volume with a physiologic crystalloid solution is generally recommended. Some authors advocate infusion of colloid-containing fluid to replace intravascular volume deficits. Since an increase in pulmonary capillary permeability accompanies septic shock, attempts to replete volume with colloid-containing fluid in this condition may result in a detrimental increase in extravascular pulmonary water.

Fluid therapy is best managed with the use of Swan-Ganz catheter monitoring of pulmonary artery wedge pressures and cardiac output. Insertion of a Foley catheter for measurement of the hourly urine output is also necessary. Many patients with sepsis and shock will develop pulmonary insufficiency necessitating endotracheal intubation and assisted ventilation. Inadequate tissue oxygenation is a consistent factor in shock, and therefore efforts to maintain a normal oxygen hemoglobin dissociation curve should be undertaken. Alkalosis, decreased pCO_2, decreased hemoglobin concentration, decreased 2, 3-diphosphoglycerate, and the presence of carboxyhemoglobin are all factors which increase the affinity of the hemoglobin molecule for oxygen and thereby inhibit delivery of oxygen to tissue.

Vasoconstrictive drugs are seldom used to raise blood pressure as they have a deleterious effect upon tissue blood flow. Agents such as epinephrine and norepinephrine support the circulation by a combination of a beta 1 adrenergic cardiac effect and alpha 1 adrenergic peripheral vasoconstrictive effect. The usual dose of epinephrine is 0.5 mg IV. Norepinephrine is usually administered in the form of a continuous intravenous infusion of D5W containing 8 mg per liter at a rate of 2-3 cc per minute or higher if needed to achieve the desired hemodynamic effect. These agents are used only when volume-restorative measures have failed to provide adequate blood pressure to perfuse vital organs. When volume-restorative measures are ineffective, low dose dopamine infusion may be helpful in maintaining renal perfusion, but only as an adjunct to fluid infusion. Dopamine is thought to dilate renal and splanchnic vasculature by its action on the dopaminergic receptors. The usual intravenous "renal" dose of dopamine is 3-5 $\mu g/kg/min$ given as D5W containing 200 mg/250 ml. This dosage can be increased for beta 1 adrenergic cardiac stimulation, and when given in doses greater than 10 $\mu g/kg/min$, commonly causes alpha stimulation and vasoconstriction that provide additional hemodynamic support in a deteriorating patient.

TABLE 7.—*Choice, Mode of Action, Spectrum, and Dosage of Antibiotic Agents*

Agent	Mode of Action	Antibacterial Spectrum of Clinical Importance	Dosage
Penicillin G	Bactericidal; interferes with bacterial cell wall synthesis	Streptococci, Pneumococci Clostridia, Neisseriae, Corynebacteria, Pasteurella multocida, Actinomyces, Treponema, Listeria	30 mil units IV/day every 2-4 hours
Ampicillin	Bactericidal; same as above	Hemophilus influenzae, Proteus mirabilis, Salmonallae, Shigellae and some E. coli. Gram-positive organisms as with Penicillin G	8 gm IV/day every 6 hours
Gentamicin	Bacteriostatic; inhibition of bacterial protein synthesis	Klebsiella sp., Aerobacter sp., Pseudomonas aeruginosa, Serratia, indole positive Proteus sp, some Methicillin-resistant Staphylococci	5 mg/kg/day every 8-12 hours
Metronidazole	Bacteriocidal	Gram-negative anaerobes especially Bacteriodes fragilis. Also effective against several protozoa.	2 gm IV/day every 4 hours
Cefoxitin (2nd generation cephalosporin)	Cell wall systhesis inhibitors; stable to staphylococcal beta lactamases	Sames as above plus Bacteroides fragilis; not active against Enterobacter spp.	12 gm IV/day every 6 hours
Clindamycin	Bacteriostatic; inhibits protein synthesis	Gram-positive and Gram-negative anaerobes, Gram-positive aerobic cocci, Streptococcus faecalis, Clostridia	1200-2700 mg IV/day every 6-8 hours

PART III

General Considerations of
Wound Management

CHAPTER XII

Sorting of Casualties

GENERAL CONSIDERATIONS

Sorting, or triage, implies the evaluation and classification of casualties for purposes of treatment and evacuation. It is based on the principle of accomplishing the greatest good for the greatest number of wounded and injured men in the special circumstances of warfare at a particular time. The decisions which must be made concern the need for resuscitation, the need for emergency surgery, and the futility of surgery when the intrinsic lethality of certain wounds is clearly overwhelming. Sorting also involves the establishment of priorities for treatment and evacuation.

Military medical activities differ from those in the civil sector in that they must adapt to the special circumstances of a tactical combat situation. Combat hospitals must be not only mobile but also capable of receiving and treating large numbers of casualties that arrive simultaneously, the so-called mass casualty situation. The facility should be designed and staffed with these contingencies in mind. The medical officers, nurses, and support personnel must be well trained in the medical tactics necessary to cope with the ever-present possibility of receiving an overwhelming number of casualties presenting within a short period of time. During such situations, conventional standards of medical care cannot be delivered to all casualties. Some of the very seriously wounded will not receive the same degree of care they would have received had they presented as a single admission. Others may receive no immediate care except to insure that they are made as comfortable as possible under the circumstances.

In all mass casualty situations, there are logical categories into which all casualties can be classified. Some will have sustained critical injuries, but will have a high potential for survival with prompt treatment. These should have a high priority for treatment, while others, with mortal wounds, are not salvageable no matter what degree of medical care resources are expended upon them. Certain others do not require immediate lifesaving procedures and will tolerate reasonable delays while the more critical are being cared for. The group with minor injuries will survive with directed self care or no care at all.

TRIAGE

In order to cope effectively and efficiently with large numbers of battle casualties that present almost simultaneously, the principles of triage, or the sorting and assignment of treatment priorities to various categories of wounded, must be understood, universally accepted, and routinely practiced throughout all echelons of collection, evacuation, and definitive treatment. This practice enables us to effectively provide the greatest amount of care to the largest number of soldiers, which in turn will salvage the greatest number of lives and limbs. The ultimate goal of combat medicine is the return of the greatest possible number of soldiers to combat and the preservation of life and limb in those who cannot be returned.

The casualty with multiple life-threatening wounds and a poor prognosis, who requires many surgeons and the expenditure of hours of operating room resources, may divert care from those with less serious, but more rapidly treatable, injuries and a better prospect for recovery. Not uncommonly, the most gravely injured are the first to be evacuated from the collection points. They will also be the first to arrive at the definitive care facility. The receiving surgeon (triage officer) must guard against overcommitting his resources to those first arrivals prior to establishing a perspective of the total number and types of casualties still to be received.

It is easier to assign priorities of care to individual casualties if the medical officer has a feel for the usual anatomical distribution of war wounds. Survivors present with a reasonably consistent pattern of wound distribution. Fortunately, the largest proportion of injuries affect less critical areas, such as the upper and lower extremities.

TABLE 8.—*Anatomical distribution of battle wounds*
Percent

Location	WWII	RVN
Multiple	11%	20%
Head/Neck/Face	12	14
Chest	8	7
Abdomen	4	5
Upper Extremities	26	18
Lower Extremities	39	36
	100%	100%

One can predict from the Table 8 that the majority of wounded is not likely to require urgent resuscitation or immediate surgical intervention. At the other extreme are those with maxillofacial or head wounds with airway destruction, those with wounds of the chest (ventilation compromise and hemorrhage), and those with abdominal wounds (uncontrollable hemorrhage), all of which require much more urgent intervention. Sometimes the time lag between wounding and hospital presentation is of such duration that those who temporarily survived the initial impact of their injury are no longer salvageable, further narrowing the group which requires urgent attention upon arrival. With experience, the forward surgeon comes to recognize this recurring pattern and the relatively consistent distribution of wound types and locations in groups of battle casualties. A small number of casualties will require urgent resuscitation and prompt operative intervention, whereas the majority of the wounded will tolerate varying degrees of delay prior to operation. Application of the following criteria makes the receipt, triage, and treatment of large numbers of simultaneously arriving casualties more manageable, while at the same time minimizing the confusion and calamity that otherwise could prevail. Again, it should be emphasized that every effort should be made to insure that the existing resources are expended upon the maximum number of salvageable soldiers. Simple lifesaving procedures which can be rapidly performed should be given the highest priority. Life takes precedence over limb, and functional repair over cosmetic concern.

PRIORITIES OF TREATMENT

Sorting is the process of prioritization or rank ordering wounded individuals on the basis of their individual needs for surgical intervention. The likely outcome of the individual casualty must be factored into the decision process prior to the commitment of limited medical resources. Casualties are generally sorted into five categories or priorities, These priority groupings are discussed in decreasing order of surgical urgency.

URGENT. This group requires urgent intervention if death is to be prevented. This category includes those with asphyxia, respiratory obstruction from mechanical causes, sucking chest wounds, tension pneumothorax, maxillofacial wounds with asphyxia or where asphyxia is likely to develop, exsanguinating internal hemorrhage unresponsive to vigorous volume replacement, most cardiac injuries, and CNS wounds with deteriorating neurological status.

Therapeutic interventions range from tracheal intubation, placement of chest tubes, and rapid volume replacement to urgent laparotomy, thoracotomy, or craniotomy. Shock caused by major internal hemorrhage will, in these circumstances, require urgent operative intervention to control exsanguinating hemorrhage.

If the initial resuscitative interventions are successful and some degree of stability is achieved, the urgent casualty may occasionally revert to a lower priority. The hopelessly wounded and those with many life-threatening wounds, who require extraordinary efforts should not be included in this category.

IMMEDIATE. Casualties in this category present with severe, life-threatening wounds that require procedures of moderately short duration. Casualties within this group have a high likelihood of survival. They tend to remain temporarily stable while undergoing replacement therapy and methodical evaluation. The key word is temporarily. Examples of the immediate category are: unstable chest and abdominal wounds, inaccessible vascular wounds with limb ischemia, incomplete amputations, open fractures of long bones, white phosphorous burns, and second- or third-degree burns of 15-40% or more of the total body surface.

DELAYED. Casualties in the delayed category can tolerate delay prior to operative intervention without unduly compromising the likelihood of a successful outcome. When medical resources are overwhelmed, individuals in this category are held until the urgent and immediate cases are cared for. Examples include stable abdominal wounds with probable visceral injury, but without significant hemorrhage. These cases may go unoperated for eight or ten hours, after which there is a direct relationship between the time lapse and the advent of complications. Other examples include soft tissue wounds requiring debridement, maxillofacial wounds without airway compromise, vascular injuries with adequate collateral circulation, genitourinary tract disruption, fractures requiring operative manipulation, debridement and external fixation, and most eye and CNS injuries.

MINIMAL OR AMBULATORY. This category is comprised of casualties with wounds that are so superficial that they require no more than cleansing, minimal debridement under local anesthesia, tetanus toxoid, and first-aid-type dressings. They must be rapidly directed away from the triage area to uncongested areas where first aid and non-specialty medical personnel are available. Examples include burns of less than 15% total body surface area, with the exception of those involving the face, hands, or genitalia. Other examples include upper extremity fractures, sprains, abrasions, early phases of symptomatic but unquantified radiation exposure, suspicion of blast injury (perforated tympanic membranes), and behavioral disorders or other obvious psychiatric disturbances.

EXPECTANT. Casualties in the expectant category have wounds that are so extensive that even if they were the sole casualty and had the benefit of optimal medical resource application, their survival still would be very unlikely. During a mass casualty situation, this sort of casualty would require an unjustifiable expenditure of limited resources, resources that are more wisely applied to several other more salvageable individuals. To categorize a soldier to this category requires a resolve that comes only with prior experience in futile surgery that ties up operating rooms and personnel while other more salvageable casualties wait, deteriorate, or even die. The expectant casualties should be separated from the view of other casualties; however, they should not be abandoned. Above all, one attempts to make them comfortable by whatever means necessary and provides attendance by a minimal but competent staff. Examples: unresponsive patients with penetrating head wounds, high spinal cord injuries, mutilating explosive wounds involving multiple anatomical sites and organs, second- and third-degree burns in excess of 60% total body surface area, convulsions and vomiting within twenty-four hours of radiation exposure, profound shock with multiple injuries, and agonal respiration.

Exposure to radiation or biologic, and chemical agents when presenting in conjunction with conventional injuries will alter the above categorization. The degree to which such agents compound the prognosis is somewhat variable and difficult to specifically apply to a mass casualty situation. A safe practice is to classify the exposed casualty at the lowest priority in his category. It has been stated that those in the immediate category with radiation exposure estimated to be 400 rads be moved to the delayed group, and those with greater than 400 rads be placed in the expectant category. Those with convulsions or vomiting in the first 24-hours are not likely to survive even in the absence of other injuries. Mass casualty situations are highly probable when troops have been exposed to radiation or chemical or biological agents. There must be areas set aside within the hospital to safely isolate these types of patients, and special procedures must be established to safeguard the attending medical personnel.

PAST EXPERIENCE

In World War II, the lines of combat were relatively discrete and fixed, allowing the echelons of medical support to be structured and upgraded in a logical manner. The most seriously wounded casualty received care as close to the front as possible; those less seriously wounded and more transportable were moved to the more fixed installations in the rear. Battalion aid stations were generally situated about 500 yards behind the front. Triage was performed here and medical evacuation for further rearward evacuation was located here. The main thrust was to render the casualty transportable after all vital systems were evaluated. Airways were cleared, adequate ventilation assured, and accessible hemorrhages controlled. Dressings and splints were applied as necessary, fluid replacement initiated, and pain medication administered. Those with the most critical injuries were considered the first priority and were evacuated about one mile to the collecting station, where further lifesaving treatment was administered. Further to the rear (five-miles) at the division clearing station, casualties were once again triaged, and those with the highest priority injuries (urgent and immediate) were taken to the adjacent field hospital for immediate surgery. The remainder, who could better tolerate delay and further transport, continued on to general or evacuation hospitalization deeper within the rear area. The bulk of the extensive lifesaving procedures was provided at the forward hospital, where the wounded were operated upon, held until stable, and then transferred to the rear echelon hospitals.

By contrast, the Vietnam conflict consisted of sporadic small unit engagements which were widely dispersed geographically and seldom lasted more than six hours. Major battles, such as those fought at Hue and in the A Shau Valley, were measured in days, fought with mobile units, and accounted for the greatest number of mass casualty situations. Major medical support was not mobile and remained fixed within relatively secure centrally-located military compounds. Although labeled as semimobile, hospitals were generally Quonset-type structures, bolted to concrete slabs and provided with permanent electrical and plumbing connections. The inflatable "MUST" hospitals, while capable of mobility, required unacceptable levels of fuel for power generation and also became relatively fixed. Since the forward hospitals could not go forward to the casualty in those campaigns, the air ambulances went forward and brought the casualties to the hospitals. Fortunately, air superiority was never in doubt.

FACILITY DESIGN

To facilitate efficiency and optimize triage, evaluation, and definitive care under mass casualty conditions, certain features should be incorporated into the combat hospital's physical plant. The design should promote smooth casualty flow through all areas of the facility. At no time should the normal progression of care or casualty flow be allowed to have a reverse direction. A casualty should not be carried off to X-ray and then returned from whence he came. Traffic should not enter and exit through the same portal. Flow against the grain must be held to an absolute minimum.

These principles should apply regardless of the nature of the construction whether it be Quonset, tentage, or modification of already existing permanent structures. Figure 21 illustrates this concept.

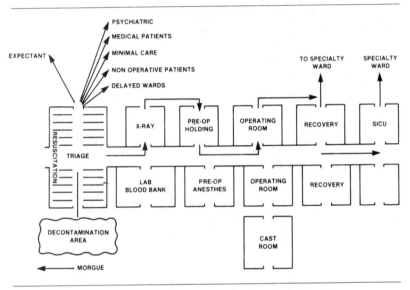

FIGURE 21 — Proposed Scheme for Mass Casualty Flow

HELIPORT. Ideally, the helipad should be close enough to the hospital's receiving area to preclude the need for intermediate motorized surface transport.

DECONTAMINATION AREAS. A decontamination area should be set up under shelter, and provided with temperature-controllable water and drainage away from the hospital. If prevailing winds exists, this area should be downwind from the hospital. A separate area nearby is required for the collection and disposal of contaminated uniforms, equipment, weapons, and personal items.

TRIAGE AREA. Adequate space in this area is of the utmost importance. Overcrowding contributes to confusion and unacceptable noise levels, and detracts from careful casualty evaluation. Each patient station must be accessible from all sides. Multiple stations consisting of litters placed on sawhorse frames should be in place and ready. Shelving or cabinets should be installed along the walls to supply the required consumable supplies: IV fluids, administration sets, venipuncture sets, tetanus toxoid, antibiotics, dressings, evaluation forms, identification tags, etc. There should be an ample supply of IV poles or an overhead cable or rail from which to suspend IV solutions and blood.

Each casualty should pass into the decontamination and triage areas one at a time. It is a mistake to have two or more helicopters discharging casualties simultaneously, although this is sometimes unavoidable when tactical aircraft assist in the evacuation. This leads to confusion and competition among litter bearers for doorways and stations, and a critical casualty may pass by the triage officer unnoticed.

Those deemed urgent and requiring resuscitation should be taken to that specific area equipped for their evaluation and management. Type O-negative or O-positive low-titer blood should be available, as well as airway management equipment, suction, and closed thoracotomy setups.

Each litter station is attended by one medical officer, usually a surgeon, and one nurse. Here the casualty undergoes evaluation, fluid administration, tetanus toxoid injection, and assignment of an appropriate priority of care by the triage officer. When appropriate, the immediates will pass through X-ray and into the preoperative area, where they are further triaged and assigned to operating teams. This cycle is repeated until all casualties have been operated. When the number of patients exceeds the bed space, convalescing patients are triaged for further evacuation to make beds available.

To ease congestion and confusion, ambulatory casualties should be evaluated in a separate area designated for minimal care. If the triage area needs to be cleared for new arrivals, wards should be made available to receive the spillover. The delayed casualties are often held in designated wards until the preoperative area is clear of the more seriously injured. One must remember that triage is a dynamic process. The initially-assigned priority may change as the individual's condition changes or with the receipt of additional casualties.

Above all, the dead must not be introduced into the triage area. Not uncommonly, a casualty will expire enroute, and, not infrequently, a unit commander will demand that his dead be evacuated in air ambulances along with the wounded. In either case, the litter bearers must halt outside and request guidance or pronouncement from the triage or some other medical officer.

OPERATING ROOMS. The surgical suites are most often configured with operating tables in a single large room. The arrangement functions very efficiently, in spite of an increased noise level.

PERSONNEL. After the intial notification of the anticipated large influx of casualties, a timely alert is passed along the chain of responsibility, and the triage officer insures that all stations and services are prepared. Personnel should be well drilled in their responsibilities and remain at their stations unless otherwise directed.

The triage area will rapidly develop into the site of greatest activity, usually attended with some degree of initial hyperexcitability and confusion among the staff. Access to this area should be restricted to the assigned medical officers, nurses, corpsmen, litter bearers, and those administrative personnel required to assist with patient identification, custody of personal belongings, and registration. Overcrowding with nonessential personnel is common and can become an impediment to efficient progress. Once the litter bearers discharge their patient, they should revert to the pool for further assignment. The tendency is to stand around in an observer status. All hospital personnel, no matter how well intentioned, should stay clear of the active areas unless their presence is requested.

TRIAGE OFFICER: The triage officer, usually the Chief of Surgery, must be the most experienced of the surgeons, and must exercise absolute authority in all decisions involving the sorting and assignment of casualty priorities. He must continually monitor each patient's status while simultaneously managing and committing his resources. He will direct the activities of the evaluating teams in the triage room and the preoperative holding area, and the eventual movement and priority of patients proceeding into the operating room. He will designate the number of operating teams necessary and will mobilize pools of medical officers and other personnel as necessary to assist in the total effort. He must continually reassess the hospital's ability to sustain momentum while simultaneously providing routine care to

patients already hospitalized. When his resources are all committed, he must request the diversion of additional workload to some
other medical treatment facility.

As the exercise proceeds, the triage officer must continually
evaluate and reevaluate the status of his resources, fatigue level of
his personnel, bed availability, and the surgical backlog. Not infrequently, a patient in the delayed category will deteriorate and
require more immediate attention. Once those in the initial immediate category have been operated and stabilized, others from
the delayed category are funneled into the surgical treatment
channels on a prioritized basis.

THE FINAL PHASE. As the casualties finally clear the
operating room suites, the pace will slow for the surgeons. The
recovery room and intensive care units will become crowded, nursing shifts will have to be extended, and fatigue will rapidly
become a hospital-wide factor. Numerous authors state that after
the first 24 hours of a mass casualty ordeal, the activities of the
personnel must be decreased by one half to allow for rest for the
participants, and a new rotation must be established to sustain a
modified but continuous effort.

Once the press is over, personnel must be encouraged to rest
rather than to socialize. Rest must be enforced since the entire
scenario may recur at any time.

COMMANDING OFFICER'S RESPONSIBILITY. The
medical facility commanding officer must be kept informed of
the tactical situation, the likelihood of extended combat in his
area, the security of his hospital, and the possible need to divert
patients to other medical facilities. He must know the status of his
resources and must support or modify the activities of the triage
process depending on the reserves within his hospital, the threat
from without, and the capacity of his personnel. He must have
knowledge and control of all the support activities involved in the
effort, including such services as feeding those unable to adhere
to the standard schedule; resupply of urgently needed items, such
as blood, plaster, or medications; and the status of his staff. His
wisdom may be required when wounded prisoners are introduced
into the triage situation, not an uncommon situation in Vietnam.
During such episodes when his unit is under maximal stress, his
role should be one of total involvement and his primary concern

should be to provide an environment in which his surgeons, nurses, and support personnel can function at the maximal level of productivity.

CHAPTER XIII

Aeromedical Evacuation

INTRODUCTION

As the intensity of combat operations varies, so varies the flow of wounded and the strain placed upon all echelons of medical care. At the same time, the ever-present requirement of maintaining available bedspace for additional incoming casualties creates the constant requirement for evacuation of those occupying the system's forward beds. The provision of optimal, individualized surgical care, in concert with the efficient utilization of resources, necessitates close coordination between the direct care providers at all levels and those responsible for the administration and operation of the full spectrum of medical evacuation.

Aeromedical evacuation is a modern, complex transportation system designed to move casualties rapidly. Appropriate utilization of this system markedly reduces the time lapse from initial wounding to definitive care. That such rapid movement of patients results in overall decreases in morbidity and mortality has been demonstrated repeatedly in recent conflicts. This holds true regardless of the category of patients considered.

At the point of initial wounding, where medical capability is limited to first-aid measures, dedicated rotary-wing air ambulances are utilized to provide rapid transfer of the casualty to an area providing first-line resuscitation capability. Triage is accomplished at each echelon of medical care. Patients are evaluated at aeromedical evacuation battlefield collecting points and categorized as to their relative needs and general stability. From these collection points, and with an awareness of each casualty's individual clinical needs and personal stability, further retrograde movements are programmed. Patients may be removed from the evacuation chain at any medical facility along the evacuation route when it is the professional opinion of the evaluating surgeon that patient safety will be compromised by continued transfer.

AIRCRAFT

Helicopters are versatile, maneuverable aircraft normally utilized to evacuate injured patients short distances rapidly. The flying time of currently deployed helicopter ambulances is about three hours with a range of 250–300 miles. Utilization of these aircraft results in the casualty reaching well-equipped medical facilities in a matter of minutes. Casualties with grave injuries that would have been fatal without the utilization of rapid air transportation reach operating rooms. The foregoing was repetitively demonstrated in Vietnam where, due to the relatively short distances involved, the battalion aid station was for the most part overflown, with direct evacuation from the battlefield to definitive care facilities having surgical capabilities.

The effects of this rapid field aeromedical evacuation system were twofold. On the one hand, many casualties, who in previous conflicts would have died of their wounds while awaiting or undergoing surface medical evacuation, reached definitive care facilities and were salvaged. Without taking anything away from the superb performance of corpsmen, nurses, and surgeons, this very substantial salvage of human life was in large measure directly attributable to the gallant, selfless professionalism of the "can do" air ambulance flight crews.

On the other hand, rapid field aeromedical evacuation of fresh battle casualties attributed at least in part to the slightly increased hospital mortality experience in Vietnam. For example, in World War II, with no field aeromedical capability, 4.5% of those wounded in action (WIA) and subsequently hospitalized died of their wounds. In the Korean conflict, with its limited utilization of field aeromedical evacuation but better medical-technical capabilities, the hospital mortality of this same group of casualties declined to 2.5%. However, in Vietnam, with its even further advanced medical-technical capabilities but almost universal application of rapid field aeromedical evacuation, hospital mortality of WIAs increased to 3.5%. This increased WIA hospital mortality rate is thought to be due, at least in part, to early hospital presentation of a small but significant number of casualties with mortal wounds. These represent casualties that would never have arrived alive at medical treatment facilities in previous conflicts.

With the availability of helicopter evacuation from the battlefield, the decision to fly casualties directly to hospitals depends on five variables: the clinical status of the casualty, the flying time, the weather conditions, the casualty generation rate or load, and the tactical situation. Where casualty generation is heavy and helicopter resources are limited, casualties can be transported by air or by land from the battlefield to nearby clearing stations. After triage and initial resuscitation, they will be moved to more definitive facilities in order of their clinical priority. Even when the hospital is relatively close to the battlefield, the division clearing station can serve as a buffer when casualty loads temporarily overwhelm a hospital's capability. It must be constantly borne in mind that the availability of rapid transportation by air does not alter, in any way, the necessity for correct application of surgical principles. Experience has shown that field aeromedical evacuation functions most efficiently and reliably when these assets are dedicated to their medical mission and are under direct medical command and control.

INTRA- AND INTERTHEATER MEDICAL EVACUATION

Intratheater medical evacuation moves patients from one hospital to another within the theater of operations. This includes evacuation between combat zone hospitals, between communication zone (COMMZ) hospitals, or from combat zone hospitals to COMMZ hospitals. Out-country, or intertheater medical evacuation moves patients from hospitals located within the theater of operations to designated casualty-receiving Medical Treatment Facilities (MTFS) located in the Continental United States (CONUS) or in host nations outside the theater. This complex evacuation system consists of two interrelated processes: patient regulation and patient movement. Whereas the medical officer is always responsible for any decision that impacts on the clinical welfare and stability of his patient, the patient administrator and the medical regulating officer (MRO) provide invaluable assistance by communicating up and down the echelons of the combat health care delivery system to facilitate the provision of safe, timely, and efficient movement of casualties. MROs at each echelon function as the gatekeepers and facilitators who achieve an even distribution of cases, assist in minimizing surgical backlogs, maintain an adequate number of available beds for current and anticipated needs, route patients requiring specialized treatment to the proper facilities, and coordinate the smooth, safe

retrograde movement of casualties. This system is designed to ensure both the efficient and safe transfer of patients, often over
great distances, in such manner that the welfare of the patient is
second only to the success of the tactical mission. To achieve these
objectives, MROs must maintain current information on the tactical situation, the availability of all types of transportation, the
location and capacity of facilities with special capabilities, the current bed status of treatment facilities, surgical backlogs, the
number and location of patients by diagnostic category, the location of airfields and seaports, and, most important of all, the individual patient's suitability to withstand evacuation.

Fixed-wing aircraft of the nonmedical variety are utilized to
transport personnel and supplies into the theater of operations.
After off loading, these same aircraft can be quickly converted and
internally reconfigured to accommodate both litter and ambulatory patients. With the exception of aircraft specifically
designed to transport patients, most aeromedical evacuation is
performed in reconfigured standard military transport aircraft.
These aircraft and their medical teams are selected carefully in
consideration of the patient's needs. Jet-powered aircraft are
capable of rapid patient movement in smooth air at high altitude
in pressurized comfort. These movements can be accomplished
for short or long distances as required. Overnight rest stops can
be provided along the way, depending upon the patient's clinical
status and the distances involved.

SPECIAL CONSIDERATIONS

Individual patients, each with his own peculiar problems, will
require special considerations. Scheduling the evacuation, managing the patient in transit, arranging special attendants and equipment, programing rest stops, and determining appropriate
destination hospitals are all vital considerations in the safe, rapid
movement of the battle casualties.

Although the exigency of a given situation may require a patient
to be evacuated earlier and for longer distances than ordinarily
would be deemed advisable, the rule should be to await adequate
clinical stability prior to subjecting the patient to what could turn
out to be an arduous, clinically risky, prolonged trip.

1. Tracheostomy care: Tubes should be of proper size. When
mechanical respirators are to be used, cuffed tracheostomy tubes

are usually required. Because of the low humidity of the aircraft cabin atmosphere, the use of a humidification device is recommended to avoid the production of dry mucous plugs and to assure proper tracheal care during flight. Humidity levels in the pressurized cabin are around 5–20%. At these levels, insensible losses and drying of the tracheobronchial tree, especially in those with tracheostomy, are considerably increased. The ultrasonic nebulizer is the most efficient apparatus at this time. A heat aerosol nebulizer is probably the second-best apparatus.

Mucous plugs and encrustations must be removed promptly to avoid respiratory distress and obstruction. The use of tracheostomy tubes that do not have cleaning cannulae should be avoided. Rubber and plastic tracheostomy tubes normally do not have cleaning inner tubes or cannulae. The periodic instillation of 2 ml. of sterile isotonic saline solution into the tracheostomy with prompt aspiration enhances the cleansing of the airway.

In emergency situations during transit, endotracheal intubation is usually safer and quicker than tracheostomy and is well tolerated by the patient. Prompt use of such tubes usually eliminates the need for tracheostomy. A T-tube, if available, should be attached to the endotracheal tube or tracheostomy tube during evacuation to provide humidity and reduce the likelihood of mucous plugging and encrustation. The balloon of a cuffed tube should be inflated with air, not water.

2. Cranial tongs: Special attention should be paid to the proper seating of the tongs. Traction must be maintained by a closed system, preferably with a spring device such as the Collins' spring. In the absence of a spring device, traction may be maintained by heavy rubber tubing tied to the litter frame. To prevent sudden jerking of the tongs, free hanging weights must not be left attached during flight.

3. Skin traction: Stockinette glued to the skin can be utilized to maintain traction during evacuation. Traction is maintained by rubber tubing interposed between the stockinette and a plaster-incorporated wire loop. The surgeon who orders the evacuation of the patient is responsible for removing weights and substituting a self-contained traction device before aeromedical transfer.

4. Chest tubes: Ideally, patients should not be evacuated by air with chest tubes in place, nor should they be evacuated within 72 hours after removal of the tube. Absence of pneumothorax must be demonstrated by a chest roentgenogram just before movement.

On the other hand, when necessary, chest tubes may be left in position during evacuation but should be equipped with functioning valves, such as the Heimlich valve. Pressurization of the aircraft to ground level is desirable if such patients must be moved. Thoracic patients that require assisted ventilation should not be placed in air evacuation channels.

5. Nasogastric tubes: All patients requiring nasogastric suction at ground level should have similar protection during flight. The combination of one's basic medical problems coupled with air swallowing due to anxiety or pain, and the reduced barometric pressure at high altitudes results in hollow viscera gas expansion that can cause complications. Failure to decompress the stomach can result in pain from distention of hollow viscera, dehiscence, and, most significantly, vomiting and aspiration with serious pulmonary complications. Increased abdominal pressure under a restricting body cast can also result in vomiting and aspiration.

6. Plaster casts: When evacuating patients with circular plaster casts, all such casts should be appropriately bivalved before movement. This allows for swelling of soft tissue, permits rapid emergency access to secondary hemorrhage, and may facilitate escape through emergency hatches in the event of an emergency. It is helpful to evacuation chain personnel when casts are labeled. Such inscriptions should include the date and type of injury, the date of surgery and cast application, and a simple sketch of the bone injury.

7. Stryker frame: Such frames may be used for transfers by air. Patients should be turned during travel as ordered by the referring surgeon.

8. Catheter care: Indwelling catheters in use before transfer should be left in place during transfer. Instructions for specific care enroute both at the staging area and aloft should be provided to the medical evacuation teams. Every attempt should be made to maintain urinary output above 1,500 ml per day.

9. Hypothermia blankets: Patients requiring hypothermia blankets before evacuation should have this therapy continue enroute. Equipment is normally available aboard the aircraft to continue such treatment. Convulsions, high fever, and respiratory distress can be expected to develop if this principle is not followed.

10. Circulating blood volume and oxygenation: The hematocrit is not a reliable indicator of the adequacy of circulating blood volume. The casualty is most likely to be hypovolemic or hyper-

volemic during the first 3–4 days post injury. Homeostatic mechanisms have usually restored the circulating volume to normal after this period. Oxygenation problems at ground level will be increased at higher altitudes. Patients having hematocrits of 30% or below should not be transferred under any but the most urgent situation. If transfer must be accomplished, proper supplies for transfusions should accompany the patient with orders for the use of blood enroute. Measurement of pO_2 should be used as a criterion of air evacuability in the seriously ill patient. Levels below 60 mm Hg are considered a contraindication to movement. It has been demonstrated that wounded patients can have dangerously low arterial pO_2 at sea level without any clinical indication of hypoxia. One U.S. Air Force casualty study revealed that none of the casualties with an arterial pO_2 of 35–40 mm Hg and normal pH was cyanotic, although some were mildly tachyneic. At this level of pO_2, arterial saturation was approximately 70%; however, many of these patients did not have enough reduced hemoglobin (5 gm/100 ml) to become cyanotic. This sort of situation at sea level is particularly dangerous in flight. At altitudes of 35,000 feet, the cabin is pressurized down to about 8,000 feet equivalent, or 564 mm Hg. At this pressure, alveolar air pO_2 is about 69 mm Hg, or 33% less than sea level. An arterial pO_2 that was 50 at sea level is dangerously low at 8,000 feet.

11. Cerebrospinal leak: A wound draining cerebrospinal fluid at ground level will drain slightly faster at higher altitudes. These wounds are not a contraindication for transfer.

12. Abdominal surgery patients: Experience shows that premature evacuation of casualties shortly after abdominal surgery carries a high morbidity. Patients with wounds and injuries of the abdomen are best retained at the facility in which they have undergone their initial surgical care until complications have been controlled, bowel functions have returned, and the wound is healing. These requirements are seldom met in fewer than seven days.

13. Vascular injuries: Patients with vascular injuries require special attention and immobilization. Casts should be bivalved to provide emergency access to the area. When circumstances permit, primary repair or graft cases should not be transferred for 14 or more days after repair, unless the wound has been closed and is healing without evidence of infection. Patients should have the repair date and type of repair inscribed on the cast or dressing.

14. Burns: Burn patients may be transferred at any time during their care; however, as in all severely wounded patients, transfer is unwise until the blood volume has been restored and the patient's condition is stable. The best time for this category of patient to travel is 4–7 days postburn, when diuresis has begun and the complications of fever and infection have not yet presented. Burns greater than 40%, or lesser burns associated with severe injuries, ordinarily should have a surgeon in attendance. Preparation for transfer should include:

a. Airway assurance by whatever means necessary.

b. Functioning intravenous pathway.

c. Adequate urinary output.

d. Fresh burn dressings.

e. Immobilization of associated injuries as indicated.

f. Functioning nasogastric tube if any gastrointestinal dysfunction exists.

g. Complete medical records, particularly accurate fluid balance sheets.

15. Maxillofacial Injuries: During transportation, these patients should be placed in a semiprone position on the litter. If there are upper respiratory difficulties, or if they are likely to develop during transportation, tracheostomy should be performed before evacuation. If tracheostomy or endotracheal intubation is not performed, the patient with a maxillofacial injury must be evacuated with an attendant especially instructed in the possibilities of respiratory obstruction and in techniques for dealing with it.

Patients with major maxillofacial wounds require special preparation before evacuation to the intermediate or reconstructive care facility. If possible, infections should be under control, no significant fever should be present, and the patient's general condition should be sufficiently stable to withstand the evacuation. All packing should be removed before evacuation, or specific instructions should accompany the patient concerning location, number, and types of packs with recommendations for time of removal. If intermaxillary fixation has been utilized, the patient should be retained for several days after surgery, taking a liquid diet, and tolerating fixation well before evacuation. If intermaxillary elastics are utilized, some type of pullout cords are indicated. In an alert patient who has a tracheostomy or absence of several anterior teeth, there is little likelihood of aspiration of emesis; therefore, any type of suitable fixation is acceptable.

16. Dressing changes: A patient who has had a debridement of a combat wound is considered to have a clean wound. The dressings should not be changed without good reason except in an operating room at the time of probable delayed primary closure. Contamination of the open wound may occur when the dressing change is conducted under less-than-optimal conditions. Neither the odor nor the staining of a dressing from blood or serum is an indication for a dressing change. Dressing changes are indicated only for serious complications, such as bleeding, unusually high fever, increasing pain, or swelling. The decision for a dressing change should be made by a physician.

17. Medications: Certain medications, such as antibiotics, narcotics and analgesics, should have a recorded "stop order" to avoid an undesirable extension of this course of therapy. It is essential that the physician ordering evacuation complete the flight tag accurately to assure antibiotic therapy continuation on schedule or discontinuation as required. Some medications are not normally available in standard supply, and when these are to be continued during patient transfer, an adequate supply must accompany the patient.

18. Medical attendants: Medical attendants, assigned to accompany seriously ill patients, should accompany those patients to the destination hospital. The attendant, in addition to providing clinical services enroute, is a vital link in the continuity of care between medical echelons. This is best accomplished by personally interfacing with the receiving medical officers and providing those clinicians with well-documented and complete medical records.

CHAPTER XIV

War Surgery Within the Division

INTRODUCTION

Physicians assigned to the unit and division levels may have the most arduous duties of any medical officer. From a medical treatment standpoint, the environment is relatively austere and the spectrum of responsibility broader. However, medical service at this level can result in great personal and professional satisfaction. Although much emphasis is placed upon the ability of the unit and division level medical officer to perform life-sustaining resuscitation during combat casualty care, the nature of combat wounds is such that the actual potential for such intervention is usually not great. The medical officer at the unit or division level will find that the major contribution to combat casualty care during battle will be to control the flow of casualties by effective triage and preparation of casualties for evacuation.

Triage of casualties at the unit and division levels is designed to recognize three categories of casualties: first, those who need immediate resuscitation and surgical intervention (e.g., shock from internal hemorrhage); second, those who have incapacitating but not immediately life-threatening injuries and are unlikely to return to duty (e.g., fractures); and third, those who can be promptly returned to duty (e.g., minor soft tissue fragment wounds).

About 10% of all wounded can be expected to be in frank shock. Three percent have severe dyspnea arising from thoracic wounds, about 1% have upper airway obstruction resulting from facial or neck wounds, and about 1% require airway management because of severe neurologic trauma. About 15% of all casualties leaving the battlefield require immediate resuscitation or surgery. Perhaps one-half of the remaining casualties will also require evacuation beyond combat zone medical treatment facilities. Assuring the stability and relative comfort of these casualties is an important part of the unit and division medical officer's duty. Casualties who have the potential for return to duty within the specified time constraints of the evacuation policy should be segregated from casualties with more severe wounds. The American experience in Vietnam was that casualties who could return to duty within a few days constituted the largest single fraction of the total combat casualty population. The unit and division level medical officer makes an important contribution to the conservation of our fighting strength by preventing the overevacuation of such casualties.

Certain basic tasks need to be performed on every casualty arriving at the aid station or medical company. First and foremost, a determination needs to be made whether the casualty constitutes a threat to the medical troops or other casualties. This is true not only when chemical or biological agents have been employed, but also in conventional warfare in which there is a need to be certain that the casualty is not carrying explosive ordnance. Sufficient clothing should be removed to allow the medical officer to inspect the wounds and to determine whether immediate life-threatening conditions such as airway obstruction, inadequate breathing, or hemorrhage are present. The level of consciousness, blood pressure, pulse, respiratory rate, and the time should be recorded on the field medical card. The time, dose, and route of administered narcotics, if any, should be noted. The prevalence of dehydration in combat casualties must be appreciated. If necessary, dressings and splints should be applied and preparations made for evacuation to the next echelon. Figure 22 is a flow diagram depicting some of the important combat casualty care decisions that need to be made at the unit or division level.

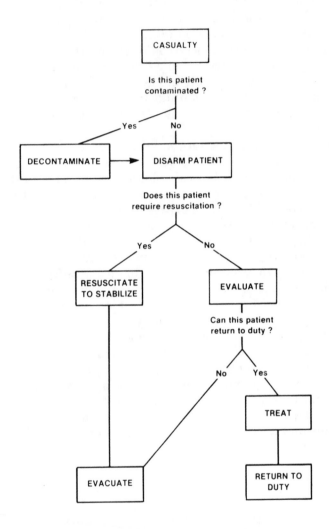

FIGURE 22.—Casualty care decision tree at the division level.

ORGANIZATIONAL AND OPERATIONAL ASPECTS

One essential prerequisite for the effective discharge of the unit and division medical officer's medical duties is a knowledge of the tactical deployment of the units the officer supports and the current level of intensity of their operations. The following text covers several of the more important functions of medical platoons and companies. Although emphasis is placed upon the function of the battalion surgeon, most of this information is also applicable to the division level medical officer. Medical officers must not forget that what they are able to do and how they do it can be profoundly influenced by current operational doctrine and by the prevailing tactical situation. The latter will dictate whether or not medical evacuation is possible and by what means it can be accomplished.

The battalion surgeon has two primary missions:

(1) Insure the health of the command
   - apprise the commander of ways to improve or preserve the health of the command
   - conduct disease surveillance
   - educate on preventive measures
   - inspect the state of health, morale, and hygiene of subordinate units
   - assess the medical threats for planned operations

(2) Provide combat casualty care
   - provide the commander with medical annexes to operational plans
   - supervise the battalion aid station
   - triage casualties
   - train combat medics
   - supervise evacuation and extraction of casualties
   - conduct medical reconnaissance*
   - prevent overevacuation of those only slightly injured who can be quickly returned to duty

*This includes map or terrain reconnaissance to determine the most secure lines of evacuation and potential location of secure casualty treatment areas near the battle areas. This should be accomplished before the battle and is part of the medical annex to the operational plan.

The battalion surgeon is responsible for the location, operation, and deployment of the battalion aid station. This involves movement to a properly located site, usually co-located with battalion headquarters and battalion trains, as well as distribution of medical elements of the battalion aid station to the rifle companies.

Two factors must be balanced against one another in selecting a site for the battalion aid station. One considers the security of location versus its nearness to supported forces. The battalion aid station is austere in both equipment and personnel and *must* rely on the other elements of the battalion trains (maintenance, supply, communications, and other battalion headquarters troops) to provide the necessary security for the battalion aid station. Cover, concealment, and the choice of a position in defilade to direct enemy fire contribute to the security of the battalion aid station as well as its ability to perform the medical support mission. Many other factors are considered when deciding where to site the battalion aid station: proximity to lines of drift of sick or wounded troops, proximity to water, ease of ingress and egress by ambulances, protection from the elements (this can include the use of commandeered structures when available, i.e., barns, houses, shops), ease of abandonment of position to keep pace with the supported unit, ease of access by next higher echelon of medical care, and a landing zone for air ambulances. To take advantage of the protection afforded by the Geneva Convention, the battalion aid station site must be suitably marked.

The battalion aid station does not necessarily require shelter unless weather or night operation light discipline mandate cover. The battalion aid station should be considered an area rather than a facility. After an appropriate site is chosen, it must be further divided into functional areas: triage, immediate treatment, delayed or minimal treatment and sick call, expectant casualties, battle stress casualties, and morgue. Ease of casualty flow in either a linear or circular manner is an essential consideration. Each area of the battalion aid station should be marked with signs and the entrance to the battalion aid station must be obvious.

Battalion aid station medical equipment should be functionally arranged. The triage and immediate casualty areas must have life-saving equipment and supplies near at hand. The sick call chest should be maintained near the minimal and sick call area, well clear of the triage and treatment area. Litters should be at the entrance to the battalion aid station for exchange by litter teams or for use by exhausted walking wounded casualties. All sections must have Field Medical Cards to insure appropriate and necessary recordkeeping.

Even though the tactical situation may allow the position of the battalion aid station to become relatively fixed and upgraded by physical improvements, it must always be prepared to rapidly advance or withdraw. Practiced and efficient set-up and take-down of the battalion aid station makes for responsiveness and mobility which allow the aid station to move more efficiently with changes in the tactical situation. This ability to respond to changes and move rapidly keeps the medical support close to those being supported.

ECHELONS OF CARE

The battalion surgeon is responsible for first echelon medical care. This equates to responsibility for supervision of the line medics assigned directly to infantry platoons as well as operation of the battalion aid station. The surgeon must be certain that all of his medics, whether assigned to rifle platoons or to the aid station, are trained and maintained to the highest possible standards achievable. Only by continual training of the medical personnel can the surgeon provide efficient and effective combat health care.

The ambulance section transports casualties from the battlefield to the aid station. Higher echelon ambulances, either ground or air, will move the casualty from the aid station to a higher level of care or, depending on the circumstances, may evacuate directly from the battlefield to a surgical facility.

Medics are all formally trained to the same level; however, their duties and subsequent practical experience will vary. The medic in the field will be primarily concerned with the provision of first aid, dealing with the airway, applying compression dressings for hemorrhage, stabilizing fractures, and initiating intravenous fluid administration. The aid station medics assist the battalion surgeon with sick call and with combat casualty care. Aid station combat casualty care consists largely of resuscitative measures as described in other chapters of this text.

POSITION AND ACTIONS OF THE SURGEON
DURING ENGAGEMENTS

The battalion surgeon must be apprised of the battle plan and the changing tactical situation. Only with this knowledge can the surgeon plan the best possible medical support and have the medics in the right place at the right time. The battle plan, evacuation capabilities, proximity, and readiness of a surgical care facility will determine where the surgeon is best utilized.

When battle lines are fluid and air evacuation difficult or impossible, surgeons may be best placed at aid stations where they can receive, triage, resuscitate and evacuate casualties emerging from the battle zone. This implies a far forward location of the aid station and the constant ability to move with the troops to avoid encirclement and capture.

If air evacuation capability exists, the surgeon may choose to follow the battle with the battalion commander in the tactical operations center. When large numbers of casualties are generated, the surgeon may be dispatched by aircraft to the battle scene to provide on-site triage. Casualties requiring urgent life-saving surgical intervention may be triaged directly to a surgical care facility. Other casualties are moved to the aid station and may be accompanied by the surgeon. As an alternative, the surgeon may elect to send the senior medic or physician assistant to the scene to provide the triage and direct casualties to the aid station or to the surgical facility.

If distances to surgical care are great and air evacuation is not possible, the surgeon may request a surgical team to augment aid station personnel and to perform resuscitative surgical procedures.

Much of the guidance referable to the tactical deployment of the battalion aid station is also applicable to the medical company. The medical company must be readily accessible, as it represents the major site of triage in the evacuation chain. It is also the first level at which there is a limited holding capability for casualties. Being responsible for clearing casualties from the brigade area requires proximity to and the ability to move with the maneuvering elements. The fact that in some units the medical company is organic to the support battalion rather than an element of a division medical battalion may place certain constraints upon carrying out the medical mission. These can be resolved only when the medical officer in command actively participates in planning and decision making. Overall, none of these factors will adversely affect the triage functions but they may limit both the sophistication of the medical care and the holding capability of the unaugmented medical company.

Not surprisingly, medical officers at the division level will find that their most difficult challenges result from the requirement to move the treatment facilities in accordance with the flow of the battle. In the attack, it is essential that the medical company be in proximity to the battalion aid stations. The medical company must move as far forward as the tactical situation allows. In deep penetrations, elements of one medical company or, ideally, two or more medical companies can be sequentially deployed or echeloned so as to provide continuous medical support. During withdrawals, medical companies or their elements deploy to the rear of each successive delay position, where they set up to receive casualties. Withdrawing medical elements "leapfrog" past them to more rearward positions where they in turn set up. Clearly, coordination with higher command levels, especially for the purpose of allocating additional medical assets, is essential. The unit and division level medical officer should be aware that the history of war contains many examples in which nontransportable casualties have by necessity been left to be taken prisoner. The decision to leave casualties behind is a command, not a medical, decision, and one that requires a decision as to how many and what types of medical personnel must remain with the casualties.

It is likely that forward surgical facilities will be co-located with selected medical companies in support of heavily engaged brigades. Surgical teams are also likely to be attached to the medical companies of airborne or air-assault divisions. In either situation, the medical company triage officer will be responsible for determining which casualties will be treated locally rather than being evacuated to the corps level for surgical care.

There are two broad indications for local surgical intervention: casualties in immediate danger of dying and casualties who will be significantly affected by a prolonged delay in evacuation occasioned by an unfavorable tactical situation. Casualties at risk of dying are those with abdominal or chest wounds who are in shock, those who are not responsive to resuscitation, those with closed head injuries showing rapid neurological deterioration, and those casualties with extremity wounds requiring a tourniquet for control of bleeding. Casualties with the second indication include those with open comminuted fractures of the femur and extensive soft tissue wounds in which anaerobic sepsis is likely to develop.

It is essential that the medical company triage officer be very selective in triage. Past experience indicates that, as a rule, no more than 5–10% of the total casualty population requires immediate surgery. At the other extreme of the injury spectrum are those casualties with minor wounds and the potential for rapid return to duty. This group is typified by a casualty with one or more superficial fragment wounds or a perforating gunshot wound of the extremity with small wounds of entrance and exit and no evidence of bone or neurovascular injury. Individual judgment must be exercised, but overevacuation of such casualties must not occur.

THERAPEUTIC ASPECTS

Emergency life-saving interventions are described in the appropriate sections of this manual. Relevant skills consist of the ability to create a surgical airway in the casualty with a severe facial wound, the insertion of an intercostal tube in the casualty with a hemo- or pneumothorax, the occlusion of a sucking chest wound, the ability to tamponade bleeding from major extremity arteries, and the infusion of therapeutic volumes of resuscitation fluids in those in shock.

Cricothyroidotomy, as shown in Figure 23, is an expeditious way to create a surgical airway. It is performed by palpating upward in the neck with the tip of the index finger to identify the cricoid cartilage. Place the tip of the index finger into the cricothyroid dimple just superior to the cricoid cartilage. By grasping the thyroid cartilage which lies just superior to the dimple, maintain the thumb and middle finger in place to steady the larynx. Stab the cricothyroid fibro-cartilaginous membrane with a #20 blade. The stab wound must be extended slightly to either side to accommodate an appropriately-sized tube.

Five to ten percent of battle deaths result from extremity exsanguination in which first aid could have controlled bleeding. Death due to hemorrhage from an extremity wound is preventable by simple direct compression. Medics must be taught to arrest high-grade hemorrhage by pressing the hand or dressing at the source until other means of control are established. A pressure bandage accomplishes this ideally when applied as a broad band of uniform tightness. If the tails of the battle dressing are tied too tightly, arterial flow may be occluded. Once immediate control of the hemorrhage has been accomplished and prior to the applica-

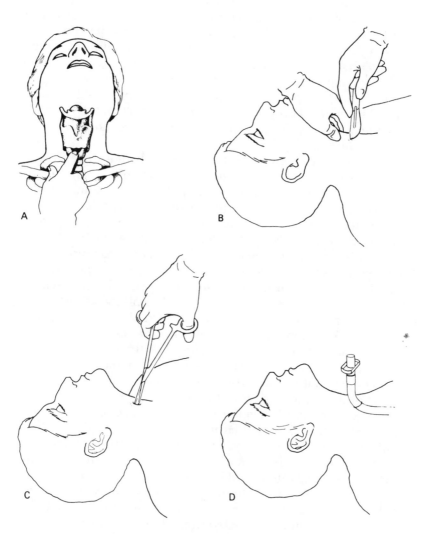

FIGURE 23.—Technique of cricothyroidotomy

tion of the pressure dressing, distal pulses should be assessed. Use of pressure points is a temporary measure to control severe bleeding while the pressure dressing is applied. Only two pressure points are of practical value for field use: the femoral artery in the groin and the axillary artery against the humerus. If the first dressing becomes soaked, a second dressing should be applied over the first applying greater pressure. Increased pressure is provided by tying the knot over a wad of material directly on top of the wound. One attempts, when possible, to preserve the distal pulse. The medical officer should bear in mind that the standard individual field dressing, when completely soaked, holds less than 250 cc of blood.

When pressure dressings fail to control the hemorrhage and the bleeding vessel is visible, a hemostat may be applied and incorporated into the dressing. Blind clamping is almost always futile. A tourniquet may be required to control hemorrhage, especially for the casualty with a traumatic amputation. A properly applied tourniquet, while endangering the limb, can save the life. An improperly applied tourniquet threatens both life and limb. A common mistake is inadequate compression which fails to occlude the artery but does occlude venous return. This results in an increased rate of blood loss. The tourniquet should be placed as distally as possible, just proximal to the wound. Once in place and adequately controlling hemorrhage, it should not be released until the casualty reaches a definitive care facility. The time and site of tourniquet application should be recorded clearly on the field medical card, and evacuation should be accelerated.

Intra-abdominal and intrathoracic hemorrhages require surgical intervention. When the intrathoracic bleeding is from the pulmonary circulation, it will usually be significantly diminished by tube thoracostomy and reinflation of the lung. Intra-abdominal bleeding may be diminished by application of a pneumatic antishock garment and inflation of both the extremity and abdominal compartments to at least 40mm Hg. Higher pressures have been employed, but there is no good evidence that they are advantageous and may in fact be deleterious if utilized for prolonged periods. The therapeutic effectiveness of the antishock garment is still very much open to question.

In the context of combat casualty care, there is very little hope for the exsanguinated, pulseless casualty. The salvage rate of traumatic cardiac arrest in the field approaches zero. Under these circumstances, the casualty that arrests after initial volume restoration and ventilation should be considered dead.

The civilian emergency medical doctrine which dictates that all trauma victims with possible injury to the cervical spine should have neck immobilization performed prior to transportation is not necessarily applicable to combat casualties. The overwhelming majority of combat casualties with penetrating wounds involving the head, neck, or upper chest who survive long enough to be treated do not have spinal cord injury or spinal injury which might predispose to a cord injury. There is likely to be little potential benefit from field immobilization of the combat casualty who does not have frank evidence of neurologic impairment. Bearing in mind the lethality of the battlefield with the resultant very substantial risk of performing time-consuming field medical procedures, medical personnel need to be selective in deciding which casualties need neck immobilization prior to evacuation from the battlefield.

Most often the medical officer's combat surgical practice does not involve managing acute life-threatening problems, but rather the splinting of extremity fractures and the dressing of soft tissue wounds. The earliest possible parenteral administration of antibiotics is mandatory in all casualties with penetrating abdominal injuries, open comminuted fractures of extremity bones, and extensive soft tissue wounds. Cefoxitin, 2gm IM or (preferably) IV is an appropriate antibiotic in such circumstances.

CONCLUSION

Unit and division level medical officers are the most forward physicians on the battlefield. As such, their role is to facilitate accomplishment of the mission of the tactical elements to which they are assigned or support. Their greatest contribution to mission success is usually the maintenance of the health of the command. The efforts of all members of the combat health care delivery team must be ongoing at all times and not just during episodic battles. In war, the unit and division level medical officer's impact on the army's fighting strength is determined more by his efforts to maintain the health of the command than by his efforts to save life and limb. To accomplish this objective, unit and division level medical officers must establish direct dialogue with their line unit commander, as failure to communicate can result in an inordinately high loss of duty days and jeopardize the mission. In summary, unit or division level medical officers must go to whatever lengths possible to be certain that they and their medics are well trained; that their equipment is adequate, appropriate, and well maintained; that resupply is available; that medical support planning for tactical operations is meticulous; and that they and their unit are flexible in their responses to rapidly evolving tactical situations.

CHAPTER XV

Anesthesia and Analgesia

In order to achieve the best results in emergency surgery for battle wounds, anesthetic management must be provided by thoroughly trained and proficient anesthesiologists and nurse anesthetists. Therefore, it is imperative that the most experienced anesthetists available be assigned to forward surgical units in which lifesaving procedures are accomplished. In these instances, the choice and application of anesthesia carry the greatest risks and can be the most dangerous factors in that individual's total care.

The most experienced anesthetists, however, may be assisted by anesthetists of more limited training and experience, who can work under qualified supervision. Nurse anesthetists are employed throughout the U.S. armed forces and frequently outnumber anesthesiologists, as they do in many civilian hospitals in this country. Under emergency conditions when qualified anesthesia providers are scarce, other medical and dental officers without special training in anesthesiology may be employed for this purpose if instructed and supervised. In past conflicts, only a small portion of anesthesiologists deployed to combat areas were fully trained and/or board certified. With the progressive increase in the total number of physicians and with a different conceptual application toward anesthesia care, anesthesia will be delivered or directed by anesthesiologists who are fully trained and have attained expertise in trauma care as well as intensive care.

Enlisted paraprofessionals should be used only as technical assistants to maintain equipment, prepare patients, take vital signs, etc. Throughout the remainder of this chapter, the term "anesthetist" will refer to either physician anesthesiologists or nurse anesthetists.

In wartime, anesthetists in forward surgical units may be called upon to perform resuscitative measures, direct respiratory therapy, and manage other aspects of perioperative care in addition to the administration of anesthetics. The success of surgical treatment of the severely injured largely depends on the effectiveness of these efforts.

It is equally important that the quality of anesthesia care be evaluated on a regular basis to record morbidity and mortality as it relates to that care. Periodic evaluations of ongoing policies, drugs, and equipment are essential to assure appropriate care of the wounded.

The most significant alterations in the physiology of the trauma patient usually involve the circulatory and respiratory systems. Since basic resuscitative treatment will frequently have been initiated soon after wounding, the anesthetist should, before instituting additional measures, have a record of the events which occurred from wounding until arrival at the hospital. The patient's field medical card will usually provide this information. In particular, the anesthetist should know what fluids have been administered, what other resuscitative measures have been necessary, and the dosages and routes of administration of narcotics, sedatives, and other drugs.

Intraoperative management includes monitoring and restoration of homeostasis, maintenance of an operating environment, and measures to relieve pain and block noxious autonomic reflexes. It must also be ensured that an effective airway is maintained, secretions are evacuated, and supplemental oxygen is provided. The anesthetist is responsible for the anesthetic drugs, blood and blood products, plasma volume expanders, and electrolyte solutions during the surgical procedure. He institutes all other required supportive measures and directs the immediate postoperative care.

Prior to the patient's transfer to an intermediate or minimal care ward, the anesthetist must be certain that the vital signs have stabilized, that essential reflexes have returned, and that drug depression has abated satisfactorily.

ANESTHESIA EQUIPMENT

The demonstrated capability for more rapid evacuation of seriously wounded casualties from the battle area has resulted in an increase in the complexity of surgery performed at installations in the combat zone. These changes have mandated a similar complexity of anesthesia equipment and techniques. Without the appropriate equipment, management of the seriously injured patient is impossible for even the most competent anesthetist.

Anesthesia equipment in a forward installation should include standard apparatus for administration of inhalation, intravenous, and regional anesthetics, as well as for oxygen supplementation and ventilatory support. An austere environment imposed by the tactical situation or geographical location may demand innovative approaches to what are normally routine clinical problems. For example, the scarcity of medical-grade compressed gas may require the anesthetist to use draw-over vaporizers, intermittent flow machines, or other techniques not in common practice in the U.S. There are many examples in the literature of improvised equipment and techniques that have served well in such difficult situations.

Complete airway equipment, including apparatus designed for pediatric use, should be readily available. An adequate suction, a defibrillator, and appropriate resuscitation drugs are required in any anesthetizing location. This is equally important regardless of whether general or regional technique is planned. It is also prudent to have a large-bore intravenous cannula or similar device handy to establish an emergency airway by cricothyroid puncture in the event of total upper airway obstruction. It should be kept in mind that ventilators are essential components of anesthesia delivery systems so that anesthesia personnel can resuscitate during surgical procedures. Experience has shown that the anesthetist must be prepared to treat local civilian casualties, sometimes including substantial numbers of children and neonates.

Appropriate adapters and delivery systems, such as nonrebreathing circuits and pediatric circle systems, are essential for proper anesthetic management.

In medical facilities dedicated to definitive care, anesthesia equipment should be as close to state-of-the-art as time and the local situation permit. Once this sophisticated equipment is in place, it must be checked and calibrated on a routine basis to assure its safety. Support personnel with mechanical knowledge of anesthesia equipment, its calibration, and its maintenance will be vital to safe application of care. Replacement units and spare parts should be in the theater supply system.

MONITORING

Since the typical battle casualty is young and healthy prior to wounding, sophisticated invasive monitoring techniques are not routinely indicated in this patient population. However, during prolonged hypoxia or myocardial contusion, cardiac disease can be present in formerly young healthy adults. In these specific situations, CVP and the pulmonary artery catheter become valuable monitors. Electrocardiogram, blood pressure, and heart sounds are routine measures for every patient. Urine output and such physical signs as pulse rate and volume, skin temperature, and capillary refill are useful indicators of the adequacy of intravascular volume.

If the operative procedure were to involve a major chest wound, major blood loss, or a vascular injury with the potential of major bleeding, direct arterial pressure monitoring is indicated. Disposable transducers are available and may be a reasonable approach. If the tactical situation or geographical location will allow, pulse oximeters, capnographs, and automated arterial blood pressure apparatus should be considered necessary anesthesia equipment.

Respiratory gas and pH measurements of arterial and mixed venous blood were shown to be major indicators of pathology in Vietnam, and are early indicators of life-threatening pathophysiology, as well as reliable guides to therapy. In the absence of instruments for arterial blood gas analysis, measurement of urine pH with indicator paper has been used successfully as a guide for treatment of metabolic acidosis. The vigilance of the anesthetist is the most effective monitor of all.

PREOPERATIVE PREPARATION

In the most severe cases of massive hemorrhage, immediate surgical control of bleeding is the only means of saving life. In cases of massive ongoing hemorrhage, laparotomy or thoracotomy oftentimes may have to be performed on an inadequately resuscitated patient. With cases such as these, the patient is intubated, paralyzed, ventilated with oxygen, given life-supporting fluids and amnestics with analgesia added, while control is obtained over bleeding as blood pressure and perfusion indices allow. As blood volume is replaced, the patient will require additional anesthesia. Using these approaches, the patient who has lost more than 50% of his total blood volume can be salvaged.

During less drastic trauma care, the anesthesiologist in

consultation with the triage physician can establish priorities as to when it is safe to induce anesthesia. During mass casualty periods, the anesthesiologist is usually too busy to spend a major portion of time in the triage area and must rely on the triage team. The latter requires a highly experienced surgeon with excellent executive ability. In every case, open communication and consultation between surgeon and anesthetist is essential. The evaluation of the efficacy of resuscitation and timing of operation in such casualties has been detailed previously (Chapter IX).

There is no assurance that either evacuation of gastric contents via nasogastric tube or induced emesis can lessen the hazard of aspiration in the trauma patient. Therefore, any battle casualty must be regarded as having a "full stomach," and the airway secured with a cuffed endotracheal tube by awake intubation or a rapid sequence induction.

Narcotics, sedatives, and other depressant drugs must be used cautiously in forward areas. Intramuscular or subcutaneous administration is not advised since drug absorption may be uncertain or erratic. Depressant drugs given to the head-injured casualty may confuse neurological evaluation and depress respiration, and are therefore contraindicated. Barbiturates, narcotics, and benzodiazepines are frequently useful as supplements to regional or local anesthetic techniques. They allay apprehension in most patients and may also elevate the seizure threshold in cases of local anesthetic toxicity. With the use of modern general anesthetic agents, the routine administration of anticholinergic medications preoperatively is probably not necessary.

If it is necessary at all, preoperative medication is best given intravenously in the operative room just before induction. For patients in severe pain, judicious doses of intravenous narcotics can be given. It is imperative that suction apparatus, ventilating equipment, and airway management equipment be readily available in the triage area. Judicious IV doses of narcotics in a 70 kg person would be in the range of 3-5 mg of morphine, 0.05 mg of fentanyl or 30-50 mg of meperidine.

ANESTHETIC TECHNIQUES

The three categories of anesthetic techniques are local, regional, and general.

LOCAL ANESTHESIA

While local infiltration techniques should be reserved for only the most minor of injuries, they do offer a fast and effective method to clean, suture, and remove small foreign bodies in forward facilities. These techniques allow early return to duty. Lidocaine, 0.5-1.0%, is the most popular agent. All of the local anesthetics shown in Table 9 can be used satisfactorily. In a medical facility overwhelmed with casualties, there is a temptation to perform an excessive number of operations under local anesthesia. Caution must be exercised in patient selection to avoid infiltration of toxic doses of local anesthetic under such circumstances. Local infiltration is seldom satisfactory for extensive debridement required to properly manage major wounds. Table 9 lists the common local anesthetics and their dosages.

Local anesthetics can be absorbed into the systemic circulation and, in excessive doses, can cause myocardial depression, hypotension, apnea, and seizures. Seizures should be treated with a rapidly acting benzodiazepine; respiratory depression by oxygenation and ventilation; and hypotension by intravenous fluid resuscitation and use of vasopressors.

It should be remembered that life support equipment such as oxygen, ventilation apparatus, airways, laryngoscopes, endotracheal tubes, adequate suction devices and muscle relaxant paralyzing drugs are minimum requirements in the event that a patient receives an overdose of local anesthetic or has an allergic reaction. Epinephrine, steroids, benadryl, intravenous barbiturate, and benzodiazepine medication should be readily available. All medications necessary to support a successful cardiopulmonary resuscitation must be available before any anesthetic is begun.

TABLE 9.—*Local Anesthetic Agents*

Anesthetic Agent and Application	Commonly Available Dosage Forms·	Recommended Maximum Dosage[1]
Subarachnoid Block[4]		
Tetracaine	1% solution or 20 mg ampule of soluble crystals	20 mg
Lidocaine	5% solution in 7.5% dextrose	100 mg
Bupivacaine	0.75% solution in 8.25% dextrose	15 mg
Infiltration, Epidural, and Major Nerve Block[2,3,4]		
Bupivacaine	0.25%, 0.5%, and 0.75 solution	3 mg/kg
Chloroprocaine	2% and 3% solution	15 mg/kg
Lidocaine	0.5%, 1%, 1.5%, and 2% solution	7 mg/kg
Mepivacine	1% and 2% solution	7 mg/kg
Prilocaine[5]	1% and 2% solution	8 mg/kg
Intravenous Regional Block		
Lidocaine	0.5% (or more dilute) solution	3 mg/kg
Prilocaine	0.5% (or more dilute) solution	3 mg/kg
Topical Anesthesia		
Cocaine	1%-4% solution	2.5 mg/kg
Dyclonine	0.5% solution	3 mg/kg
Lidocaine	2%-5% solution, ointment, jelly, or viscous solution	3 mg/kg
Tetracaine	0.2%-1% solution	1 mg/kg

Notes:

(1) These are general guidelines only. The smallest total dose necessary to accomplish satisfactory anesthesia should always be used. Consider patient age, physical status, debility, etc. , in determining dosages.

(2) Dosage limits for infiltration, epidural, and major nerve block are calculated assuming epinephrine is added to solutions. Reduce dosage by approximately 50% if using plain solutions.

(3) Plasma levels vary widely within anatomical site of nerve block or infiltration. Consult standard texts for specific limits.

(4) Only single-dose, preservative-free preparations should be used for subarachnoid or epidural administration.

(5) Do not exceed 600 mg in the adult.

REGIONAL ANESTHESIA

Regional anesthesia can be a valuable and efficient technique in combat surgery. In a mass-casualty situation, the busy anesthetist may be able to safely administer more than one anesthetic at a time, with monitoring delegated to lesser-trained personnel. Shortly after establishment of the block, the anesthetist's attention can usually be directed intermittently elsewhere without jeopardizing the safety of the patient. The advantages of regional anesthesia include the absence of nausea, vomiting, aspiration, and other pulmonary complications, and decreased bleeding.

Major nerve blocks are particularly appropriate for isolated extremity injuries. Regional anesthesia is not normally satisfactory for intra-abdominal exploration. The anesthetic level required to block sensation from visceral manipulation in such cases is usually dangerously high, necessitating both circulatory and ventilatory support.

Subarachnoid or epidural anesthesia is contraindicated in patients whose intravascular volume is inadequate or uncertain. It may be administered cautiously when fluid losses have been corrected by appropriate resuscitative measures. The sympathetic block from a subarachnoid or epidural anesthetic may be advantageous for the patient with a vascular repair of the leg, while a brachial plexus or stellate ganglion block may provide the same benefit to those with vascular injuries of the arm or hand. Another advantage of these techniques is that they often provide long-acting postoperative analgesia without the use of depressant medications.

The intravenous regional or Bier block is a very useful technique for extremity injuries because of its ease of administration, reliability, and relative safety. It is not a satisfactory technique if the limb has multiple puncture wounds or jagged foreign bodies are embedded. Postoperative analgesia is usually of only brief duration.

Table 9 lists commonly available anesthetic agents and dosage forms. The maximum recommended dosage limits shown must be tempered by modifying factors such as patient size, condition, and site of incision.

GENERAL ANESTHESIA

Anesthetic drug requirements in the critically injured patient will usually be much less than under more normal conditions. Often intraoperative management is primarily a matter of achieving hemodynamic stability, optimizing oxygenation, and supporting ventilation. If the patient is in profound shock, oxygenation, fluid resuscitation, and muscle relaxation may be the only 'anesthesia' administered. Such patients rarely have recall of intraoperative events. In addition, blood flow is preferentially distributed to the heart and brain in the hypotensive patient, which may further decrease anesthetic requirements.

INDUCTION OF ANESTHESIA

Time constraints and the risk of aspiration usually dictate that induction be rapid and controlled. Several intravenous agents are available which are in common use in the trauma setting. These include the rapidly acting barbiturates (such as thiopental), the benzodiazepines, rapidly acting narcotics, etomidate, and ketamine. The overriding factors in the decision as to which drug is best relate to the adequacy of blood volume, history of allergic reaction, or recent food intake. If the patient is markedly hypovolemic and there is insufficient time for fluid resuscitation, it is best to modify dosages of induction agents or use less cardiovascular depressant drugs, such as narcotics, etomidate, or ketamine. "Normal" dosages become lethal doses in the hypovolemic patient.

Some of the more important induction agents are:

Thiopental. This rapidly-acting barbiturate is quite familiar to most present day anesthetists. It has the advantages of fast onset, short duration, and good patient acceptance. However, normal induction dosages may cause disastrous hypotension in the hypovolemic patient. An induction dose is 3-4 mg/kg intravenously, given over one minute in a solution of 2.5% or less in normal saline. This drug can be a potent cardiac depressant and can produce hypotension. It can cause laryngospasm immediately after or during induction, is a poor analgesic, and produces poor muscle relaxation. This drug is best used in combination with a muscle relaxant paralytic drug.

Etomidate. This drug usually preserves cardiovascular stability in the intact elective surgical patient but probably has no advantage over thiopental in the case of hypovolemia. It also produces localized pain and myoclonic movements on rapid injection.

Ketamine. This agent is also fast acting, has analgesic properties, and supports the blood pressure by sympathetic stimulation. However, one must still be wary in the severely hypovolemic patient in whom sympathetic outflow may already be near maximal intensity. In these cases, the direct depressant effect on the myocardium may produce decreased cardiac output. Postoperative excitement and dysphoria, which is produced at times by this drug, may be minimized by using lower dosages or giving small amounts of benzodiazepines in combination with ketamine.

Narcotics. Rapidly acting narcotics, such as sufentanil, in conjunction with benzodiazepines are an alternative induction technique. If newer agents, such as the narcotic alfentanil, and the benzodiazepine midazolam prove safe in trauma cases, they should be considered also.

Regardless of the induction agent chosen, the risk of aspiration during induction (and emergence) remains a critical consideration. Drugs such as histamine receptor blockers, metaclopramide, and nonparticulate antacids offer promise as prophylactic measures; however, these agents will not be available on the battlefield, and the rapid and secure control of the airway remains the primary means of preventing this grave complication.

The anesthetist must ensure that an adequately functioning suction apparatus is close at hand and operational prior to induction or emergence.

MAINTENANCE OF ANESTHESIA

Inhalation Agents. These agents have the advantage of being relatively easy to titrate, thereby facilitating changes in anesthetic depth. There is a considerable body of experience in the use of inhalation anesthetics in trauma surgery. Halothane was used to a great extent during the Vietnam conflict. However, one must remember that all potent halogenated agents depress the respiratory and cardiovascular systems and that such effects are even more pronounced in the presence of hypovolemia. Often sub-minimal alveolar concentration (MAC) dosages are adequate to provide analgesia and amnesia in the critically injured casualty. Of the potent halogenated agents in current usage, isoflurane appears to offer the advantages of very limited metabolism and a lesser degree of cardiac depression than halothane or enflurane. These three halogenated drugs are potent bronchodilators and therefore are useful in the asthmatic patient.

Isoflurane has a MAC of 1.15 in oxygen; 0.5 in 70% nitrous oxide. Inspired levels must be maintained at 40% higher than MAC. For induction, one should use inspired gas concentrations 3-4 times the maintenance. This drug is a potent respiratory depressant, decreases peripheral vascular resistance, produces hypotension with little cardiovascular depression, can cause malignant hyperthermia, has good muscle relaxant properties, and allows rapid recovery due to low solubility. Nitrous oxide is usually safe, provided adequate oxygen is administered. Therefore, an in-line oxygen analyzer should be used in the circuit when nitrous oxide is given. The tendency for nitrous oxide to expand in any closed space in the body (e.g., pneumothorax, pneumocephalus, bowel obstruction) should also be kept in mind. Although diethyl ether has had widespread use as a battlefield anesthetic in the past, its flammability and lack of familiarity to most recently-trained anesthetists make it a less attractive choice. Cyclopropane, in addition to being highly explosive, is, like diethyl ether, no longer in common use and neither one should be used in modern combat anesthesia.

Intravenous Agents. Narcotics, such as fentanyl and morphine, are good analgesics and in adequate dosage are effective in blocking autonomic reflexes generated by noxious stimuli during operations. The combined use of nitrous oxide, muscle relaxants, and amnestics in a balanced anesthetic regime produces a "complete" anesthetic. Although considerably less depressant than the potent inhalation agents, narcotics should be carefully titrated in the unstable patient.

Fentanyl is a short-acting narcotic. One hundred mcg (2 ml) is equivalent to 10 mg of morphine. This drug may be given as intermittent bolus injection of 1-2 mcg/kg or as a continuous infusion of 2-50 mcg/min as titrated against blood pressure, pulse, or evidence of reaction to pain. Side effects of fentanyl include respiratory depression, bradycardia, bronchoconstriction, vomiting, and muscle stiffness. The muscle stiffness may need to be treated by intravenous muscle relaxants. Fentanyl has minimal effect on blood pressure.

Newer agents, such as sufentanil and alfentanil, in conjunction with short-acting muscle relaxants, may provide effective short-duration anesthesia and be successfully used in outpatient surgical procedures. These can be especially useful when recovery ward or ICU staffing is limited. The newer agonist-antagonist type of opiate drugs, such as nalbuphine and butorphanol, have also proved to be effective trauma anesthetics.

Ketamine is an effective analgesic and dissociative maintenance agent which can be used either in incremental doses or as a continuous infusion. To prevent recall in a lightly anesthetized patient, anterograde amnesia can be induced with scopolamine or small doses of a benzodiazepine.

After an intravenous dose of 1-2 mg/kg rapid induction of anesthesia (within 30 seconds), an intense analgesia is produced. An endotracheal tube may not be required, but one must remember that respiratory depression, apnea, coughing, and laryngospasm are possible at any time. Ketamine produces increased salivation and tracheal secretions, and can cause unwanted tachycardia, hypertension, increase in intraocular and intracranial pressures, and eye movements.

This is an effective drug for treating bronchospasm that is resistant to commonly used bronchodilators. It is an excellent agent for induction of anesthesia in the asthmatic.

Ketamine's intense analgesia makes it useful in the treatment of the burn patient for repeated debridement and dressing changes.

Postoperative excitement and dysphoria, which is produced at times by this drug, may be minimized by using lower dosages or giving small amounts of benzodiazepines in combination with ketamine. A continuous infusion can be used to reduce the total dose required for an anesthetic. A solution of 1 mg/ml can be infused at a rate of 1-25 ml/min. A loading dose of 50 mg should be used in the adult.

Midazalam, a new short-acting benzodiazepine, is probably the intravenous agent of choice to reduce ketamine emergence reactions.

MUSCLE RELAXANTS

Succinylcholine is the most commonly used relaxant for rapid sequence intubation, although appropriate doses of nondepolarizing agents will also provide good intubating conditions reasonably quickly. Intravenous injection is followed by fasciculations and muscle cramps and after one minute a flaccid paralysis that requires ventilatory support and has a duration of 5-15 minutes. This drug may cause hyperkalemia in patients with burn or crush injuries but is usually safe in the acute injury situation and for the first several days post-injury. Hyperkalemia, cardiac arrythmia and arrest can occur in these patients after 48 hours and in patients with renal failure, spinal cord injuries, and severe sepsis. One must be aware that this drug can produce a rise in intraocular pressure, and (rarely) vomiting and aspiration secondary to abdominal muscle contraction, bradycardia, salivation, postoperative muscle pain, malignant hyperthermia, and prolonged apnea.

Pancuronium produces an atropine-like tachycardia that is normally not a problem in the young and healthy trauma patient, but may confuse the differential diagnosis of a rapid heart rate intraoperatively. This drug has an onset of paralysis in three minutes and a duration of forty minutes or longer. The initial dose for adults is 0.04-0.1 mg/kg intravenously.

D-Tubocurarine can cause significant histamine release and a resultant hypotension, which limits its usefulness in the hypovolemic patient. D-Tubocurarine and Pancuronium usually need to be reversed by neostigmine or edrophonium in combination with an anticholinergic drug intravenously.

Atracurium and Vecuronium are newer, short-acting, nondepolarizing muscle relaxants which have an onset time of 2-3 minutes and a duration of 20-40 minutes. These drugs can be used by single injection for short procedures or as a continuous infusion. These agents are not vagolytic and do not support the tachycardia or hypertension seen with pancuronium. They can be used to replace succinylcholine for rapid-sequence intubation. These drugs are metabolized by routes other than the kidney and therefore are useful in renal failure patients. Atracurium can cause a small amount of histamine release, but this is usually not hemodynamically significant. Vecuronium is relatively free of cardiovascular side effects. The usual dose of vecuronium is 0.1 mg/kg, and for atracurium 0.3-0.4 mg/kg intravenously.

Use of a nerve stimulator to monitor the degree of neuromuscular blockade will facilitate the management of muscle relaxants and should be considered standard procedure.

POSTOPERATIVE MANAGEMENT

Hospitals dedicated to advanced resuscitation and surgical care must anticipate the sequelae of trauma, anesthesia, and operation. As a result of thoracic trauma, the likelihood of overhydration, or surgical manipulation, many of these patients will be unable to breathe adequately and will require mechanical ventilatory support. Ventilators used for these applications should be volume-cycled machines capable of delivering inspired oxygen concentrations up to 100% and of providing positive end-expiratory pressures. Ideally, they should have the same alarms, adjustments, and options (such as intermittent mandatory ventilation) as ventilators in current critical care applications.

Narcotics and analgesics must be judiciously managed in the postoperative surgical patient. Small doses administered intravenously are usually most effective in the immediate recovery period. Changes in position and the adjustment of pads, braces, pillows, etc., may do much to make the patient comfortable and decrease the need for pharmacological intervention. The use of regional blocks should provide effective analgesia while avoiding depressant medications. It must be borne in mind that restlessness and agitation may be signs of hypoxia rather than true pain.

Anesthetic techniques using short-acting narcotics, hypnotics, and muscle relaxants may reduce recovery room problems, but it still may be necessary to reverse narcotics or use additional muscle relaxant reversal drugs. It is equally important to be sure that each recovery site offers the safety of an oxygen supply in the event that a patient must be ventilated, as well as effective suction apparatus. Wherever logistically possible, the ability to measure blood gases should be available. Measurement of arterial or central venous oxygen tension gives the physician a working knowledge not only of lung function but also of metabolism, cardiovascular stability, and effectiveness of resuscitation. The addition of trained and experienced specialists in critical care medicine to forward medical facilities will enhance the quality of care provided and will free anesthesia personnel to concentrate their efforts in the operating rooms.

MASS CASUALTY MANAGEMENT

Anesthesia personnel should prepare for mass casualty

situations by becoming involved in the planning for such functions as staffing, organization, and logistical support for the triage/preoperative area. Attention to details such as adequate electrical and oxygen outlets, suction devices, emergency airways, and supplies of intravenous fluids is mandatory. When the initial influx of patients begins, anesthetists may assist in fluid resuscitation, airway management, ventilatory support, and other critical measures. Once these procedures are in progress, they must usually dedicate themselves to their areas of primary responsibility, the operating and recovery rooms.

The anesthesiologist must serve as a continuous resource and consultant to assure safe pre-, intra-, and postoperative care. A theater consultant in anesthesiology with on-site knowledge of patient care, who is informed by periodic reports specifically related to anesthesia problems, will make valuable contributions to the quality of care given.

CHAPTER XVI

Wounds and Injuries
of the Soft Tissues

To maximize the preservation of life and minimize the attendant morbidity of battle wounds, the surgeon attempts to localize or isolate the deleterious effects of injury and to optimize healing. This objective is best accomplished by removal of all foreign material and detached or severely disrupted muscle from the wound, by the establishment of open drainage of the wound's recesses, and by maintaining adequate capillary perfusion of the injured tissues. Early institution of systemic antibiotic therapy plays more than an ancillary role in the management of these contaminated war wounds. If these management objectives are achieved, the risk of further local tissue destruction and systemic invasion by pathogenic micro-organisms is reduced to a minimum.

The emphasis of this chapter is on the management of damaged muscle. Surgical management of other soft tissue and bone injuries is dealt with in other chapters. Two separate mechanisms are responsible for the injury caused by the passage of missiles through tissues. As the projectile punches through muscle, it destroys the tissue in its direct path by crushing it. Temporary cavitation forces, which present about one millisecond after passage of the projectile, stretch the tissues adjacent to the permanent missile track and result in additional injury or destruction.

Crushed Muscle: The amount of crushed muscle resulting from a single bullet or single fragment is closely related to the presenting cross-sectional area of the projectile. The gross anatomy of muscle will be much more severely disrupted by multiple penetrating projectiles striking in close proximity to each other, as is the case with explosive device injuries, deforming or fragmenting rifle projectiles, or any rifle projectile that strikes bone. Some remnants of muscle crushed by penetrating projectiles will generally be seen as a frayed edge along the missile track. Detached pieces of muscle, partially detached muscle flaps, and muscle islands surrounded by perforations should be regard-ed as nonviable. They would most likely act as foreign bodies that will potentiate infection in an already contaminated wound.

Stretched Muscle: Temporary displacement of muscle by cavitation (see Chapter II) can cause petechial hemorrhages from torn small vessels (contusion), thrombosis of other small vessels, and patchy broken muscle fibers. Cavitation follows the path of least resistance, which is most often to separate muscle between parallel fibers and bundles. Gross radial splits are sometimes seen in muscle but not nearly to the extent that they are seen in skin. Although both bullet yaw and bullet deformation appreciably in-crease the dimensions of both the permanent and the temporary cavities, the effects of bullet fragmentation are by comparison devastating, and may result in an injury that is multiplied by several orders of magnitude in muscle that has been weakened a millisecond earlier by the creation of multiple radial fragment tracks.

DEBRIDEMENT

Where one draws the line in excising muscle surrounding a missile path has been the subject of intense debate in wound ballistics. The 5th CINCPAC War Surgery Conference (Tokyo 1971) stated "...the surgeon must choose between leaving tissue of ques-tionable viability or causing morbidity by removing viable and functional tissue." Most other opinions of the past two decades have held that "complete excision of all devitalized tissue is man-datory," "bold removal of all devitalized muscle is imperative" (NATO Handbook, 1975), and that deformity or dysfunction resulting from such "bold" operations is justified.

Development of life-threatening gas gangrene is the complica-tion most often cited to justify recommendations of "radical debridement" or wide excision of muscle. Of 224,080 wounded in France in WW I, those with soft tissue injury and no bone frac-ture developed gas gangrene in only 1.0% of cases and less than half of these were fatal. A streptococcal bacteremia was by far the most common cause of death. Many of the less than 0.5% of the deaths attributed to clostridia were suspected to have been due, in reality, to undetected streptococcus. Streptolysin, excreted by the virulent Streptococcus species, breaks down the fibrin that has been deposited by the body in its attempt to wall off collections of pathological bacteria. This made generalized streptococcal spread impossible to control in the pre-antibiotic era. Since the discovery of antibiotics, streptococcal bacteremia has all but disappeared from the battlefield *because of antibiotics,* a fact overlooked by those who suggest that antibiotic therapy is only an ancillary measure in the management of combat wounds.

Debridement should be rational rather than radical. The recommendation is not to excise the wound to the extent that viable muscle is intentionally excised circumferentially, but rather to open the wound such that drainage is assured, while at the same time excising that muscle which is severely damaged or disrupted and therefore devitalized. The surgeon must aggressively incise the wound, but should not empirically excise tissue more widely than clinical judgment would normally dictate. It should be borne in mind that debridement of the wound is intended to relieve excessive tension within the wound, to rid the wound of dead tissue and massive hematoma, and to provide excellent drainage. Some would say that the relief of tension is the single most important element of wound debridement.

WOUND DYNAMICS

From the time a wound is inflicted until healing is complete, the surrounding area is in a state of constant change. In the first few hours after an extremity is exposed to the violent temporary cavity stretch of the AK-74 wound, a marked vasoconstriction of these tissues is revealed by skin blanching for a distance of 6–8 cm from the skin edges. Marked hyperemia appears around the blanched area and gradually encroaches upon it, eventually replacing it entirely in about four hours. Although less dramatic than the skin changes, increasing perfusion of muscle surrounding the missile path has been clearly demonstrated for up to 72 hours after wounding.

Since blood flow in the muscle around the projectile path is changing, it is difficult at best for the surgeon, at any point in time, using any set of guidelines, to be certain of excising only (but all of) the nonviable muscle, and not viable muscle. Writings in the past two decades have demanded this judgment of our young surgeons when even the most experienced combat surgeon was not always certain. This was demonstrated in the Vietnam conflict when some wounds, which were treated in accordance with the conventional "4 c" guidelines (color, contraction, consistency, circulation) were noted on arrival at another hospital, a few days later, to have obviously necrotic muscle. Some surgeons at this higher echelon of care concluded that the initial debridement had been done improperly. The 5th CINCPAC War Surgery Conference in 1971 corrected that misconception by stating that the later appearance of necrotic tissue in a wound "does not necessarily mean that the original debridement was improperly done," but rather was the result of the transitory dynamics of wound physiology at the time of the original debridement.

From a practical standpoint, the question is not whether or not to excise devitalized tissue, for there is good agreement here, but rather how to accurately differentiate muscle that is injured but will heal from that muscle which is nonviable and should be excised. Generations of surgeons have accepted the assumption that nonviable muscle can be identified by its dark color, its "mushy" consistency, its failure to contract when pinched with forceps, and the absence of brisk bleeding from a cut surface (the 4c's). The surgeon inclined to err in the direction of radical excision should bear in mind that in all studies in which animals were kept alive long enough to observe and measure wound healing objectively or to evaluate the pathology around the missile wound microscopically, there was less lasting tissue damage than estimated from observation of the wound in the first few hours after the wound was inflicted. The foregoing notwithstanding, the surgeon must base judgment on decisions made at the table at the time of operation. The majority of combat surgeons continue to utilize the 4 c's as guidelines and consider it prudent to excise muscle of questionable viability.

TREATMENT RECOMMENDATIONS

Establish an adequate blood level of penicillin or an antibiotic with a similar spectrum as soon as possible after wounding. Make generous incisions of the wound to relieve mechanical pressure and establish open drainage. Remove easily-accessible foreign bodies and detached pieces of muscle, and irrigate the wound copiously. The wound track is then inspected and any additional muscle whose gross architecture is severely disrupted is excised. At the conclusion of the procedure, complete hemostasis must be achieved to preclude the subsequent development of collections within the wound that would impede capillary perfusion of borderline tissues. The technique is shown in Figure 24.

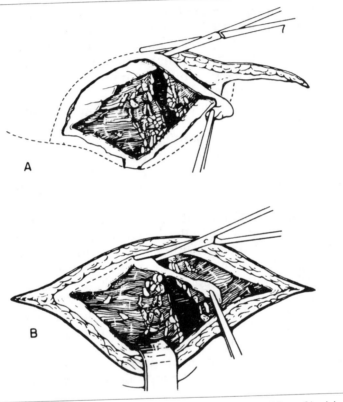

FIGURE 24.—Technique of debridement in soft-tissue wounds. A. Line of incision and excision of traumatized skin. B. Excision of traumatized fascia.

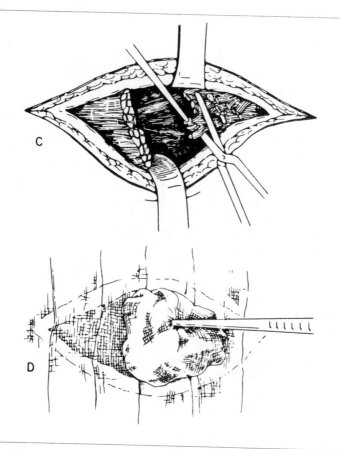

FIGURE 24.—Continued. C. Excision of devitalized muscle. D. Technique of wound dressing.

1. Excise entrance and exit wounds with a narrow margin of skin oriented parallel to the underlying muscle fibers. This excised skin margin should include, in continuity, the underlying subcutaneous tissue. These incisions should be generous, such that optimal surgical exposure and adequate subsequent drainage will be achieved.

2. Through these openings, generously incise the fascia parallel to the muscle fibers in both directions. The underlying muscle surrounding the missile tract should be opened in the direction of its fibers to the degree necessary to achieve exposure adequate to

inspect the track, remove foreign bodies, and excise non-viable muscle. These maneuvers are performed at both the wound of entry and the exit wound. The muscle surrounding the central portion of the track can usually be dealt with through the entry and exit wounds. For example, a mid-thigh, through-and-through wound of the soft tissues can generally be surgically managed by working through the excised and extended wounds of entry and exit. This approach precludes the necessity of cutting across good muscle groups as is generally the case when one elects to connect the two wounds. Appropriate drainage of war wounds is often easier said than done. Liberal incisions tend to facilitate drainage from the wound's deeper recesses. Whereas excision of skin, fascia, arteries, nerves, veins, and bone is conservative, the excision of muscle should be more liberal.

3. As a dressing, dry sterile gauze should be laid lightly in the wound. This should be no more than a wick. In no case should gauze be "packed" into the wound since this additional pressure can cause necrosis of any tissue that already has its blood supply partially compromised.

4. The single most important principle in the management of battle wounds is their nonclosure following debridement. The surgeon must not give in to the temptation to primarily close certain "very clean appearing" war wounds. Such closure is ill advised and inappropriate and can only be condemned. All wounds must be left widely open with the following exceptions:

   a. Sucking chest wounds
   b. Joint capsules
   c. Wounds of the dura
   d. Some head and neck wounds; however, with severe contamination it may be safer to leave these open.

5. The delayed primary wound closure is usually performed in a communication zone hospital 4–10 days after debridement, but occasionally may be performed at the forward hospital when evacuation has had to be delayed. The indication for delayed primary closure is the clinically clean appearance of the wound. Whereas most wounds are closed in the operating room utilizing the interrupted wire technique and local or general anesthesia, some may be very amenable to tape closure. This technique can be initiated 4–6 days post debridement. Approximation of the skin edges is accomplished with micropore paper tape or wide "butterflies" applied in overlapping diagonal "basket weave"

fashion after the skin has been degreased with acetone, and tincture of benzoin has been applied and allowed to dry thoroughly. Edges of the wound may not come completely together with the first tape application. This is not a problem, as they will come progressively closer together with each reapplication of tape, done at 48 hour intervals. Tape closure offers some advantages over suture closure. Even compression of wound edges decreases skin edema, and the problem of cutting needles causing additional tissue damage is avoided. The wound edges are very vascular and needle passage can cause hematomas. Since tape closure is, in reality, a gradual "encouragement" of the skin toward closure rather than a total closure from the beginning, a great margin for error is added and the potential complication of wound breakdown, sometimes seen after suture closure, is almost completely avoided. No anesthesia is needed for this procedure and it can be performed by supervised ward nursing personnel.

It should be recognized that even though the surgeon diligently attempts to excise all devitalized tissue, the dynamics of wound physiology and the imperfections of one's ability to absolutely identify nonviable tissue are such that some devitalized muscle may be left behind or evolve over time in the wound. In the appropriately drained wound, this minimal amount of devitalized tissue will be absorbed or extruded. A small percentage of these wounds will require a second debridement prior to delayed primary closure. At worst, in the absence of adequate drainage, an abscess that requires subsequent drainage may develop. In this situation, antibiotics localize or isolate the deleterious effects of the injury to the site of injury, thereby precluding systemic, life-threatening sepsis.

TREATMENT PRIORITIES

Whereas all of the foregoing is felt to represent optimum management of war wounds, battlefields of the future may present medical officers with constraints beyond their control that preclude optimum casualty management. The lack of air superiority may deny aeromedical evacuation from forward areas. Tactical encirclement or weather may compel the forward maneuver element to hold its wounded. Battalion surgeons or physician's assistants may find themselves in a position where they are denied the option of moving casualties to definitive care facilities.

Medical personnel or equipment shortfalls may be the limiting factor. A resource-workload mismatch may result from a casualty generation rate that overwhelms medical capabilities. In situations such as these, the battalion surgeon and the medical treatment facility chief surgeon must be prepared to limit treatment in consonance with their capabilities and certain treatment priorities.

1) The forward medical officer should observe the general principles of resuscitation to the extent possible. The inability to surgically control high-grade hemorrhage may necessitate the prolonged use of tourniquets.

2) The early institution of systemic antibiotics is of prime importance, especially when war wounds cannot be promptly treated surgically. Tetanus toxoid and morphine analgesia are given.

3) If any surgical and anesthetic capability exists, operative treatment of wounds is usually limited to local anesthesia and wound incision to improve drainage. Under these circumstances, if wound incision is elected in the absence of blood transfusion capability, care should be exercised to avoid hemorrhage.

4) It is possible that even the larger definitive care facilities may find themselves overwhelmed by casualties or understaffed due to combat losses of their personnel. The area medical regulating officer may not be able to divert casualty excesses to other facilities. Under circumstances such as these, appropriate care may have to be limited to wound incision and antibiotics.

5) Simple non-occlusive dressings should be utilized. These dressings should allow, to the extent possible, egress of drainage from the wound.

CHAPTER XVII

Crush Injury

GENERAL

The "Crush Syndrome," or traumatic rhabdomyolysis, is a syndrome resulting from skeletal muscle injury, and the resultant release of muscle cell contents into the general circulation. This syndrome was first described in World War II air raid victims who had been trapped under fallen masonry. During peacetime, the syndrome may be seen in association with natural disasters such as earthquakes and mine cave-ins, or occasionally with vehicular disaster. Present-day terrorist activities utilizing high explosives and military operations in urbanized terrain represent current causes of the syndrome. Any individual who has been crushed beneath debris or run over, or whose limbs have been compressed for any reason for an hour or more, is at risk of developing the crush syndrome.

The collapse of a building due to an explosion causes immediate death among the majority of the victims due to the blast effect, the direct effects of the falling debris, the fire, or compression by the rubble. Immediate death is mainly caused by severe damage to vital organs. The survivors whose extremities are pinned under heavy rubble, thereby trapping them, are the ones at risk of developing the syndrome.

PATHOGENESIS

Sustained compression of a limb impedes perfusion, which results in hypoxia progressing to anoxia, muscle injury, and increased capillary permeability. The crush syndrome is a reperfusion injury. When the extremity is extricated from the compressing rubble, the damaged muscle liberates muscle pigment, potassium, creatinine, lactic acid, and other intracellular substances into the general circulation. The trapped victim may also be suffering from other severe injuries that contribute to or of themselves result in shock. After release from compression, the extravasation of plasma results in swelling of the affected part. When this happens, oligemic shock is precipitated or aggravated. Untreated oligemic shock contributes to acute renal insufficiency. Liberated myoglobin, which accumulates in the renal tubules, also contributes to the development of renal failure. Liberated phosphate and uric acid aggravate an already developing metabolic acidosis. Hyperkalemia can result in sudden cardiac arrest and death. Coagulopathies not uncommonly develop. This combination of hypovolemic shock coupled with myoglobinuric acute renal failure carries a grave prognosis.

CLINICAL CONSIDERATIONS

A clear history of crush injury is not always available in wartime, and the syndrome sometimes develops insidiously in patients who appear well when they first present. Crush injuries of the trunk and buttocks can be overlooked if a complete physical examination is not performed.

Although the compressed region may appear normal when it is released from pressure, paralysis caused by the compression is sometimes present. Erythema may appear at the margin of the affected area early after release, and the adjacent skin may blister. These signs are sometimes the first evidence of damage.

Shortly after release from compression, swelling caused by extravasation of plasma appears in the part. The loss of plasma initiates or aggravates oligemic shock, and the patient's condition rapidly deteriorates. The blood pressure, which was at first maintained by vasoconstriction, falls rapidly as plasma loss continues. The damaged part, which is usually a limb, becomes swollen, tense, and hard. If it is incised, serous fluid oozes from it. The distal pulses tend to disappear. When the fascia is opened, swollen or friable muscle, which in the later stages is very pallid, bulges out. Later symptoms and signs may include anorexia, hiccups, dryness of the tongue, and drowsiness or mental disturbances as the blood urea and blood pressure mount.

In favorable cases, diuresis ensues 6–8 days after injury and the patient improves clinically, although renal dysfunction may persist for months. In less favorable cases, death may occur promptly from shock or from pulmonary edema, aggravated by the unwise forcing of fluids in the presence of renal shutdown.

Later death may be attributable to cardiac arrest caused by the hyperkalemia of uremia. In untreated cases, renal insufficiency almost always occurs within a few hours of release of compression.

Laboratory findings reveal an elevated hematocrit reflecting the state of hemoconcentration. Serum potassium and uric acid levels are elevated. The blood area nitrogen levels are unchanged. Free myoglobin may be detected. The serum creatinine phosphokinase (CPK) is markedly elevated to at least five times normal. The first urine specimen, because it was collected in the bladder before injury, may be normal. Later, urine becomes dark due to the presence of myoglobin. It will have an acid pH.

LOCAL MANAGEMENT

The early splinting of major soft-tissue injuries and fractures is urgently important in crush injuries to minimize hypotension. To reduce tissue metabolism, the limb is kept cool by exposure to air. Unnecessary dressings and unnecessary movements of the limb are hazardous, as they cause the release of deleterious substances, particularly potassium in potentially lethal amounts, into the general circulation.

A tense and swollen limb should be decompressed immediately by liberal incision of the fascia. This measure is particularly urgent when the pressure of extravasated fluid impairs circulation. An early amputation is indicated when the limb is so severely crushed that it is obvious that function cannot be restored or when it is the only emergency procedure that permits extrication of the victim from under unmovable rubble. Debrided wounds and fasciotomy incisions should not be closed primarily.

GENERAL MANAGEMENT

Intravenous therapy should be initiated immediately after extrication or even, when possible, while the casualty is still trapped. Glucose-saline is the solution of choice; however, Ringer's solution may be used. The early objective is to achieve a constant diuresis of at least 300 cc's per hour with a urine pH of greater than 6.5. An indwelling urinary catheter is inserted. A central venous or pulmonary artery wedge pressure catheter should be utilized to guide fluid infusion and reliably monitor central pressures.

1. In the presence of an appropriate urinary response,

crystalloid solution is administered at the rate of 500 cc/hour. Bicarbonate, 44.5 mEq, is added to the crystalloid solution every other hour.

2. Urine volume and pH are monitored hourly.

3. Serum electrolytes, osmolality, and arterial blood gasses are evaluated at six hour intervals.

If the urinary volume is less than 300 cc per hour, mannitol (1.0 g per kilogram body weight) should be given intravenously. If the arterial pH reaches 7.45 or the urine pH is below 6.5, 250 mg acetazolamide should be given intravenously. This therapy should continue until myoglobin disappears from the urine. It usually takes about 60 hours to achieve this goal.

The earlier one starts intravenous therapy, the better the chance of preventing acute renal failure. When fluid therapy is delayed for six hours following extrication, acute renal failure is almost assured. If the desired urinary output cannot be achieved, the use of diuretics, preferably furosemide, should be considered. The majority of crush injury victims who do not receive intravenous therapy early enough and who do not respond to enforced alkaline diuresis go on to develop renal failure and the requirement for hemodialysis. If renal failure develops, prompt reduction in fluid administration is indicated.

Infection, which contributes to the development of acute renal failure, should be prevented by all possible means. Wide-spectrum antibiotics, including agents which are effective against anaerobic microorganisms, are indicated. Tetanus toxoid should be given according to the casualty's state of immunization.

The clinical features of crush syndrome may not become evident until just before the patient is to be evacuated on the basis of his other injuries. If renal insufficiency seems to be developing, the patient should be evacuated, as soon as the other injuries permit, to a medical facility that is capable of monitoring and treating the condition with renal dialysis.

CHAPTER XVIII

Vascular Injuries

In recent wars, vascular injuries of the extremities have only comprised about 1-2% of all major injuries seen in living casualties. However, major vascular injuries are always life threatening and may result in significant morbidity among survivors. Advances in peripheral vascular surgery over the last thirty years have made it possible to repair major arterial and venous injuries not only in the civilian trauma setting but also in the combat zone hospital. Dramatic results following vascular repair can be expected if proper surgical facilities and experienced personnel are available. On the other hand, the performance of major vascular operations requires a significant commitment of time and resources. When surgical facilities are inadequate or overrun by large numbers of casualties, the performance of major vascular procedures is inappropriate. Under such unfortunate conditions, amputation rather than vascular repair may be more appropriate. Under these circumstances, experience and mature judgement are required to make the proper decision for each patient.'

TABLE 10.—*Arterial wounds and associated injuries, Vietnam, 1965-1970*

Location	Total #	Nerve #	Nerve %	Vein #	Vein %	Bone #	Bone %
Axillary	59	54	91.5	20	33.8	16	27.1
Brachial	283	202	71.3	54	19.0	96	33.9
Iliac	26	3	11.5	11	42.3	2	7.6
Femoral, common	46	7	15.2	18	39.1	9	19.2
Femoral, superficial	305	61	20.0	139	45.5	72	23.6
Popliteal	217	81	37.3	113	52.0	87	40.0
Total	936	408	43.5	355	37.9	282	30.1

Major vascular injuries almost always require prompt surgical intervention if the tissues supplied are to be salvaged. Diagnosis and preliminary management should begin in the field, and these patients should be evacuated promptly to a definitive treatment facility. Operational conditions may have a profound influence on the ultimate outcome of vascular injuries. During the Vietnam conflict, for instance, helicopter evacuation allowed many who might have otherwise expired to reach the hospital alive. Whether or not similar circumstances will exist in future conflicts remains to be seen.

GENERAL PRINCIPLES

As in the civilian sector, the majority of combat-incurred vascular injuries that are amenable to surgical repair involve peripheral vessels. The majority of those with central vascular injuries or injuries of the thoracic or abdominal aorta usually do not survive to reach a surgical facility capable of dealing with these injuries. The penetrating and perforating vascular wounds of the battlefield, as opposed to those of the civil sector, are more likely to have been caused by high-velocity projectiles. High-velocity missiles more often cause secondary damage to adjacent tissues as a result of temporary cavitation. Secondary fragments resulting from either fragmentation of the projectile or from fragmentation of bone will cause additional damage. Temporary cavitation can result in thrombosis of an artery even though the missile does not actually strike the artery. This results from intimal disruption, subintimal dissection of blood, and intimal prolapse and subsequent thrombosis.

The use of various fragmentation devices in military operations creates the potential for multiple vascular injuries (as well as other major nonvascular wounds) in the same individual. The multiplicity of wounds must be taken into account in the overall management of the patient.

Although the surgical repair of vascular injuries is usually urgent, it must not be done precipitously. Every surgeon confronted with a casualty with obvious major vascular injury must also determine what other injuries are present and formulate the best overall management plan. Priority of care must be established for each injury. The ability of the patient to tolerate the additional operative time required for vascular repair must also be considered. Finally, adequate resuscitation usually must be accomplished before the reparative vascular procedure is attempted. In some cases, the control of hemorrhage will be part of the process of resuscitation. Failure to observe these basic precautions may result in loss of life as a result of overzealous attempts to salvage a limb.

DIAGNOSIS

Injuries to blood vessels consist of several types. Among these are lacerations, transections, avulsions, and contusions. The latter may or may not be associated with intimal injury. All can result in spasm, thrombosis, expanding hematoma, and distal thrombus embolization. Full-thickness injuries may result in false aneurysm, arteriovenous fistula, and life-threatening hemorrhage. Neurological symptoms may develop secondary to ischemia, associated nerve injury, neural compression by expanding hematoma, or a compartment syndrome.

Diagnosis of vascular injury is sometimes difficult. This is especially true when a missile track is near a major vessel but distal pulses are still intact. Classically, a cold, pulseless extremity results from an arterial injury. Similar physical findings can occasionally be the result of environmental exposure, shock, arterial spasm, or crush injury. At times, an accurate diagnosis is not possible until exploration is undertaken. In most instances, however, the following signs and symptoms (commonly referred to as the 5 Ps) may be taken as presumptive evidence of arterial injury: pain, pallor, pulselessness, paresthesia, and paralysis. Additional findings may include contracture, mottling, and cyanosis. Anesthesia or external hemorrhage may or may not be present. In some cases, the injured limb may be clearly larger than the uninjured limb due to the presence of a large subfascial hematoma.

For the most part, the surgeon will have to rely solely on clinical skills in diagnosing and evaluating postoperative patency of arterial repairs. However, during the Vietnam conflict, it was shown that the Doppler instrument could be used effectively in the combat setting. Nowadays, sturdy, lightweight, and inexpensive instruments are widely available, and will in all likelihood be available in combat zone hospitals.

SURGICAL TIMING

The management objective of arterial injuries is restoration of arterial flow at the earliest possible moment. As the time lag from injury to repair increases, so increases the failure rate of arterial repair. While the best results are obtained when blood flow is reestablished within six hours of injury, it remains impossible to define the precise time beyond which successful repair can be expected. Thus, there is no inflexible time limit beyond which arterial repair is absolutely contraindicated.

When occlusion of a major artery occurs as a result of trauma, limb viability depends on collateral circulation. Whether or not operation can be delayed in such cases is dependent upon the adequacy of collateral blood flow. Irreversible muscle damage may occur within a few hours if collateral circulation is inadequate. On the other hand, limb survival may occur without arterial repair in some cases solely on the basis of collateral blood flow. In such cases, false aneurysms and arteriovenous fistulae may present as delayed manifestations of the acute injury. Since it is usually not possible to determine the irreversibility of ischemic damage by clinical means, repair of major blood vessel injuries should be performed even in questionable cases if support is available. Although the entire limb might not be salvaged, a more distal level of amputation may result.

PRINCIPLES OF TREATMENT

Control of Hemorrhage

In most instances, hemorrhage from peripheral arterial and venous injuries can be controlled by a well-placed compression bandage. If a tourniquet must be placed as a lifesaving measure, it should be as distal as possible on the extremity and it should be tight enough to control both arterial and venous hemorrhage. Once applied, for control of arterial hemorrhage, the tourniquet should be left in place until removed by a medical officer, usually at the hospital in an operating room.

At the time of operation, direct pressure over the traumatized artery both proximally and distally by an assistant usually provides adequate temporary control of hemorrhage until direct control can be obtained with vascular clamps. An anatomical approach to provide adequate exposure to the injured vessels should be used regardless of the location of the wound. In large wounds, the ends of the artery may already be visible. In such cases, the severed ends can be controlled directly with clamps. When the vessel ends are not exposed, proximal and distal control is usually obtained through normal tissue planes by application of umbilical tapes, silastic loops, or vascular clamps. Intraluminal control using balloon-tipped catheters is also effective and is particularly useful in the repair of false aneurysms. These devices, originally developed and field tested during the Korean War, are available in combat zone hospitals.

Noncrushing vascular clamps should be used to control hemorrhage. If crushing clamps were placed under emergency conditions, they should be replaced with noncrushing clamps, and the crushed portion of artery should be resected prior to definitive repair. If noncrushing clamps are not available, atraumatic control can be achieved with double-looped cotton or silastic tourniquets or with Rummell tourniquets.

If an extremity arterial injury is distal enough to permit the use of a pneumatic tourniquet, a great deal of time and blood loss can be saved during exposure and control of the injured vessel. The tourniquet should not be inflated until it is actually needed, and it should be deflated as soon as the injured vessel is under control to allow flow through collaterals.

Debridement and Evaluation of Patency

After gaining control of the injured artery, rapid wound debridement is accomplished in the standard fashion. Excision of devitalized tissue should be complete, including any damaged artery. Debridement of the artery itself should be as conservative as possible. Only grossly injured artery should be excised. Although microscopic changes have been found in the normal-appearing artery adjacent to the obviously traumatized segment, there is no evidence that resection of normal-appearing artery on either side of an injured segment is necessary.

Distal arterial patency may be evaluated before repair by careful passage of a balloon tipped catheter. One cannot be certain of distal arterial patency based on the presence of or the rate of back bleeding, as back bleeding simply indicates patency to the level of the first major collateral. Only operative arteriography or reestablishment of distal pulses after repair can be considered proof of distal arterial patency.

The possibility of additional arterial injuries, either close to or at some distance from the recognized injury, should be considered and demonstrated either by intraoperative arteriography, if practical, or by direct exploration. Failure to repair a second arterial injury usually leads to a poor result regardless of the adequacy of repair of the initially recognized injury.

Conservative Management

Some arterial injuries may be treated in the acute stage without operation. When an artery is severed, there may be little or no external hemorrhage because of vessel retraction and arterial compression by an expanding hematoma within the associated musculofascial compartment. As the compartmental pressure approaches that in the damaged artery, hemorrhage stops and a stable pulsating hematoma develops. As encapsulation of the hematoma occurs, a false aneurysm forms. Some of these false aneurysms may be missed in the acute stages and will require repair when recognized later.

When both the artery and vein are injured, an acute arteriovenous fistula may result. Patients with well-established arteriovenous fistulae who present without secondary hemorrhage, and whose extremities are viable, have a low priority for operation in the combat zone. This is also true for pulsating hematomas when recognition of the arterial injury has already been delayed and viability of the limb has been preserved by collaterals.

One must use caution in electing not to operate emergently on the above-mentioned vascular injuries. When surgical capabilities are adequate, there is little justification for nonoperative management of arterial injuries. Delay of operation in hopes of development of a false aneurysm or arteriovenous fistula with concomitant adequate collateral circulation can be rationalized only when the capability to perform arterial surgery is nonexistent or marginal.

Surgical Repair

Lateral suture repair is suitable for small, clean-cut lacerations of large arteries. For larger tangential wounds, an autogenous vein patch should be used to prevent stenosis of the repair site. If damage to the affected artery is extensive or irregular, the damaged segment should be excised and continuity reestablished by end-to-end anastomosis or an interposition graft.

After the artery has been adequately debrided, noncrushing vascular clamps are applied at about one centimeter from each end of the transected vessel. At this point, it is determined if the ends can be anastomosed without tension. Undue tension must be avoided as it is likely to result in dehiscence and hemorrhage, or anastomotic narrowing and thrombosis. In any case, undue tension will doom the repair to failure. The surgeon readily develops judgment concerning the amount of tension which can be safely applied to a vascular repair. When too much tension exists, further dissection is carried out proximally and distally. A moderate amount of dissection may compensate for a defect as long as two centimeters but rarely for one longer than this. Branches of the damaged artery generally should not be sacrificed since this practice gains little length while at the same time sacrificing important potential collaterals—collaterals that could be of critical importance should the primary repair fail.

Direct anastomoses are most often performed using a running technique. A continuous suture is placed through the full thickness of the vessel wall with individual passes about 1.0 mm back apart and 1.0 mm from each cut end. In vessels the size of the radial, ulnar, or tibial arteries, an interrupted suture technique should be used. Although care should be taken to avoid pulling adventitia into the lumen as the needle passes from the outside to the inside of the vessel, it is not necessary to perform a formal excision of the adventitia, as doing so weakens the repair. To assure preciseness of coaptation, the vessel ends can be held in a constant relationship to one another by lateral stay sutures as the continuous anastomosis is performed. Synthetic monofilament vascular sutures of 5-0 or 6-0 on cardiovascular needles are most commonly used for venous and arterial repairs. Aortic injuries are more commonly repaired with 3-0 monofilament synthetic sutures. Braided arterial silk lubricated with sterile mineral oil or by passage through subcutaneous fat may be used if synthetic suture is not available, as may braided synthetic sutures with an external plastic coating which approximates the characteristics of a monofilament suture.

During repair, the lumen of the vessel should be inspected to assure that no local thrombi are present. If present, thrombi should be removed by flushing with heparinized physiologic saline (10 units/cc).

Small leaks from the suture line are usually controlled by pressure alone. Topical hemostatic agents, such as gelfoam, collagen powder or topical thrombin are also useful in controlling minor suture line leaks and leaks from needle holes. Larger leaks are best managed by carefully placed figure-of-eight or mattress sutures.

Management of Associated Injuries

Unstable fractures can compromise vascular repairs. Bone length should be regained and fractures should be rapidly realigned and stabilized prior to vascular repair. Internal fixation is contraindicated, because of the risks of infection. External stabilization by skeletal traction or rapidly applied external fixation devices should be utilized. Dislocations, which result in ischemia due to distortion or compression of the associated artery, should be reduced immediately.

Concomitant nerve injuries which may occur in association with any vascular injury are more common in the upper than in the lower extremity. Repair of nerve injuries is generally not recommended in the combat zone. If nerve ends can be found expeditiously, they should be tagged with a nonresorbable suture for delayed elective repair.

Injuries to major veins should be repaired whenever possible. This is particularly true of injuries of the iliac, common femoral, superficial femoral, and popliteal veins. Occlusion of these veins frequently results in significant edema and late sequelae similar to the post-phlebitic syndrome. In some instances, simple closure techniques such as lateral repair may be possible. In others, more complex repairs using panel or spiral vein grafts may be needed. In such instances, the greater saphenous vein from the opposite, rather than the ipsilateral, extremity should be used. Preservation of the ipsilateral greater saphenous vein preserves an important source of venous outflow, should the venous repair fail.

Choice of Conduit

When major arteries or veins require patching or replacement, the surgeon must decide which patch material or conduit to utilize. Conventional wisdom is that the greater saphenous vein is the material of choice. It should be harvested from the uninjured extremity whenever possible to avoid compromising venous outflow from the injured extremity and wound healing problems should an arterial repair fail and result in marginal ischemia. When the greater saphenous vein is not available, the lesser saphenous vein is the next best choice, as its histology is similar to that of the greater saphenous vein. Upper extremity veins are another available source of patch material or conduit, but have thinner walls and are thus more prone to degeneration and aneurysm formation. Neck veins should not be used because they are too thin walled to withstand arterial pressure. In the trauma setting, autogenous arteries and synthetic conduits should be used only under extreme circumstances, when no other vascular substitute is available. Synthetic conduits of all types are prone to infection. In the rare event that a synthetic conduit is needed, poly-tetrafluoroethylene (PTFE) is preferable to Dacron, as it appears to have a better chance of resisting and withstanding infection.

POSTOPERATIVE CARE

After arterial repair, the injured limb should be kept at or slightly above the level of the heart. If the extremity has been flexed, gradual extension over a period of several days is encouraged to avoid development of a contracture. Equinus deformity of the ankle is prevented by assuring that the ankle is splinted in a neutral position. Active muscle exercises are begun in the early postoperative period. As soon as other injuries permit, ambulation is encouraged and progressively increased.

When arterial continuity has been restored in situations where there is questionable viability of muscle tissue, the patient must be observed closely for (1) a decrease in urinary output, which is evidence of acute renal insufficiency; (2) increasing temperature and pulse rate as evidence of wound infection; and (3) increasing pain, confusion, fever, and tachycardia. These latter signs of toxicity may be evidence of clostridial myositis. Myoglobinuria may result from muscle necrosis. Development of any of the above are indications for debridement of necrotic muscle or for early amputation of a clearly nonviable extremity. If the vascular repair fails, but none of these complications develops, amputation of the nonviable extremity can be deferred until a clear line of demarcation is established.

If fasciotomies were not performed at the time of arterial repair, the patient must be carefully observed for development of a compartment syndrome. Fasciotomy should be seriously considered at the time of arterial repair when there has been a concomitant major venous injury, when there has been a delay of greater than six hours between arterial injury and repair, when there has been an associated crush injury or muscle maceration, and when significant edema is already present at the time of operation. Therapeutic fasciotomies should be performed at the first clinical evidence of an increase in compartment pressures as manifested by loss of previously present pulses, or the development of paresthesias or anesthesia in the distribution of the major nerves supplying the affected part. In the upper extremity, additional clinical signs suggesting the need for fasciotomy include pain on passive motion of the fingers and thumb, and spasm of the wrist and finger flexors leading to a persistent flexion attitude of these structures. In the lower extremity, the first nerve to suffer is the deep peroneal, as manifested by pain on passive motion of the ankle and great toe and decreased sensation in the dorsal web space between the great toe and the second toe.

If compartment pressures are measured, a pressure between 30–40 mm Hg should increase one's vigilance and should lead to fasciotomy if signs and symptoms develop. A compartment pressure greater than 40 mm Hg represents a recognized indication for fasciotomy. In the lower leg, adequate decompression of all four compartments can be obtained through two incisions. One posteromedially-placed incision is used to open the superficial and deep posterior compartments. A second incision placed anterolaterally is used to open the anterior and lateral compartments. The vertical skin incisions should measure 10–12 cm in length and should be left open for delayed primary closure or skin grafting, if necessary. The fascia can be opened all the way to the ankle using either a fasciotome or scissors.

Fasciotomy of the forearm and hand requires four incisions. Two are placed vertically on the dorsum of the hand between the second and third and the fourth and fifth metacarpals, respectively. A third incision is placed vertically on the dorsum of the forearm. The final incision is used to decompress the flexor compartment of the forearm and the palm of the hand. This incision is a lazy-S which starts on the proximal ulnar forearm, curves across to the radial flexor forearm, returns to the ulnar forearm, then extends to the mid-palm just ulnar to the thenar crease.

ADJUNCTIVE THERAPY

Intravenous broad spectrum antibiotic therapy should be initiated as soon as possible after injury. This should be continued throughout the operation and for roughly 24 hours thereafter, assuming there is no continued source of contamination. In most instances, a cephalosporin provides effective prophylaxis.

Anticoagulation of the distal arterial tree is acceptable during operation, but one must be aware that, because of collateral flow, locally injected heparin ultimately becomes systemic. For this reason, relatively small doses of heparin (1500–3000 units at a concentration of 100 units per cc of physiologic saline) are used for anticoagulation of a lower extremity. Systemic anticoagulation is usually not advisable because of the presence of associated injuries. There is rarely, if ever, an indication for postoperative anticoagulation. Adjunctive agents, such as low molecular weight dextran, may be used and may be of value particularly after small artery repairs; however, dextran must be used with caution to prevent volume overload. In most instances, vascular repairs will be successful if the tissues are adequate, the repair is done well, and the hemodynamic and volume status of the patient are kept within normal limits postoperatively.

Although preoperative arteriograms are rarely available in the combat setting, single-shot hand-injected intraoperative arteriograms can be easily obtained and are helpful to rule out additional arterial injuries, distal thrombosis, and inadequacy of the repair. Injection of full-strength contrast (Radio-Conray 60) through a 19 gauge needle usually results in an excellent study.

Fifteen to 20 cc is usually all that is needed. The film should be exposed while the contrast material is still being injected. At times, run-off may be so rapid that the contrast is washed out by the time the film is exposed. Should this occur, a second injection with inflow occlusion will usually provide adequate visualization. Sympathetic blocks and sympathectomy are of no value in the management of acute arterial injuries. Sympathectomy, as a delayed procedure, may occasionally be helpful to the patient who has had a suboptimal result from arterial repair.

COMPLICATIONS

The most serious of the common complications after repair of arterial injuries are infection and hemorrhage. Infection of a wound harboring an arterial repair frequently results in disruption of the suture line or degeneration of the conduit used for revascularization. Either may result in life-threatening hemorrhage. Secondary repair should not be attempted within the infected wound site. Occasionally it may be possible to bypass the infected wound and revascularize the extremity using an extraanatomic route. In other instances, this will not be possible, and proximal and distal arterial ligation with removal of the infected conduit will be required. This will, of necessity, result in a high percentage of amputations.

Thrombosis at or distal to the vascular repair is another potential complication. It may be necessary to perform a second operation in the early postoperative period if thrombosis occurs and viability of the limb is threatened. However, if limb viability is maintained by collaterals, additional operations in the combat zone should be avoided, as repeated operations under field conditions are followed by a higher incidence of infection which jeopardizes life as well as limb. If chronic arterial insufficiency develops, secondary vascular operations should be performed electively at a higher echelon of care.

A limb that is profoundly ischemic after arterial injury may develop ischemic contracture. This complication can be prevented if perfusion is restored within a reasonable period of time. When circulation is restored, muscle groups may swell, necessitating fasciotomies to prevent compartment syndrome and small vessel occlusion, which can cause myonecrosis even in the presence of a successful arterial repair. These changes are most prone to occur in the flexor compartment of the forearm and in the anterior compartment of the leg. Under some circumstances, prophylactic fasciotomies, as discussed earlier, may be indicated to prevent delayed development of compartment syndrome.

RESULTS

Prior to the Korean conflict, major vascular injuries were routinely treated by arterial ligation. This resulted in a 50% amputation rate. Combat zone arterial repairs, rather than routine amputation, were first accomplished in Korea. This practice was continued in Vietnam, where thousands of arterial repairs were performed. Amputation rates after acute arterial repair were lowered to 13.7%. Popliteal arterial injury continues to be associated with a higher amputation rate. Rapid evacuation and resuscitation of the wounded in future conflicts should continue to result in high rates of salvage of both life and limb.

CHAPTER XIX

Wounds and Injuries of Bones and Joints

The frequency of extremity injuries in combat invariably generates significant numbers of bone and joint injuries. These injuries may be closed (simple) but are usually open (compound). Closed injuries are treated as they might be under other conditions, with the exception that elective surgical procedures should not be performed in forward medical facilities. The management of the open injury begins exactly as for open soft-tissue injuries (Chapter XVI). The immediate objectives in the treatment of these injuries are the preservation of neurovascular function and the prevention of infection. Complete wound healing and return to full function constitute the long-term goals. Staged wound management consisting of thorough debridement and delayed wound closure will convert an open injury to a closed injury in a high percentage of cases. Historically, failure to adhere to this basic principle of management has consistently yielded an unacceptably high incidence of infection and has frequently resulted in catastrophic functional loss.

GENERAL PRINCIPLES

The forward surgeon should manage open injuries of bones and joints according to the following general principles:

1.   Evaluation. One must initially determine the extent of the wound and of the structures involved. In high-velocity missile wounds, tissues and structures at some distance from the actual wound tract may be damaged and require debridement.

2.   Prophylaxis. Parenteral antibiotic treatment and tetanus prophylaxis should be initiated at the earliest opportunity. In

general, broad spectrum antibiotic coverage for both Gram-negative and Gram-positive organisms is recommended. Since all open war wounds are contaminated and present a risk of developing tetanus, all of these individuals should receive a 0.5 cc IM tetanus toxoid booster injection. Antibiotics and tetanus coverage should never be construed as a substitute for adequate wound cleansing and debridement.

3. Debridement. Generous incisions should be the rule. Such incisions permit better exploration of the wound, facilitate removal of foreign material (clothing, soil, vegetation, accessible metal fragments), and allow more complete excision of all devitalized tissue. In general, small, detached bone-chip fragments should be removed, but major in situ fragments with significant soft tissue attachments should be retained. Copious irrigation of the wound, with pulsatile lavage if possible, is mandatory. Properly performed debridement provides the basis for prevention of infection and the success of all future treatments, including reconstructive surgical procedures. Definitive surgery, primary closure of wounds, relaxing skin incisions, and nerve and tendon repair have no place at this stage of treatment.

4. Arthrotomy. Penetrating joint wounds require arthrotomy irrigation, thorough surgical exploration, and debridement.

5. Vascular repair and fasciotomy. These are the only appropriate definitive procedures performed at the time of initial wound surgery. Vascular injuries should be addressed through "wounds of election" and fasciotomies should be routinely performed following vascular repairs. If possible, an attempt should be made to cover the vascular repair with viable soft tissue; however, the wound should be left open.

6. Leave wound open. Perhaps the most important principle after debridement of war wounds is to leave the wound open. Bleeding points are controlled, but otherwise no attempt at wound closure is made, and drains are usually not necessary.

7. Nonocclusive dressing and immobilization. The wound is covered with a sterile, bulky, nonocclusive dressing and the extremity appropriately immobilized by plaster splints or a plaster

cast which is immediately bivalved. In some cases, external skeletal fixation may be utilized.

8. Documentation. It is important to document in the medical record all operative findings, particularly vascular, neural, tendon, or muscle damage, in addition to the more obvious skeletal injury. This information is vital to subsequent care providers as the patient progresses through the evacuation chain. If a plaster dressing is used, this information can also be briefly documented with a marking pen on the plaster itself.

Adherence to these general principles at all treatment levels will substantially enhance the likelihood of functional recovery and minimal morbidity.

MANAGEMENT BY FIELD MEDICAL PERSONNEL

The combat medic's main objective in the initial management of the casualty is to do no further harm and to evacuate the patient rapidly to a definitive treatment center. Wounds are covered with sterile dressings and hemorrhage is controlled by local compression. Rarely, a tourniquet may be necessary but normally should be avoided. If used, the tourniquet should not be released before arrival at a definitive surgical facility. Extremities with fractures should be gently aligned and splinted; no attempt should be made to reduce these injuries. Fluid replacement should be initiated.

MANAGEMENT AT THE FORWARD HOSPITAL

Following resuscitation, antibiotics should be started immediately according to the principles outlined in Chapter XI.

At operation, a properly applied tourniquet is a definite aid in locating and controlling sites of major hemorrhage. Attention to accepted tourniquet usage principles is mandatory. In almost every case, the tourniquet, if used, should be released after two hours. It is also an absolute necessity that any tourniquet used during the procedure be released at the conclusion of the procedure prior to dressing to ensure appropriate hemostasis. Wound debridement should be carried out through generous incisions generally in the long axis of the extremity, avoiding the crossing of flexion creases at right angles.

Incisions should be planned such that the option to extend them is maintained. One should attempt to place the incision such that later reconstructive surgery is not compromised. The full extent of the wound including the deep fascia, should be widely exposed to facilitate the complete removal of foreign material, devitalized muscle, and other nonviable tissue (Chapter XVI). Small fragments of bone without soft-tissue attachment should be discarded, but larger fragments, particularly those contributing to length and circumferential integrity and those with significant soft tissue attachments, should be retained. Large, completely detached fragments should be cleaned thoroughly and replaced as near to their anatomical positions as possible. The wound should be copiously irrigated with pulsatile lavage containing an antibiotic solution whenever possible. Irrigation is an extremely important aspect of wound debridement, and with major injuries should optimally consist of approximately 10 liters of solution. Vascular repairs are accomplished as indicated in the acute phase, but nerve and tendon repairs should not be performed at this stage of treatment of battlefield casualties.

As has been said, the wound must not be closed. No attempt should be made to effect wound coverage. Relaxing incisions, pedicle flaps, or any other definitive plastic type of wound approximation techniques are contraindicated at this time.

The wound should be dressed with a single layer of fine-mesh gauze followed by bulky fluffed gauze, then wrapped. Packing of the wound, which impedes drainage and capillary flow, should be avoided (Chapter XVI).

FRACTURES

In the early stages of treatment, certain principles of war wound management should be adhered to:

1. The neurovascular status of all injured extremities must be accurately established and recorded.

2. All open fractures require open debridement and irrigation.

3. The fractures should be reduced and aligned as accurately as possible and initially splinted in some fashion. As previously stated, the neurovascular status of the extremity must be established and care must be taken not to compromise the vascular status of the extremity. If fracture reduction results in circulatory

insufficiency, the fracture must be repositioned and/or the cause of circulatory insufficiency delineated. Biplanar radiographs are desirable to optimally treat any fracture. It should be kept in mind that the primary objective in management of extremity wounds is to optimize the situation such that early wound healing can be obtained, infection prevented, and function restored.

4. Internal fixation of fractures resulting from war wounds is generally contraindicated in the initial stage of wound management. While there are some exceptions, this should be considered a generally universal principle. Fractures in extremities where vascular repairs have been performed are no exception; past combat experience has demonstrated that traction or other forms of external immobilization can be utilized with vascular repairs. The addition of internal fixation material to a wound containing a vascular repair results in an unacceptably high risk of infection and breakdown of the vascular repair.

5. Fractures can be stabilized by the use of splints, circular dressings, pins incorporated in plaster casts (Figure 25A), or external fixators (Figure 25B). An external fixator should only be applied only by a surgeon familiar with its indications, application, and potential complications. The fixator can be extremely useful in the management of large open wounds in which there has been considerable bone or soft tissue loss or where vascular repair is to be performed. The advantages in these types of situations are rapid application, ability to maintain length and position, the ease of access to the wound for dressing changes and repeat wound debridement, and control of pain because of the stability provided. The rigid fixation attained frees adjacent joints that would be immobilized in plaster casts and eliminates the additional weight of the cast, allowing crutch ambulation or transportation in a sitting position in many patients who would otherwise be litterbound. Additional uses are the control of hemorrhage in displaced pelvic fractures, and the care and mobilization of patients with humeral, pelvic or femoral fractures with associated chest or abdominal wounds. Sufficient rigidity can be obtained in most long-bone fractures with the use of a single frame configuration, consisting of one longitudinal bar attached by two or three pins distal and proximal to the fracture, to allow early care and transportation. The use of half-pins, which pass through the soft tissues on one side to engage the bone but do not penetrate the soft tissues on the opposite side, minimize the risk to adjacent nerves, vessels,

and muscles. Predrilling the bone with a drill bit and daily local pin care minimize the complications of pin loosening and pin tract infection.

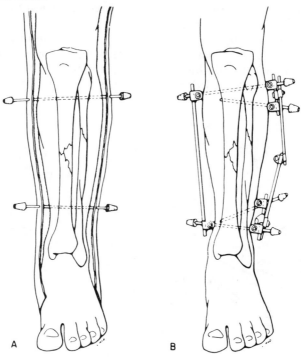

FIGURE 25.—External fixation of fractures. A. Pin and plaster technique. Cast must be bivalved. B. External fixator.

6. A circular plaster dressing (cast) is applied for immobilization of the joints above and below a fracture. Once applied it must be immediately bivalved to the skin. A monovalved cast has no place in the early treatment of a combat casualty. Bivalving the cast for transportation and evacuation is mandatory. Plaster casts should be marked with identifying information pertinent to the underlying injury and the date of cast application for use during transit and by receiving personnel. In general, plaster splinting is inadequate for anything other than temporary field immobilization. If a spica cast is constructed, one should avoid making the cast much wider than a standard litter; this will facilitate movement during medical evacuation.

7. When skeletal traction is employed, Steinmann pins are

preferable to Kirschner wires. They can be easily incorporated into the plaster cast for evacuation and are less likely to bend. In
general, the larger diameter pins should be utilized to prevent
loosening and pin traction infection. Incorporation of traction
bows into the cast is unnecessary.

8. Fractures of the humerus or injuries to the shoulder girdle,
with or without brachial artery repairs, are best transported in a
Velpeau dressing with the extremity strapped across the chest; a
"sling and swath" can be substituted if necessary (Figure 26).

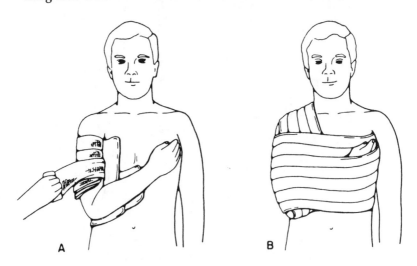

FIGURE 26.—Immobilization of upper extremity. A. Position of arm and forearm.
B. Immobilization effected by binding arm to chest.

9. Elevation of an injured extremity facilitates venous return
and minimizes swelling. Ice, when available, can also be applied
in the early injury phase to help control swelling and make the
patient more comfortable. The neurovascular status of the extremity should be carefully monitored after treatment, and in injuries of both the forearm and the leg the surgeon must be constantly alert to insure early recognition of compartment
syndrome.

10. When plaster casts or splints are utilized, particularly in the
patient with impaired sensation, vigilance must be maintained
to prevent skin breakdown from excessive cast pressure. Complaints of pain under the cast must not and cannot be ignored.
Patients in spica casts should be turned at intervals to prevent

pressure sores over the sacrum and other bony prominences. Cast pressure can be minimized by the use of properly padded and applied plaster.

11. The possibility of fat embolization should be considered in all patients with long-bone fractures. This is particularly true in patients developing signs of cerebral or pulmonary dysfunction. Adequate oxygenation is fundamental in the treatment of fat embolism syndrome and frequently requires the use of mechanical ventilation and positive-end-expiratory pressures. At the present time there is no hard evidence that validates the efficacy of intravenous alcohol, heparin, or steroids in the treatment of this primarily respiratory syndrome. Treatment consists of supporting the patient's respiratory function.

12. Preferred regional splinting is as follows:

a. The shoulder joint and humerus, depending on the injury, can be splinted or immobilized in several manners. As previously noted, a sling and swath or Velpeau-type of dressing is satisfactory for many injuries. A well-padded, plaster shoulder spica for more significant injuries provides better support during transportation. The shoulder spica cast is extended to include the forearm but not the wrist. An external fixator applied on the lateral aspect of the humerus with half-pins is a useful alternative to the shoulder spica or in those with associated chest wounds.

b. The elbow joint and forearm is normally immobilized with a plaster cast, with the elbow at approximately 90° of flexion and the wrist and forearm in a neutral position. The plaster extends from the proximal palmar crease to the axilla. A sling or a collar and cuff should be used to support the cast and will increase patient's mobility and comfort.

c. If the injury is limited to the wrist itself, the plaster extends from just below the elbow to the proximal palmar crease (short arm cast). The wrist should be held in a position of approximately 30° of dorsiflexion. If the thumb is incorporated, it should be positioned such that the digits can oppose the distal thumb. The hand should be immobilized with the metacarpal-phalangeal joints flexed and the interphalangeal joints extended when possible. An unaffected digit should not be incorporated into the splint or dressing. An external fixator or pins incorporated in a short arm plaster cast are especially useful to prevent shortening in severely comminuted fractures and those with bone loss.

d. To immobilize the hip joint or a femoral fracture, a

bilateral plaster spica extending from the axilla to the toes on the affected side can be used. The knee should not be immobilized in hyperextension nor should it be immobilized beyond 10-15° of flexion. The spica extends to just proximal of the knee on the unaffected side. When the spica includes the foot, care must be taken that the normal arch of the foot is maintained and that the foot is not held either in inversion or eversion. When a cast includes the toes, plaster must be trimmed away on the dorsum of the foot to a point just proximal to the base of the toes, thereby permitting the toes to move freely and protecting them from further injury. This precaution permits periodic evaluation of the distal neurovascular status. An external fixator applied on the lateral aspect of the femur with half-pins is especially useful in open femoral fractures. In fractures of the pelvis or hip associated with abdominal or perineal injuries, a pelvic frame alone, or one attached to a femoral frame, greatly aids nursing and wound care.

e. To immobilize the lower leg and ankle extend the cast from the groin to the toes. The knee is immobilized with slight flexion avoiding hyperextension or full extension. The foot is placed in neutral dorsiflexion (at a right angle to the leg). The same care is taken with respect to the foot as was described in the paragraph above. A single frame applied to the anterior tibia with half-pins allows mobilization of the ankle and knee with crutch ambulation, while maintaining length and easy wound access.

f. A plaster cast for the foot and ankle is applied from just below the knee to include the toes as previously described (with the foot in neutral). Care must be taken that excessive pressure is not placed on the peroneal nerve which courses just below the lateral aspect of the fibular head.

13. Joints not immobilized should be actively exercised on a frequent basis.

JOINT INJURIES

A penetrating wound of a joint has a high potential for infection which can often be avoided or at least minimized by appropriate surgery. In addition to the previously described techniques of wound surgery, the following specific principles are applicable to open joint injuries:

1. For all penetrating injuries of a joint, a formal arthrotomy

is required. While this sometimes can be accomplished through the actual wound itself by extending it as necessary, a separate standard arthrotomy incision may be required. The extremity should be draped in a manner that allows movement of the joint as necessary to facilitate exposure. Arthrotomy should be done as soon as possible after injury in an operating room. If applicable, the use of a tourniquet is recommended.

2. All loose bony fragments, detached or badly damaged cartilage, foreign bodies, clots, and devitalized tissue should be removed. Biplanar radiographs are desirable.

3. The joint should be thoroughly explored utilizing appropriate retractors.

4. The joint should be copiously irrigated with an antibiotic-containing solution, utilizing pulsatile lavage when possible.

5. The wound should be left open. The same principles apply to joint injuries as to open fractures with respect to wound closure. Depending on the degree of contamination, it may be possible to close the synovium leaving the capsule or soft tissue open. However, closure of the synovium is not absolutely necessary provided an occlusive dressing is applied.

6. If the synovium or capsule cannot or should not be closed because of joint contamination, the open joint should be dressed carefully with a single layer of fine-mesh gauze and followed by fluffed gauze and a wrap. Depending on the degree of damage of the articular surface, appropriate immobilization may be instituted. Early motion should be considered in those injuries where the joint surfaces are not significantly involved.

7. Penetrating wounds of the lower abdomen and pelvic area should be evaluated carefully for involvement of the hip joint. Any evidence that the hip has been penetrated requires arthrotomy, exploration, irrigation, and drainage. Frequently these procedures coincident with the abdominal operation. Posterior arthrotomy may be necessary to adequately accomplish the surgical goals; care should be taken with respect to the posterior blood supply of the femoral head.

8. Joint injuries thus treated should be dressed and immobilized as previously delineated for fractures.

COMPARTMENT SYNDROME

Compartment syndrome in the leg and forearm is a potentially devastating complication. The pathophysiology is at the microvascular level, and failure of early recognition of the syndrome can led to severe functional loss or amputation. The surgeon must have a high index of suspicion. An open fracture does not necessarily decompress the compartments and in fact, because of the high energy associated with the injury, may increase the risk of such a syndrome. The classic findings of pain, paralysis, pulselessness, and paresthesia usually present is too late to successfully intervene. Patients with significant trauma, who have been treated and splinted but continue to have unremitting pain in the involved extremity, particularly with passive motion of the digits, should be considered to have a compartment syndrome until proven otherwise. Compartment syndromes are progressive problems that may develop insidiously, thereby requiring repetitive examinations of the extremity. Diagnosis is clinical and the treatment is decompression, i.e., surgical fasciotomy. Appropriately-timed fasciotomy makes the difference between amputation and a viable extremity.

REDEBRIDEMENT AND WOUND CLOSURE

After the wound has been debrided, irrigated, and appropriately dressed, it is not inspected for 4-10 days unless the clinical course dictates an earlier appraisal. Intervening dressing changes are not indicated unless the clinical course indicates that there is continued hemorrhage, vascular changes, or infection. This inspection of the wound should be performed in the operating room. At that time, if there is significant devitalized tissue or purulent drainage, redebridement is accomplished. If the wound is clean and without evidence of infection, a delayed primary closure is performed. The wound should not be closed with undue tension, nor with extensive development of flaps. Wounds that cannot be easily closed should be dressed for subsequent split-thickness skin grafting at the next echelon of surgical care. Any wound closed by the delayed primary technique should be followed carefully for evidence of inflammation or infection. If signs of infection develop, the wound should be reopened. If the patient is not to be retained at the forward hospital so that he can be followed for several days, it is advisable to defer delayed primary closure to those personnel in the evacuation chain who are able to provide proper continuing follow-up.

INFECTED BONE OR JOINT INJURIES

Early medical evacuation from the battlefield provides access to the casualty before frank infection has developed. However, if the tactical situation is such that infection has already occurred, emergency operation is still indicated. Wide exposure is accomplished for excision of devitalized tissue, removal of foreign bodies, and drainage of purulent material. The wound is irrigated copiously, and systemic broad-spectrum antibiotics are utilized until an infecting organism has been identified and sensitivities determined. The use of suction irrigation as a technique in infected fractures and septic joints is somewhat controversial. Caution must be used to avoid systemic toxicity when continuous antibiotic irrigation is employed.

SPRAINS AND DISLOCATIONS

Ligamentous injuries (sprains) are frequently encountered in the combat zone. These injuries do not have the inherent seriousness of penetrating missile injuries of joints as previously described, but they may be severe and disabling in terms of combat effectiveness. Support of the joint by bandaging, splinting, or casting usually will facilitate healing. The use of immobilization and casting, particularly for lower extremity injuries, may allow the individual soldier to return to limited duty.

Closed dislocations of joints, which are encountered less frequently than sprains, are usually more disabling. Dislocated joints should be considered a surgical emergency and the joint should be reduced as soon as possible. This reduction can usually be carried out without the administration of anesthetic, with the possible exception of the hip and knee joint dislocations. The distal neurovascular status of the extremity should always be checked both before and after reduction. The post-reduction radiographs are extremely important to insure complete reduction and to rule out the presence of iatrogenic fractures.

CHAPTER XX

Wounds and Injuries of Peripheral Nerves

The majority of war wounds affecting the nerves do not require immediate operation. While soft tissue, bony, and vascular injuries associated with the neural lesion require emergency exploration, neural repair, if indicated, can be carried out electively. There are, however, important exceptions to this rule.

High-velocity missile injuries to nerves in combat are generally not neat and sharp. The nerve, if not directly transected by the projectile, is stretched by cavitation forces but remains grossly intact. Early on, there is no way to determine intraoperatively whether to resect such a lesion. Early repair of nerves transected by penetrating missiles is not satisfactory because of the difficulty associated with deciding how far back to trim the injured nerve before reaching potentially healthy fascicular tissue. As a result, acute repair under these circumstances runs the risk of anastomosing contused tissue of questionable viability. With time, however, the damage to the nerve stump will be delineated so that the amount of proximal neuroma or distal glioma requiring resection will become obvious. Ideal timing for such repairs is 2–3 weeks after injury. If a transected nerve is found during the course of debridement and/or repair of other non-neural injuries, it is best to "tack" stumps down with non-resorbable monofilament suture, to adjacent tissue planes and to place each stump at a different level. This maintains length, an important consideration since most nerves will retract after transection. By placing the stumps in different planes and, wherever possible, away from acutely repaired or traumatized vessels, tendons, bone, or muscle, neuroma formation is prevented. Sling sutures, holding the stumps together until an elective repair can be performed at a later date, are to be discouraged, since they tend to produce neuromas. These neuromas, when they occur, will require resection that often produces a larger gap than if the stumps had been left to retract. Placing the nerve stumps in a setting free of other traumatized or recently-repaired tissues minimizes the development of scar around the stumps and tends to reduce the subsequent length of required resection.

It is important to obtain a baseline neurologic assessment of the limb. The following questions must be answered: What nerve(s) is involved? What is the distribution of motor, sensory, and autonomic loss? Is the loss complete or incomplete distal to the level of the lesion? Partial losses which represent incomplete lesions tend to recover spontaneously with time, whereas complete losses probably will not, and will usually require surgical intervention. Electromyography (EMG) and conduction studies will not be of help in the first few weeks after injury since the Wallerian degenerative process takes time to produce deinnervational changes, at least for major nerves.

The suspected in-continuity lesion should be observed over time to see whether clinical or electrophysiological improvement is demonstrable prior to exploration and intraoperative evaluation by stimulation and recording of nerve action potentials (NAP). During this follow-up period, it is important to maintain motion in the injured extremity to prevent joint stiffness, tendon shortening, and pain. It is especially important to close soft-tissue wounds associated with neural damage as soon as practical so that physical therapy can be initiated early. There is no indication for putting the paralyzed or partially paralyzed limb, or the non-repaired nerve, to continuous rest. If devices such as cock-up wrist splints are used to keep the limb in a position of function, they should be dynamic and, whenever possible, removed several times a day for range of motion (ROM) exercises to the limb. If a splint or cast is necessary because of concomitant fracture(s) or acute vascular or tendon repair, then the joints both proximal and distal to the immobilized portion of the limb must be put through a full ROM at least three or four times per day. This is especially important for joints that have lost their innervation, for these tend to freeze or stiffen much more readily than normally innervated joints. ROM is also necessary for the limb with a bluntly transected nerve, since disabling joint stiffness can occur as early as two weeks after injury.

MISSILE WOUNDS LEADING TO ANEURYSM OR ARTERIOVENOUS FISTULA COMPLICATING NERVE INJURY

An expanding mass in the shoulder and arm, the presence of a thrill and/or a bruit, and progressive loss of function with severe pain should alert the clinician to this possibility. The pain is almost like true causalgia with burning paresthesia and electric shocks, but usually presents without automatic manifestations. The patient, unlike the individual with true causalgia, usually permits manipulation of the distal extremity. To be accurate, traumatic aneurysms are usually pseudoaneurysms arising from dissection of blood into and around the vessel wall. Thus, angiography may not demonstrate extravasation of contrast or filling of the aneurysm. When this diagnosis is suspected, immediate exploration is indicated. At exploration, an aneurysmal mass or, in a few cases, a fistula will be found compressing and stretching neural elements. This situation is especially common when axillary or posterior popliteal vessels are involved.

BLOOD CLOT OR SIGNIFICANT SOFT TISSUE CONTUSION

Occasionally missile wounds are associated with significant clot. If the clot is confined to a closed space incorporating neural elements, progressive loss of function can occur. Such closed spaces include the popliteal and knee spaces, the anterior compartment of the lower legs, and the buttocks, especially in the subgluteal space. Similar closed spaces in the upper extremity include the elbow and forearm, either beneath the lacertus fibrosis and pronator musculature, or the more distal forearm muscles. Immediate decompression and drainage are indicated for clots in these areas, while fasciotomy is indicated for extensive contusions which have resulted in a swollen, tight extremity. Nerve damage, muscle necrosis, fibrosis, and limb contracture can occur. A Volkmann's contracture, for example, can result in loss of median, radial, and sometimes ulnar function.

SHELL FRAGMENTS OR OTHER FOREIGN BODIES IMBEDDED IN NERVE AND ASSOCIATED WITH SEVERE PAIN

Shell fragments or other foreign bodies imbedded in nerve are associated with severe pain. An occasional patient will have a shell fragment come to rest within a neural element causing severe pain and paresthesia. Relatively immediate surgical removal of such an intraneural foreign body may ameliorate the pain or, failing this, may permit better control with analgesics or by a combination of Tegretol (Carbainazepine) and Elavil (Amitriptyline HCL).

TRUE CAUSALGIA

Causalgia is a severe burning pain, often associated with autonomic changes and typically relieved by sympathetic block. Aggressive management is usually required. While vasoconstriction and dryness with trophic changes of skin and nails are more common later on, vasodilation of skin vessels and hyperhydrosis predominate initially. The pain is all consuming and the patient does not tolerate the least bit of manipulation of the affected extremity. In the combat situation, close to 50% of true causalgia presents within hours to several days after wounding. This pain pattern is invariably associated with incomplete injury to a nerve, typically the median or posterior tibial. Analgesics and even narcotics provide only minimal relief. Early sympathetic blocks with a local anesthetic are preferred. If the pain pattern is relieved but then recurs despite repetitive blocks, surgical sympathectomy is indicated. Other lesser pain patterns can be treated fairly successfully with pharmacological agents, at least in the early stages.

SHARPLY TRANSECTED NEURAL ELEMENTS

Historically, close to 40% of nerve injuries cared for by the military during war have not been directly related to combat. These represent clean-cut transections of nerves by glass or sharp metal edges. These should be definitively repaired at an early date. Soft-tissue wounds due to sharp injuries and associated with complete paralysis of one or more nerves need to be closed in any case.

If, during such closure, the sharply transected and noncontused nerve stumps with neatly divided epineurium are located, there may be some advantage to acute (primary) repair. Stumps will not have had time to retract, anatomy is straightforward, and a repair under minimal tension can be readily carried out. The surgeon must have had some experience with nerve repair. The necessary instruments include magnification Loupes, a bipolar coagulator, and 6-0 suture. The surgeon should be willing and able to take the time to do a careful repair. Acute repair of transected elements is of special value for sharp transections of brachial plexus elements and the sciatic nerve where delay and secondary repair oftentimes require the use of nerve grafts because of stump retraction and scar formation.

CHAPTER XXI

Amputations

The prime indication for amputation is the preservation of life, i.e., the sacrifice of the part in order to preserve the whole. Three factors influence the decision to attempt salvage of a severely traumatized limb: the extent of the extremity injury, the general condition of the patient, and the experience of the surgeon. Every effort should always be made to save a limb. However, experience has shown that a severely disrupted extremity provides the potential for sepsis and causes a far greater drain on the patient's limited resources than does amputation. The foregoing notwithstanding, conservative surgical management of an injured extremity should always be the rule. Such management includes prompt institution of antibiotic therapy, early repair of vascular injuries, prompt debridement, and postoperative immobilization. Even under unfavorable tactical situations, every effort should be made to control hemorrhage and minimize the likelihood of infection prior to resorting to amputation. The judgmental decision to amputate should compare the risk to life associated with attempts to preserve a limb as compared to the realistic likelihood of ultimate reconstruction of a functional extremity. It is always desirable to secure the opinion of a second surgeon before amputating.

Amputations for trauma are of two types: elective and emergent. Near the front, essentially all amputations are of the emergency type. In the great majority of these emergent amputations, the surgeons simply complete a traumatic amputation by achieving hemostasis and debriding the stump. They are indicated to save life and are performed at the lowest level of viable tissues to preserve limb length. After one has performed adequate debridement of skin, muscle, and other devitalized tissues, thereby converting the injury to a clean surgical wound, the decision to amputate or attempt to retain a viable limb frequently becomes self-evident. In upper extremity injuries, especially those involving the hand, as much viable tissue as possible should be retained for subsequent reconstruction. Reasonable attempts should also be made to preserve the knee and elbow joints, even when their preservation results in extremely short stumps. Emergency amputation is rarely the definitive surgical procedure, as subsequent stump revision is usually required prior to prosthetic fitting. It should be kept in mind that long bone fractures and joint dislocations can cause elevated compartment pressures that, if allowed to progress unnoticed, can result in limb necrosis and subsequent limb loss.

INDICATIONS

The following are clear indications for emergency amputations:

1. Massive injuries in which the components of an extremity are so badly mangled that the extremity is obviously nonviable.

2. Extremities with severe involvement of skin, muscles, and bone with an anesthetic terminus and irreparable nerve damage.

3. Overwhelming local infection, which, despite adequate surgical measures and antibiotic therapy, endangers life.

4. Established death of a limb (vascular gangrene), where vascular repair has failed or has proved to be impractical.

5. Massive septic gangrene (clostridial myositis) is a most compelling indication for amputation. Anaerobic cellulitis or myositis confined to a single muscle group can be managed by resection and is not an indication for amputation.

6. Secondary hemorrhage in the presence of severe infection, even though initial wound surgery apparently may have been adequate. Included in this group are patients in whom the tactical situation precluded adequate early surgical intervention.

TECHNIQUE

In all amputations, the limb should be prepped and draped such that circumferential operative access is provided. When practical, the limb is kept elevated while prepping and draping to salvage as much of the distal venous blood as possible. A tourniquet is indicated, when practical, to prevent additional blood loss.

LEVEL OF AMPUTATION

The level of amputation is determined by the nature and extent of the injury. Amputations should be performed at the lowest possible level of viable tissues. All viable skin and soft tissues distal to the indicated level of bone amputations should be preserved for use in subsequent closure of the amputation stump. This is especially true for amputations below the knee, in which short tibial stumps can be saved with posteriorly-based flaps. Surgical principles concerning the construction and dimensions of viable flaps should be tailored to the specific need for each patient. To save length, any shape or form of a viable flap should be used.

OPEN CIRCULAR TECHNIQUES

The open circular amputation, as described below, is the most acceptable type for combat conditions:

1. A circumferential incision is made through the skin and deep fascia at the lowest viable level. This layer is allowed to retract without further dissection (Figure 27A).

2. The muscle bundles exposed are then divided circumferentially at the new proximal level of retracted skin edge. The incised muscle bundles will promptly retract, proximally exposing the bone beneath (Figure 27B).

3. The soft tissues are then manually retracted proximally to facilitate bone transection at a still higher level (Figure 27C). Periosteum should not be stripped. This technique has the appearance of a cone with the apex directed proximally.

4. The blood vessels are divided between clamps and are ligated as they are encountered. In addition, a transfixing suture is added to the cuff of large arteries. The artery supplying the sciatic nerve may require separate ligation. Temporary pressure, bone wax or thromboplastin is applied to the open medullary cavities of large bones to control oozing when necessary.

5. Major nerves are transected 2–3 inches above the amputation at the highest possible level *without resorting to traction*. Nerve stumps are neither ligated nor injected with alcohol or other chemical agents, but may be injected with a long-acting local anesthesic agent to reduce pain during the postoperative recovery period.

6. Since the amputation has been performed because of irreparable damage to a contaminated, if not grossly septic, extremity, the stump is never closed primarily.

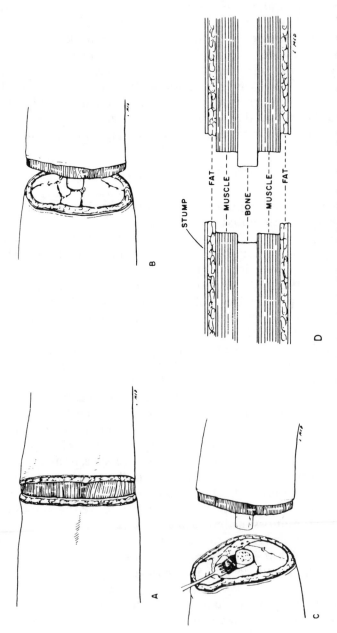

FIGURE 27.—Technique of open circular amputation. A. Circular incision of skin. B. Section of the muscles at the level of retracted skin. C. Section of the bone at the level of retracted muscles. D. The resultant surgical wound has the appearance of an inverted cone.

DRESSINGS

A layer of sterile fine-mesh gauze soaked with betadine is placed over the wound, and the recess of the stump is dressed loosely with fluffed gauze or other suitable material. A stockinette for skin traction is then applied to the skin above the open stump. A liquid adhesive (benzoin tincture) to prevent slippage of the stockinette is used. The stump is wrapped with gentle compression, decreasing proximally, and 5–6 pounds of traction are applied with weights and pulleys or with a self-contained traction device (Figure 28). Constrictive wrapping at or above joints must be avoided. Traction should be reapplied after dressing changes and maintained continuously.

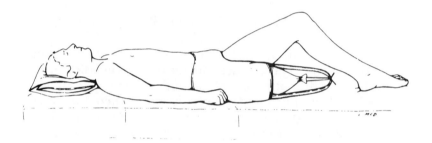

FIGURE 28.—Self-contained traction device incorporated into a plaster cast facilitates evacuation.

The amputation with preserved flaps requires individualized dressing consideration. The flaps should be held in their intended position by the dressing, although the major area of the amputation should be left widely open. No element of the flap should be suspended loosely within the dressing. No tacking sutures should be used. If possible, traction should be applied on the remaining skin elements and not on the flap.

POSTOPERATIVE MANAGEMENT

To prevent flexion contracture of the hip following transfemoral amputations, the patient should be kept in the prone position as much as possible until he has become familiar with active range of motion exercises. When he lies supine, sandbags should be used to hold the stump in position. A tourniquet should be readily available for emergency use during the first 5–7 postoperative days. It should be loosely attached to the bed or to the litter during evacuation.

Prior to amputation, or as soon as the patient becomes conscious postoperatively, the patient should be counseled that he will experience both normal and painful sensations in the phantom limb. This counseling is critical to allay apprehension and prevent fear which can drain the postoperative patient's energy for recovery. There is frequently severe causalgia-like pain in the end of the residual limb which subsides with healing. The patient should be told that this is normal and will subside soon. Adequate pain medication should be provided as required for stump pain.

STUMP WOUND CLOSURE

The timing and the method of wound closure require as great a measure of surgical judgment as did the original decision to amputate. Delayed primary closure is not indicated in open circular amputations. Continued traction will often result in the skin eventually closing over the end of the stump. If it does not, small split-thickness skin grafts can be used. A definitive revision may be necessary later, but it can be performed at higher echelons which permit immediate fitting techniques, thereby allowing more rapid prosthetic application. Delayed primary closure too often results in a chronically inflamed, edematous, indurated, and sometimes draining stump that is unreceptive to prosthetic application.

TRANSPORTATION

Traction ideally should be continuous throughout the evacuation chain. A customized traction device may be fashioned by incorporating a wire ladder splint into a cast. Rubber tubing between the wire ladder splint and the stockinette provides the traction.

GENERAL PRINCIPLES

Certain principles in the management of amputations in the forward area merit additional emphasis:

1. Amputations are performed to save lives.

2. Amputations are performed at the lowest possible level of viable tissue.

3. An obviously useless extremity should be amputated as early as possible.

4. There is no ideal or standardized level of amputation in the forward area.

5. All amputations should be left open.

6. Cold injury, per se, is not an indication for emergency amputation.

7. During evacuation, continuous traction should be provided to the amputation stump to prevent skin retraction.

8. Patients should be counseled regarding stump and phantom pain. Adequate medications for stump pain should be provided.

PART IV

Regional Wounds and Injuries

CHAPTER XXII

Craniocerebral Injury

CLASSIFICATION

Craniocerebral injuries are classified according to the type and extent of injury sustained by the scalp, the skull, and the brain and whether the injury is open or closed.

TABLE 11.—*Classification of craniocerebral injuries*

Scalp		Skull	Brain	
Open:	puncture laceration avulsion	depressed fracture comminuted fracture linear fracture	*Open*:	penetrating injury
Closed:	contusion		*Closed*:	diffuse parenchymal injury focal intracranial hematomas: extradural subdural intracerebral

In open injuries, the scalp may be punctured, lacerated, or avulsed. In closed injuries,the scalp is not penetrated but is almost always contused.

Skull fractures are classified as linear, comminuted, and depressed. If open, they are termed compound. It is rare to have comminuted or depressed skull fractures without an overlying scalp laceration. It is important to determine whether fractures cross the meningeal vascular markings or the dural venous sinuses of the skull and whether they involve the paranasal sinuses or mastoid air cells. The depth of fracture depression should be measured on tangential X-ray views.

Brain injuries are classified as open (with penetration of the brain) or closed. The category of closed injury encompasses focal intracranial hematomas (extradural, subdural, and intracerebral) and diffuse parenchymal injury. Various combinations of scalp, skull, and brain injuries often coexist.

MECHANISMS OF INJURY

An understanding of the mechanisms and pathophysiology of injury is necessary for successful treatment. The mechanisms of injury can be divided into the primary events occurring at the time of impact, and the secondary events that develop over subsequent hours to days (Table 12).

TABLE 12.—*Mechanisms and pathophysiology*

Primary:	
Open: transection, disruption	*Closed:* diffuse parenchymal injury: shearing of axons disruption of capillaries

Secondary:
  intracranial: hematomas, edema, seizures, loss of cerebrovascular autoregulation, waves of increased intracranial pressure.

  systemic: hypoxia, hypotension, hypercarbia, electrolyte imbalance.

Primary open injuries disrupt neurons, glia, and blood vessels. *Primary closed* injuries produce parenchymal damage through the shearing of axons and capillaries, particularly in the white matter, and through small pectechial hemorrhages. These may coalesce over the first week after injury into delayed focal hematomas.

Secondary brain injuries occur as a result of systemic and intracranial processes following the primary brain injury. The brain can be protected from secondary injury by prompt recognition of such systemic events as hypoxia, hypotension, hypercarbia, hyponatremia, and other forms of electrolyte imbalance. Secondary injury of intracranial origin can be reduced by the prompt detection and treatment of hematomas and of waves of intracranial pressure elevation that accompany loss of cerebro-vascular autoregulation, cerebral edema, seizures, and infection.

The causes of death after head injury can be divided into those occurring in the acute phase within a few hours of injury and those occurring in the subacute phase within a few days of injury. In the acute phase, massive sympathetic and parasympathetic discharges give rise to cardiac arrhythmias, low cardiac output, and respiratory difficulties due to ventilation/perfusion mismatches.

Patients who survive the immediate effects of coma-producing injury develop a hyperdynamic cardiovascular and metabolic condition caused by a preponderance of sympathetic overactivity. Cardiac output is often elevated to twice normal by a combination of arterial hypertension, a reduction in systemic vascular resistance, and tachycardia. The metabolic rate of the body is increased to 1.5 times normal. This state lasts 5–10 days. Dehydration therapy for the purpose of preventing cerebral edema may lead to cardiovascular collapse and should be avoided.

Death in the subacute phase is usually due to the enlargement of an intracranial mass in the form of a hematoma or parenchymal swelling. In response to increasing intracranial pressure, the temporal lobe(s) herniate through the tentorial notch, or the cerebellar tonsils herniate through the foramen magnum, causing damage to the cardiovascular and respiratory centers. The time required for casualty evacuation and triage results in the majority of neurosurgical care being delivered in the subacute phase of injury. Initial care is directed toward the prompt recognition, treatment, and prevention of secondary injuries, particularly those due to hypoxia and to focal intracranial hematomas. Definitive neurosurgical treatment is best carried out by specialist teams in fully-equipped hospital facilities.

HISTORY AND NEUROLOGICAL EVALUATION

The history should record the time of injury, the type of missile or cause of injury, and the state of consciousness immediately after injury. It is very important to make permanent records of all observations for physicians elsewhere in the evacuation chain to review. The examination should begin with evaluation of consciousness. Consciousness can be described qualitatively with the terms conscious, (awake, aware); lethargic, (conscious, but with slowed reactions); stuporous (arousable only by painful stimuli); and comatose (unarousable).

1. The neurological condition may be expressed quantitatively with the Glasgow Coma Scale (GCS), in which numerical scores quantitate to the best level of motor, verbal, and eye-opening response to standardized verbal and tactile stimuli (Table 13). Coma in the GCS is defined as absence of verbal response (V = 1) and eye-opening (E = 1), with a motor response that can vary from none to localizing (M = 5). A summed GCS of 7 or less, six hours after injury, in a patient with adequate blood pressure and ventilation, indicates severe brain injury. Survival and neurological outcome are accurately predicted by the GCS score.

2. The pupillary size and response to light should be recorded. Progressive dilation of a pupil indicates an expanding intracranial mass and transtentorial herniation that in 85% of cases occurs on the side of the dilated pupil. The oculocephalic reflex, or eye movement in response to head rotation (doll's eyes reflex), should be recorded. Loss of this reflex indicates brainstem injury. Unilateral pontine injury will produce fixed deviation of the eyes to the contralateral side; frontal lobe injury will produce eye deviation to the side of the injury.

3. Motor responses should be tested in each limb. Asymmetries between right and left and between upper and lower limb strength should be noted. Abnormal (extensor) plantar responses should be sought.

4. Blood pressure, pulse rate and rhythm, respiratory pattern (waxing and waning or Cheyne-Stokes, irregular or gasping), and body temperatures should be recorded. Frequent recording of neurological status and vital signs on a time-oriented flow chart is very helpful in revealing neurological deterioration, particularly when patients are transferred from one echelon to another with suboptimal continuity of care along the evacuation route. Although the GCS correlates well with eventual outcome, it is only a shorthand for certain aspects of the neurological examination and does not substitute for detailed notes regarding the patient's condition.

TABLE 13.—*Glasgow Coma Scale*

BEST MOTOR RESPONSE		EYE OPENING		BEST VERBAL RESPONSE	
Obeys	6				
Localizes Pain	5			Oriented, Conversing	5
Withdraws	4	Spontaneous	4	Disoriented, Conversing	4
Abnormal Flexion	3	To Verbal Command	3	Inappropriate Words	3
Extension	2	To Pain	2	Incomprehensible Sounds	2
None	1	No Response	1	No Response	1

Add the scores for each category.

A total score of 7 or less indicates a severe injury.

The most common patterns for comatose patients are M = 5 or less, V = 1, E = 1.

X-RAY AND LABORATORY EVALUATION

Skull films should be obtained in the AP, right and left lateral views in order to localize fractures and fragments. The presence of an irregular area of increased or overlapped bone density suggests a depressed fracture, and a tangential X-ray should be obtained. Stereoscopic films can help localize intracranial fragments. Lateral shift of the pineal gland if calcified (rare in young individuals) can indicate the presence of an intracranial hematoma. Cervical spine fractures may occur in association with head injury, and cervical spine films should be obtained. The presence of an intracranial hematoma can be visualized by CT scanning, which should be available where definitive neurosurgical treatment is carried out.

Lumbar puncture with a 20 or 22 gauge needle, with 3–5 cc of spinal fluid removed for glucose cells and culture, should be performed if meningitis is suspected after a penetrating wound or after basal fracture with cerebrospinal fluid (CSF) leakage or pneumocephalus.

Frequent measurement of arterial blood gases, serum electrolytes, and osmolality are of great importance in management.

MANAGEMENT

Triage

Subtle changes in neurological condition or state of consciousness can be the first or even the only sign of impending intracranial disaster. On the other hand, apparent neurological
deterioration can be the first sign of systemic problems, such as
hypoxia or shock.

As a first step, the airway must be cleared and maintained, even
if this necessitates intubation or tracheostomy. Unconscious patients must not be transferred or evacuated without airway protection. Where there is hemorrhage into the upper airway, a cuffed
endotracheal tube is imperative. The use of low-pressure cuffs
obviates many problems.

Definitive neurosurgical management will rarely, if ever, be carried out at the front lines. Patients in extremis at the front line
will not usually survive, regardless of what treatment is given. Many
considerations will enter into the priorities of triage. As a rule,
thoracic, vascular, and abdominal injuries take precedence over
head wounds. Multiply-injured patients will require evaluation
and treatment by several surgical teams simultaneously. When faced with a number of evacuated but untreated head-injured patients, the neurological surgeon will be required to make initial
triage decisions on clinical grounds. Even the decision to send a
patient to CT scan implies a commitment to a certain level of treatment. Deteriorating casualties who are not moribund are treated
first. Alert patients with the potential to deteriorate are taken next.
Among the stable patients, those with obtundation are evaluated
before those who are awake. As a rule, head injuries are more
urgent than spinal injuries.

EMERGENCY MANAGEMENT

After the airway is protected, shock is treated or prevented by
placing two large-bore venous catheters and infusing plasma, normal saline, or lactated Ringer's solution. The stomach should be
emptied and the bladder catheterized. $NaHCO_3$, 1meq/kg is
given for metabolic acidosis, and should be administered empirically when respiration has been compromised.

In the face of neurological deterioration, some time can be gained to prepare for operation upon an expanding intracranial mass by administering furosemide, 40mg IV, followed by mannitol 1gm/kg. This will result in dehydration and must be carefully watched. The osmolarity should not be permitted to rise above 305 mOsm/l. Since the value of steroids is unproven, steroids need not be administered.

Anticonvulsant prophylaxis is begun with phenytoin, 1 gm IV push over 15-20 minutes. Cardiac arrhythmias may result from too rapid administration. If given as an IV solution, phenytoin must only be diluted in 50cc normal saline, and dripped in over 20 minutes. Any other solution of phenytoin will precipitate. A maintenance dose of 400 mg/day is required.

The use of narcotics or sedation in the spontaneously breathing patient is contraindicated.

Intravenous antibiotics are administered in meningeal doses for one week. Although the efficacy of prophylactic antibiotics has not been proven, the use of antibiotics in this setting is considered therapeutic and represents a full course of treatment for contamination of injured tissue and CSF by a foreign body. Which antibiotics to use will depend on local conditions and the types of organisms that are encountered in any given situation.

OPERATIVE MANAGEMENT

Operative Management of Open and Penetrating Wounds

Treatment is carried out in the following order:

(1) The head is shaved and the wound inspected. X-rays are examined to determine the distribution of bone and metallic fragments.

(2) Endotracheal intubation and general anesthesia are preferable in most cases. Adequate blood is made available for wounds near major dural venous sinuses.

(3) The scalp is scrubbed with an antiseptic solution, preferably an iodophor. The wound is copiously irrigated with 1-2 liters of sterile saline.

(4) The patient is positioned and draped so that entry and exit wounds are accessible and a contralateral burr hole can be made if needed. The head should be elevated slightly above heart level,

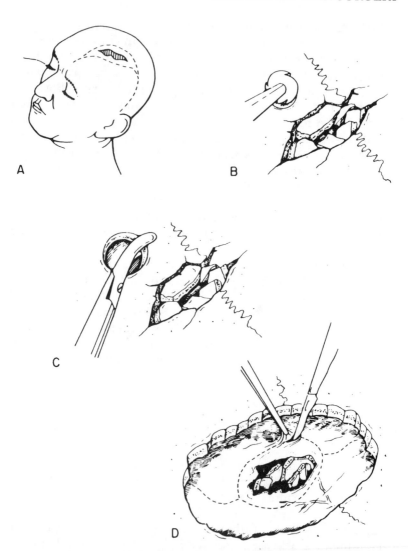

FIGURE 29.—Technique for debridement of head wounds. A. Conservative excision of devitalized skin and galea. B. Burr holes should be placed in intact bone adjacent to the area of damage. C. Bone is then removed by rongeur towards the area of contamination. D. Only minimal trimming of the dural edges is required.

to encourage venous return, but not so high as to risk air embolism.

    (5) Devitalized scalp and foreign bodies are removed. Incisions

are made along lines that can be utilized to rotate the scalp, should it become necessary to perform plastic repair of the scalp. As much scalp as possible is preserved (Figure 29A).

(6) Contaminated pericranium is removed. Burr holes are made in intact bone adjacent to the area of damage. A margin of normal dura is exposed. Bone is removed with rongeurs toward the area of contamination (Figure 29 B, C).

(7) Contaminated dura is removed, preserving as much as possible for closure (Figure 29 D).

(8) Damaged brain, blood clots, and foreign bodies are removed with gentle saline irrigation and suction. Removal of all bone fragments is of greater importance than removal of all metal fragments. The use of intraoperative ultrasound facilitates localization of fragments. The debrided track should remain open after debridement. Closure of the track suggests the presence of deeper or adjacent clot or necrotic brain tissue exerting pressure on the track (Figure 29 E).

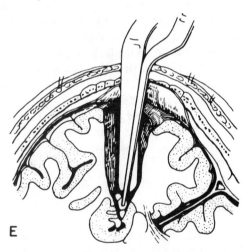

E

FIGURE 29.—Continued. E. All blood clots, devitalized brain tissue, indriven bone fragments, and visible foreign bodies are removed.

With high velocity injuries, there is more destruction at the wound of exit than the wound of entry, and debridement of the exit wound initially may provide the most rapid decompression. Complete hemostasis is accomplished before closure.

The brain is copiously irrigated with normal saline solution containing 1000u/l bacitracin at body temperature. A concentrated bacitracin solution (500u/cc) should be used to irrigate the track.

(9) Massive swelling of the brain is an uncommon but serious occurrence during operation that may represent the development of an intracerebral hematoma or a contralateral subdural hematoma. It may also represent an anesthetic complication or loss of autoregulation of the cerebral vasculature. After determining that there is no technical difficulty with anesthesia, swelling is treated in a stepwise fashion by increasing the ventilatory rate to obtain a $PaCO_2$ of about 25mm Hg, by tapping the ventricle and draining CSF, and by administering barbiturates. Pentobarbital sodium, 100–300 mg, is given intravenously. Additional doses of 100 mg may be required hourly. If the brain is swollen at the time of closure, an intracranial pressure monitoring catheter is placed, preferably intraventricularly, and the intracranial pressure is monitored in the post-operative period.

(10) The dura is closed without tension. Dural grafts may be harvested from pericranium, temporalis fascia, or fascia lata.

(11) The scalp is closed primarily without tension. Rotation of scalp flaps with closure of the secondary defect with split-thickness skin grafts or a myocutaneous pedicle flap may be necessary.

(12) Post-operative X-rays or CT scans are obtained to check for the presence of retained fragments.

(13) The need for reoperation for retained fragments is a difficult judgment call that requires much experience. It need not be done routinely if optimal follow-up neurosurgical and CT scan capability is anticipated.

Operative Management of Closed Injuries

A critical step in the management of closed injuries is the recognition of which patients require operation for evacuation of intracerebral hematomas that can cause, or are likely to cause, neurological deterioration. Recognition of the presence of hematomas may have to be made solely on the basis of deteriorating neurological status if intracranial pressure (ICP) monitoring and CT scanning are unavailable. The presence of fractures across venous channels or sinuses, the site of intracranial fragments, or a tangential wound of the skull may indicate the presence and location of an intracranial hematoma. Tangential wounds produced by high-velocity missiles should be evaluated carefully, as there is often extensive brain injury under the site of skull impact. If a compound depressed fracture has been produced by a tangential wound, a craniectomy should be performed and the dura opened to inspect for subdural or intracerebral hematoma.

If the presence of a hematoma is suspected, radiographic confirmation can be obtained by CT, cerebral arteriography, or ventriculography. Useful information can be provided by even the most simple form of arteriography, obtained by puncture of the common cartoid artery with a 18 or 20 gauge needle, injection of 10 cc of low concentration radiopaque contrast over 1-2 seconds, and exposure of a single AP X-ray film of the head. Ventricular puncture and injection of 5 cc of air can also be used to demonstrate shift of the midline of the brain.

Intracranial hematomas that produce more than a 5 mm shift of the midline or similar depression of the cortical or cerebellar surface should be evacuated, as such hematomas are capable of producing neurological deterioration. Evacuation of acute subdural and epidural hematomas will require a craniotomy. A large fronto-temporal-parietal flap can be elevated quickly and provides good exposure of the cerebral convexity. If exploratory twist-drill holes or burr holes are made prior to a craniotomy, aligning the skin incisions should be done so that they can be extended into a craniotomy incision. The frontal burr hole is placed at the mid-pupillary line and 1 cm anterior to the coronal suture; the temporal hole is made at the pterion (junction of the frontal, parietal, temporal squamosal, and sphenoidal bones).

Non-operative, Intensive Care Unit Management of Closed Injuries and Post-operative Patients

The goal of management is the prevention of secondary brain injury due to systemic and intracranial causes. Good pulmonary care is essential. How long intubated patients can be maintained before performing tracheostomy will depend on the respiratory care facilities available. In some cases, intubation can be maintained for one or two weeks without tracheal damage.

Feeding should be started via nasogastric tube as soon as bowel sounds are present. As high a caloric intake as can be accomplished without producing fluid overload is desirable. Arterial hypertension should be controlled with hydralazine and beta-blocking antihypertensive drugs if blood pressure becomes greater than 160 mm Hg systolic. Arterial blood gases, serum osmolality, electrolytes, and hemoglobin should be monitored daily, or more frequently as needed.

Prevention of secondary damage due to intracranial swelling and herniation can be accomplished most easily when the intracranial pressure is monitored. This may not be practical in the combat environment. A rising intracranial pressure indicates either (1) the expansion of a hematoma, (2) the late development of a hematoma, typically intracerebral, or (3) the presence of brain swelling. Expanding hematomas should be localized and evacuated. Brain swelling should be treated with a series of steps listed here in order of increasing complexity:

(1) Repositioning the patient to avoid neck vein compression. In general, a flat position or slight head elevation will minimize the intracranial pressure.

(2) Correction of hypoxia and hypercarbia; hyperventilation to achieve a $PaCO_2$ of about 25 mm Hg.

(3) CSF drainage via ventriculostomy.

(4) Administration of mannitol 1 gm/kg, IV.

(5) Other pharmacological measures to reduce intracranial pressure, such as lidocaine infusions or the induction of barbiturate coma, may be of benefit but should only be considered if optimal neurosurgical ICU support is available.

PROGNOSIS

The prognosis of craniocerebral injuries is good in patients who are not deeply unconscious, who respond to simple commands, and who do not deteriorate. In any head-injured patient who shows signs of deterioration, it must be determined whether or not this deterioration is due to a problem requiring surgical intervention. The prognosis is grave in patients who are rendered immediately comatose and who remain in a state of unconsciousness for a long period of time. Any improvement in the neurological condition of the acutely injured patient is significant. Restlessness and return of voluntary activity are phases which many head-injured patients go through as they recover.

CHAPTER XXIII

Maxillofacial Wounds and Injuries

The management of maxillofacial injuries is divided into immediate, primary, and reconstructive phases.

1. In the immediate phase the establishment and maintenance of the airway and control of hemorrhage have the highest priority. Appropriate protective dressings are applied and hydration is maintained. The institution of antimicrobial therapy in this phase contributes to minimizing the incidence of subsequent infection.

Penicillin is the drug of choice. If there is a question of penicillin allergy, clindamycin is an excellent alternative.

2. The primary phase consists of early definitive surgical repair of the wound and is accomplished at the first primary care facility to which the casualty is evacuated. Treatment performed during this phase of management significantly influences the subsequent requirement for or the magnitude of bony as well as soft tissue reconstruction and, therefore, the ultimate long-term functional and cosmetic outcome. Generally, both hard and soft tissues are conservatively debrided. Repair begins with reapproximation and fixation immobilization of fractured bones, application of intraoral devices, reestablishment of dental occlusion or intermaxillary ridge relationships, and finally, primary closure of intraoral mucosa and overlying soft tissues wherever possible.

3. In the third or reconstructive phase, the tertiary care center attempts to correct deformities, such as malocclusion, and to obliterate defects with grafts or prosthetic devices. Ideally, treatment is carried out in specialized units staffed by dental, oral, and plastic surgeons who work in close cooperation with specialists in otolaryngology, ophthalmology, and neurosurgery. At least 25% of casualties with maxillofacial injuries also have injuries of the head and neck. In addition, dental laboratories should be available for the fabrication of dental appliances.

DIAGNOSIS

To be certain that wounds which are not obvious are not overlooked, patients with maxillofacial injuries require careful roentgenologic and local examination, including inspection and palpation. Cervical spine fracture must be ruled out by X-rays.

Both the injured and intact sides of the head and face are examined comparatively to detect contusion, swelling, emphysema, tenderness, areas of analgesia, and distortion of bony landmarks. The surgeon should examine particularly for asymmetry of the level of the eyeballs and the presence of diplopie, periorbital hematoma, and edema, all of which are indicative of orbital floor fracture. Otorrhea and rhinorrhea of cerebrospinal fluid origin indicate fractures involving the sphenoidal and ethmoidal bones of the tegmen. Temporomandibular joint function is noted, as is the integrity of the palate and buccal sulci and the alignment of the upper and lower teeth.

Wounds within the oral cavity suggest segmental dental alveolar fractures or damage to the body of the mandible. The open-mouth or so-called gagging facies usually is caused by fractures of the mandibular ramus or by condylar dislocation, but it may also result from a horizontal fracture of the maxilla, higher level midface fractures, displaced teeth, or hematoma formation around a posterior fragment of the mandible.

INITIAL MANAGEMENT

The problems associated with maxillofacial injuries are similar to those of other injuries; that is, maintenance of the airway, control of hemorrhage, reduction of fractures, prevention of infection, and maintenance of fluid balance. Special problems arise because of mechanical interference with breathing and swallowing. A patent airway and an adequate fluid and nutritional intake are difficult to achieve in many maxillofacial injuries because of the partial or complete obstruction of the respiratory or alimentary orifices.

If patients with maxillofacial injuries require sedation, narcotics must not be used until it is certain that there is neither associated intracranial injury nor a marginal airway. Tracheostomy may be required.

RESPIRATORY OBSTRUCTION

Respiratory obstruction in a patient with maxillofacial injuries may be due to several causes, as follows:

1. Blockage of the airway by accumulated blood and secretions or by loose objects, such as broken teeth or dentures.

2. Prolapse of the tongue, which occurs frequently with injuries, especially when acute avulsion of the mandibular symphysis has occurred.

3. Injuries of the hyoid bone and its attached muscles, with resulting loss of control of the tongue-hyoid complex.

4. Swelling of the tongue and soft palate.

5. Laryngeal spasm, which may be caused by anesthetic agents.

No time should be lost in reversing hypoxia, which can rapidly progress to death. The patient is positioned to permit drainage by gravity, and the airway is rapidly cleared of blood, secretions, foreign bodies, or whatever else may be blocking it. Direct vision and strong suction are necessary. In the event that these non-invasive maneuvers fail to immediately relieve obstruction, there must be no hesitancy to perform endotracheal intubation or cricothyroidotomy. In certain laryngotracheal crush injuries and other wounds which transect the trachea, it may be necessary to perform emergency tracheostomy. Cervical spine in-line control must be maintained during these maneuvers.

SHOCK AND HEMORRHAGE

Hemorrhage is temporarily controlled by digital pressure until permanent control can be achieved by clamping and ligation. Clamping must be done under full vision, not blindly, because there are numerous important anatomical structures in this area, the damage of which could be extremely serious. Ligation of the external carotid for regional control of hemorrhage is seldom necessary.

PREVENTION OF INFECTION

Because of the contiguity of the naso-oral passages and the per-forating nature of these wounds, maxillofacial wounds are doubly exposed to bacterial contamination. The mouth, pharynx, and nose are heavily populated by a variety of pathogens. All fractures in this region, except for fractures of the ascending ramus of the mandible, usually communicate with the internal mucus membrane wound and the external skin wound.

Antibiotic therapy must begin early and be maintained if serious infection is to be prevented or controlled. Oral hygiene, with particular attention to the teeth, is also necessary. Placement of a nasogastric tube for feeding in the immediate postoperative period in the presence of extensive intraoral wounds may be desirable.

INITIAL WOUND SURGERY

The surgical field is prepared as usual, ingrained dirt being removed by gentle scrubbing with a soft brush. The eyebrows are not shaved.

Debridement. Tissues should be handled very gently, with fine instruments. The blood supply of the facial tissues is so adequate and resistance to infection so high that only the most minimal excision of skin is necessary. From 1–2 mm of the wound edges are trimmed to be certain that noncontaminated, nonbeveled edges can be accurately approximated. The trimming is done with ophthalmic scissors or a sharp No. 15 blade. The remainder of the procedure is carried out with conservation of as much tissue as possible. No bone with retained periosteal or musculovascular attachment should be removed from the wound. Only that bone which washes freely away with copious irrigation should be removed.

Primary wound closure. Maxillofacial injuries furnish one of the very few exceptions to the general rule that soft-tissue wounds should not be closed at the time of initial wound surgery. Whereas primary wound closure of facial injuries is preferred to delayed primary wound closure, this policy does not pertain to associated wounds of the neck.

Ideally, treatment of these multisystem wounds is carried out by multidisciplinary teams that include otolaryngologists, ophthalmologists, neurosurgeons, oral surgeons, dentists or plastic surgeons. This sort of coordinated team approach allows surgeons of several different specialties to make diagnostic, prognostic, or therapeutic contributions during a single general anesthetic.

Closure, which must be accomplished without tension, is begun intraorally and proceeds outwardly. When the parotid duct is found severed, primary repair should be considered. If primary repair is not deemed practical, both the distal and proximal portions of the duct should be cannulated with a plastic catheter which is securely sutured to the buccal mucosa and retained in place for 5–7 days. When the proximal portion of the duct cannot be located or is missing, the cannula should still be placed into the depth of the wound prior to closure and brought out through the distal segment of the duct intraorally. If the distal segment of the duct is missing, the catheter should be brought out into the mouth through the mucosal wound repair in order to prevent or reduce the incidence of cutaneous salvary fistulae. The foregoing guidance is more difficult to apply with injuries of the submandibular gland because of its dependent position in the floor of the mouth and the likelihood that an injured duct will become stenotic. Extensive injury to the submandibular gland duct is often best managed by removal of the gland.

The repair of severed branches of the facial nerve, identified during wound repair, should be accomplished utilizing fine suture material and magnification. All branches proximal to a vertical line extending downward from the lateral canthus should be repaired primarily. When there is bone destruction as well as extensive soft-tissue damage, it may be necessary to suture the buccal mucosa to the margins of the skin to cover the fracture site. Watertight closure over a fracture is always desirable. The oral mucosa is closed with fine chromic catgut; otherwise, the finest nylon or silk, mounted on swaged needles, should be used. Skin sutures are introduced close to the cut edge and are placed not more than 3 mm apart. Temporary application of a pressure dressing may help to prevent edema and hematoma formation.

In rare cases, when a defect is so large that closure is impossible without tension or distortion, a flap may be used. All skin flaps must be carefully approximated and held in position by suturing without tension.

FRACTURE MANAGEMENT

After conservative debridement of bone fragments has been completed, any remaining exposed bone must be covered by soft tissue. A mandibular stump can be covered by suturing mucous membrane to the skin edge. If the oral cavity has not been excluded by watertight closure, the fracture site must be drained to the exterior for 2–5 days.

Only teeth which are completely loose or fractured teeth with exposed pulp should be removed. Firmly embedded teeth are left in situ, even if they are near fracture lines. Damaged teeth are useful for immobilization of fractures. Residual molar teeth in otherwise edentulous jaws are especially valuable for fixation. Although dead, carious, or loose teeth may cause infection, they should not be disturbed at this time.

Immobilization of the jaws is necessary for accurate reestablishment of occlusion as well as early union of fractures. It also facilitates the healing of soft-tissue wounds, limits the spread of infection, and prevents deformity.

Several methods of immobilization of the jaws are practical, as follows:

1. Application of commercially-produced archbars to the labial and buccal aspect of the maxillary and mandibular teeth with simple circumdental wires (Figure 30). Fixation is then achieved either with intermaxillary wires or elastics or both.

2. Any one of several other commonly described techniques; i.e., eyelet loops, continuous loops, and Risdon wiring.

3. In the edentulous situation, the patient's dentures may be fixed by circumferential wires in the mandible and by peralveolar pins or wires in the maxilla. The dentures may then be used as anchorage for intermaxillary fixation. If dentures are not available, other options, depending upon the situation and preferences of the surgeon, include open reduction and rigid fixation with a bone plate or similar device, or the application of an external biphase splint. Construction of individualized dental splints is seldom possible or indicated in a combat zone hospital.

4. When portions of the mandible have been avulsed, the external biphase splint is an excellent and expedient technique by which the mandibular segments may be retained in good position and alignment during healing. Other types of preformed or adaptable plating and bridging devices may be used, but they require

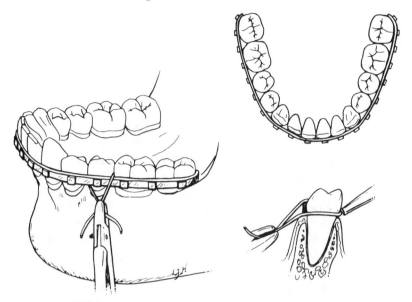

FIGURE 30.—Technique of archbar application to maxillary and mandibular teeth.

larger wound exposure and entail a greater risk of infection and therefore are not recommended for use in the combat zone.

5. Multiple and grossly comminuted fractures are most often best managed by closed reduction techniques.

POSTOPERATIVE MANAGEMENT

Patients without intermaxillary fixation may be given all ordinary fluids and soft foods which require little or no chewing. If intermaxillary fixation has been used, the diet, which must be thin enough to suck through a tube, should consist of such nourishing items as milk and milk products, any of several commercially available dietary supplements in liquid form, thin custards, and thick soups. Feedings should be at frequent intervals and in adequate amounts.

If it is necessary to protect the lips from the wires used in intermaxillary fixation, pieces of soft wax are useful. Lubrication of the lips and nostrils will help to prevent fissures and ulcers.

After repair of maxillofacial wounds, a pressure dressing is applied whenever possible and left in place for at least 48 hours. Sutures are removed on the fourth or fifth day.

REGIONAL FRACTURES

Fractures of the Mandible

Next to the nasal bone, the mandible is the most commonly fractured facial bone. Its weakest and most frequently fractured area is the neck of the condyle. Forces delivered to one side of the mandible often produce fractures of the opposite side, either at the condylar neck or at the angle, and forces directed to the chin often produce fractures at the condylar neck and parasymphyseal regions. Such fractures may, in fact, occur bilaterally and it should be remembered that nearly half of all mandibular fractures resulting from blunt trauma are multiple in nature.

Examination will reveal one or more of the following findings: restriction of the normal movements of the jaws, abnormal mobility of the jaws, crepitation upon manipulation, an open injury extending into the mouth, irregularities in alignment of the teeth, and abnormal occlusion. Swelling and bruises of the soft palate, fauces, and lateral wall of the pharynx are occasionally seen in severe fractures of the ascending ramus.

Primary treatment of mandibular fractures is dictated by a number of considerations, among which are the nature, location, and severity of the fracture and the condition of the existing dentition. Some of these fractures may be managed by dietary control only, others by closed techniques utilizing simple intermaxillary fixation, and some by open reduction and internal fixation. There is no indication for immediate bone grafting in the primary repair of mandibular fractures in the combat hospital.

FRACTURES OF THE FACIAL BONES

Zygomaticomaxillary compound fractures. Fracture dislocations involving the zygomatic bone are the third most common fractures of the facial skeleton. The zygoma forms the major portion of the lateral and inferior rims of orbit, as well as a portion of the orbital floor. Because of its complex articulation and the importance of the soft tissue structures attached to it as well as those which it supports, early reduction of these fractures is highly desirable.

Fractures of the zygoma will usually displace the lateral palpebral ligament inferiorly, and are often accompanied by an orbital floor fracture which produces enophthalmos and diplopia. Diplopia may also be caused by entrapment of the inferior extraocular muscles which restrict upward and lateral motility of the eye. Additional signs of this injury may include loss of cheek bone prominence, limitation of mandibular excursion due to impingement upon the coronoid process of the mandible by the depressed zygoma or fractured and depressed zygomatic arch, subconjunctival hematoma, sensory disturbance over the distribution of the infraorbital nerve, and a palpable bony step-off at the inferior and lateral rims of the orbit and at the lateral wall of the maxilla intraorally. Bleeding from the nostril on the injured side is frequently seen. Nose blowing should be avoided.

Special attention should be given to the eye examination. Direct ocular injury is occasionally observed, particularly hyphema, dislocated lens, retinal detachment, and rupture of the globe, which are all ophthalmologic emergencies. Occasionally many of the findings associated with this and other midface fractures are obscured by swelling, edema, and ecchymosis. Thus, a knowledge of the fracture combined with a careful clinical examination and a well-directed radiographic survey are all essential to an appropriate diagnosis.

Definitive treatment of this injury depends upon the nature and severity of the fracture. In a straight-forward and non-comminuted type of fracture, an incision over the zygomaticomaxillary region at the lateral brow is made. An appropriate elevator is passed behind and beneath the zygoma and the fracture is elevated and reduced. If stable, no interosseous wiring is necessary. An unstable fracture may require wiring both the frontozygomatic and rim fracture. Orbital floor exploration frees muscle or fat entrapped inferiorly after realignment of the fractures. Intermittent release of pressure to intraorbital tissue is mandatory. Methylmethacrylate globe protectors are preferred. Large floor defects are repaired with an implant of suitable material. Except in grossly complicated cases, the use of packing or an antral balloon in the maxillary sinus is seldom required.

Midface Fractures. Fractures of the middle third of the face most frequently are described as Le Fort I (horizontal), Le Fort II (pyramidal), and Le Fort III (craniofacial dysjunction). All result in disturbances of the dental occlusion and share certain similarities upon clinical examination. The distinction between and complexity of these injuries lie principally with the level within the midface at which fracture dislocation has occurred.

Le Fort I level fractures course through the lateral walls of the maxillary sinus, nasal fossa (including the nasal septum usually immediately superior to the floor of the nose), and the pterygoid process of the sphenoid bone posteriorly. The entire alveolar process of the maxilla containing the teeth, palate, floor of the maxillary sinuses and nose are mobilized. Upon clinical manipulation, all of these structures are mobile and, depending upon the magnitude of displacement, there will be varying degrees of malocclusion of the teeth. The fracture fragment is most often one mobilized segment, but occasionally may be fractured sagittally or into several segments. When this occurs, the ideal method of treatment is with an individualized palatal splint, application of maxillary and mandibular archbars, and intermaxillary fixation in centric dental occlusion. Sagittal and segmental fractures of the maxilla can be treated with intermaxillary fixation without palatal splints, and indeed on occasion must be so managed, but bony union and healing in malposition with significant malocclusion is a frequent sequella. Treatment for the Le Fort I level component rarely requires anything other than simple intermaxillary fixation. Blood accumulated in the maxillary sinus is ordinarily absorbed without incident. On rare occasions, additional suspension from a point above the level of the fracture may be required. A final inspection of the nasal septum is done and, if repositioning is required, it should be done at the time of primary repair.

The Le Fort II level fracture presents a more complex problem. Posteriorly, the fracture resembles that of the Le Fort I injury. Anteriorly it courses superiorly through the inferior rims of the orbits, often involving the orbital floors, then across the nasal bones separating them from the nasal process of the frontal bone. Frequently there is compounding into the anterior cranial fossa in the region of the cribriform process and crista galli of the ethmoid bone, with cerebrospinal rhinorrhea presenting as a part of the clinical findings. Clinical manipulation reveals mobility of the dentition and maxilla, which is transmitted to the infraorbital rims and to the junction of the nasal bones with the frontal bone. Periorbital ecchymosis and edema are usually more profound and the face may appear to be elongated. The latter finding results when the pyramidal midface fracture fragment is displaced superiorly in its anterior portion and inferiorly in its posterior portion. This type of anteroposterior rotational displacement in a counterclockwise direction, when viewed from the patient's right side, results in premature posterior occlusion, anterior open bite, and the appearance of increased vertical facial height.

Treatment of the Le Fort II fracture consists of repositioning the midface fragment and stabilizing it to the intact mandible by intermaxillary fixation. Depending upon the nature of the fracture, open reduction and internal wire or bone plate fixation at the infraorbital rims, implantation of the orbital floors, and appropriate suspension from a stable point above the level of the fracture may be required. If it is necessary to pack the nose for hemostasis in the presence of cerebrospinal rhinorrhea, the packing should be removed as soon as possible as it is a significant promulgator of infection, placing the patient at increased risk of developing meningitis. When cerebrospinal rhinorrhea is not at issue, nasal packing for support of fractures may be done if desired. In any case, the combination of intermaxillary fixation and nasal packing is ordinarily a clear indication for tracheostomy.

The Le Fort III fracture separates the nasal bones from the frontal bone, courses downward and backward through the medial wall and floor of the orbit, across the lateral wall and rim of the orbit, and posteriorly through the maxilla, zygomatic arches, nasal septal-ethmoid region, and pterygoid process of the sphenoid bone, thus producing a dysjunction of the facial skeleton from that of the cranium. Many of the findings and treatment considerations previously described for the Le Fort II fracture are shared by this injury, except that manipulation of the maxilla results in mobility of the midface which is transmitted to the junction of the nasal and frontal bones and at the lateral rims of the orbits.

Nasal-Orbital Ethmoid Fracture. Direct blunt trauma to the nasal region may produce fracturing and dislocation of the nasal bones and septum of varying degrees of severity. With increasing force of trauma, the resulting injury is often much more extensive. In the nasal-orbital-ethmoid fracture, the nasal skeleton is separated from the frontal bone and driven posteriorly into the interorbital region occupied normally by the ethmoid air cells. The medial walls of the orbits become laterally splayed into the medial portion of the orbits. With lateral splaying of the medial wall, the medial canthal ligament is likewise displaced or on occasion severed free.

Some commonly associated clinical signs of this injury are widening of the nasal bridge, increased intercanthal distance (normally about 34 mm in the adult white male), and an alteration in configuration of the medial palpebral fissure which has been described as "almond shaped." The injury is frequently accompanied by significant and sometimes massive edema and ecchymosis. Recognition and appreciation of the extent of the injury is therefore sometimes difficult. Evaluation by plain film radiography is often inadequate and more sophisticated studies are helpful, especially computerized axial and coronal tomography. In the final analysis, in most cases involving appreciable disruptions and displacements, accurate assessment and optimal repair are most often achieved by open exploration. The goals of treatment are:

1. Reattachment of the nasal skeleton, which is not infrequently comminuted, to the nasal process of the frontal bone.

2. Recontouring of the medial orbital walls (medial canthal ligaments are repositioned and fixed by transnasal wiring).

3. Stenting of nasolacrimal duct injuries with silicone tubing.

Superior-Orbital-Fissure Syndrome. Although uncommon in injuries of the face, direct trauma and fracturing into the orbit may produce hemorrhaging and encystation of blood or an extension of the fracture into the superior orbital fissure, impairing or directly traumatizing the III, IV, and VI cranial nerves which course through this fissure, resulting in ophthalmoplegia, ptosis of the lid, proptosis, and a fixed and dilated pupil. Sensory disturbances over the distribution of the ophthalmic division of the V cranial nerve, supratrochlear and supraorbital, complete the superior-orbital-fissure syndrome. In most instances, the treatment of choice is conservative. Ophthalmological consultation is indicated, and occasionally decompression is performed. Extension of the superior-orbital-fissure syndrome to include optic nerve involvement has been called the orbital-apex syndrome.

FRACTURES OF THE PARANASAL SINUSES

Frontal Sinuses

Simple nondisplaced fractures of the anterior and posterior walls of the frontal sinus require no specific therapy. If the anterior wall is depressed, open reduction and direct wire fixation are indicated. When the anterior wall is comminuted, it can be supported with packing material, such as medicated gauze or Penrose drains. The frontal sinus may be approached through the open wound or via a brow incision.

If the nasofrontal duct is destroyed, it will be necessary to remove the mucosal lining of the frontal sinus and obliterate the sinus, preferably with fat harvested from the abdomen. When the posterior wall of the frontal sinus is depressed and the dura is torn, resulting in CSF leak or spinal fluid rhinorrhoea, neurosurgical consultation should be sought.

Ethmoidal Sinuses

Partial ethmoidectomy may be required in the debridement of some wounds. If there is evidence of CSF rhinorrhoea, neurosurgical consultation is indicated.

Maxillary Sinuses

Simple effusion of blood into the maxillary sinuses is best left alone, as it usually is absorbed. If infection develops, nasal antrostomy and lavage is performed. Missile wounds of the maxillary sinuses are debrided through a Caldwell-Luc approach if foreign body removal is necessary.

Occasionally, it may be necessary to pack the maxillary sinuses for hemostasis or support of comminuted fractures; however, it should be borne in mind that such packing of the sinus is a source of infection that should be avoided whenever possible. All wounds and injuries of the paranasal sinuses should receive antimicrobial coverage. Empirically, penicillin is the antibiotic of choice.

EVACUATION

As previously discussed, the immediate priorities in the management of the maxillofacial casualty are airway, hemorrhage, and circulating fluid volume. Once the patient has arrived at the primary treatment facility and early definitive surgical repair of the injury has been accomplished, the considerations for movement of the maxillofacial casualty consist of the following:

1. The patient should be afebrile, without evidence of active infection, comfortable, and taking adequate nourishment by mouth.

2. If intermaxillary fixation is in place and there is not sufficient space (i.e., missing teeth) to permit autoevacuation of regurgitated gastric contents, a means of rapid removal of the fixation must be provided. At the minimum, the patient must wear scissors or wire cutters around the neck.

3. Antral and nasal packings and other drains, along with date of placement, must be clearly identified.

4. Indwelling IV catheters should be of a flexible polyethylene type, well secured, and labeled with the size and date of placement.

5. Tracheostomy tubes and cannulas:
   a. must be of proper size, and
   b. must be well secured in place with the faceplate of the outer tube sutured to skin.
   c. Instructions for humidification must be clearly written. Aircraft have notoriously low cabin humidity, and this and other instructions concerning tracheostomy care are critical.

6. If it becomes necessary to evacuate a patient who has required nasogastric suction at ground level, it will certainly have to continue to be observed during flight.

7. Cerebrospinal fluid leaks, not uncommon in maxillofacial war wounds, do not contraindicate evacuation, but increases in such drainages may occur at altitudes and it must not be impeded.

8. Clear, concise, legible orders must accompany the patient with special attention to:
   a. IV fluids
   b. antibiotics
   c. analgesics
   d. antiemetics

f. remaining packings, cannulae, drains, and tubes

g. diet

CHAPTER XXIV

Wounds and Injuries of the Eye

Under battlefield conditions, the casualty with an injured eye is usually seen first by nonspecialized personnel at a facility that has little or no specialized equipment. If his injury is minor, the soldier is treated and sent back to his unit. If it is not, he should be promptly evacuated. The distinction between minor and serious ocular injuries is not always easy to make. The most trivial-appearing injury may prove to be very serious indeed. If an injury of the eye is properly managed, a good result (or at least some salvage of vision) is often secured even in serious injuries. If improperly managed, a trivial penetrating ocular wound may be converted into a serious one; a large majority of these may result in blindness. All care providers must know how to detect, assess, and initially manage patients with eye injuries. The mandatory principles of initial management are presented in this chapter. In ophthalmic surgery, the first opportunity to repair an injury is usually the only opportunity. There is an inordinately high rate of ocular injury relative to the amount of surface area exposed to injury. Although comprising as little as 0.10% of total body surface and only 0.27% of the erect frontal silhouette, the eye is injured in nearly 10% of nonfatal casualties. The likelihood of ocular injury is further increased by various postures assumed in warfare. For example, although 25% of the projected body surface is exposed in the prone position, the eye comprises a considerable proportion of the prone silhouette. The recent introduction of laser technology to the battlefield will lead to a new class of ocular injury. These injuries are most likely to fall into two categories. The first category is that of thermal burns of the eyelids and cornea. The second category constitutes injury to the retina and vitreous body, leading to intraocular hemorrhage. Laser injuries of the eye are covered separately.

EXAMINATION AND DIAGNOSIS

As in any echeloned system of care, if the patient can communicate and combat conditions permit, an ocular examination should always begin by recording the circumstances of injury and the type of wounding agent. A penetrating ocular injury should be suspected in every wound of the eye and of the upper portion of the face until it is proved not to exist. The preliminary examination, should be conducted with the lids retracted, after loose foreign matter has been flushed out of the conjunctival sac with copious irrigations of plain water or physiologic salt solution or wiped out with a wet cotton-tipped applicator. Foreign bodies in contact with the eyeball should be removed from the lids. Since voluntary opening of the eyelids is often impossible, topical anesthesia (proparacaine hydrochloride 0.5%) and gentle lid separation with Desmarres retractors may be required for both vision testing and inspection. In the absence of available lid retractors, a pair of paperclips can be opened and bent into a curved blade configuration to serve as retractors, and any force required should be applied to the orbital bones, not the globe itself. The slightest pressure on the globe which has been lacerated or perforated may cause irretrievable loss of the vital contents.

Visual acuity, the most important parameter in evaluating the seriousness of the eye injury, should be recorded as follows: no light perception, light perception, perceives hand motions, counts fingers, or reads. In evaluating light perception, it is important to pass a very bright light alternately in front of and away from the eye. At the same time, the other eye must be completely shielded, and the patient must be questioned carefully to detect inaccurate responses. Spurious perception of light may result simply from the patient's natural desire to see, from an awareness of heat from the light, from a sensation of air movement on the skin produced by motion of the light source, or from incomplete shielding of the other eye. The other tests of visual acuity should be utilized with as much precision as circumstances permit.

It is imperative to inspect the anterior chamber of the eye with a bright light placed near the cornea and directed from the temporal to nasal side. A magnified view can be obtained by employing either a +18D refracting lens, or the high plus (black numbered) lenses on the ophthalmoscope. A marked deepening of the anterior chamber compared to the normal side, coupled with loss of the normal red reflex when the eye is illuminated and viewed in the axial direction, indicates the presence of a posterior segment penetrating injury which may be hidden and seemingly associated with only minor lid lacerations. These wounds may have actually perforated the lids and penetrated the globe. Additional findings on this inspection may include pupillary irregularities, blood within the anterior chamber (hyphema), shallowing, or even collapse of the anterior chamber, where loss of aqueous humor causes the iris to impinge directly against the posterior surface of the cornea. Lacerations of the eyelids, cornea, or sclera; foreign bodies within the eye or orbit; or disruption of the glove may be present. Gross contamination by dirt or other particulate matter frequently accompanies these injuries.

Corneal lacerations are usually evident by loss of the anterior chamber and distortion of the pupil. Iris incarceration or prolapse through the wound is common. Scleral lacerations often exhibit extruding, darkly pigmented choroid. However, small perforating wounds and even large scleral lacerations may be obscured by subconjunctival hemorrhage. More extensive prolapse of intraocular contents (vitreous humor, uvea, even lens and retina) may present within the lips of any laceration of the globe.

If the general appearance of the eye is undistorted and careful inspection reveals no site of ocular penetration, gross differences in intraocular tension may be estimated by *very gentle digital palpation*. The tips of the index fingers are used in ballottement of the globes through the upper, closed eyelids. First, test the tone of the unaffected eye, and then compare with that of the injured eye. Asymmetric tension is indicative of serious ocular injury to the softer eye.

Unless total disruption is evident, the possibility of salvaging the eye should be considered. This possibility exists even in the face of questionable light perception since vitreous hemorrhage alone may mask the perception of light. Since the advent of vitreous surgery, many eyes previously considered hopelessly damaged may now be salvaged. For this reason, the decision to enucleate any eye must be made by the most skilled specialist available. The principle goal of all others who manage the patient is to protect the eye from further damage.

MANAGEMENT

Minor Injuries

Minor ocular injuries which may be handled safely in the division area include laceration of the eyelids, subconjunctival hemorrhage, superficial foreign bodies, and corneal abrasions. Irrigation of the eyes and removal of superficial corneal foreign bodies may be performed under 0.5% Opthaine or Opthetic (Proparacaine hydrochloride 0.5%) or 0.5% Pontocaine (Tetracaine hydrochloride) anesthesia. A sharp-pointed instrument, such as a large needle or eye spud, should be used. The superficial abrasion left after the object is removed is treated by instillation of an antibiotic ointment and patching. If the particles are found to be multiple and more deeply imbedded than has been anticipated, the patient should be evacuated. Foreign bodies should be managed as previously described in the section on examination and diagnosis.

Subconjunctival hemorrhages associated with neither decrease of visual acuity nor blood in the anterior chamber (hyphema) or in the vitreous humor require no treatment. However, thorough ophthalmoscopy through a well-dilated pupil is necessary before returning the patient to duty. If blood is found in the anterior chamber or the vitreous humor, the patient should be placed on bedrest, with elevation of the head, monocular patches applied, and prepared for immediate evacuation.

Contusions of the eyelids and eyeball should likewise be examined carefully. If there is only subcutaneous and subconjunctival hemorrhage, without intraocular hemorrhage or disturbance of vision, the patient can be returned to duty.

Foreign body sensation, aggravated by blinking, and pain referred to the upper lid are characteristically found with corneal abrasion, which is usually a minor, but always painful lesion. Documentation by the use of a fluorescein strip, placed momentarily in the conjunctival fornix, may be diagnostically helpful. The abrasion can often be seen merely by focusing on the anterior corneal surface with + 8D and + 12D lenses (black numbers) using the conventional direct ophthalmoscope. The inner surface of the upper lid should be carefully examined for the presence of foreign bodies. This may necessitate careful eversion of the upper lid.

The treatment of ordinary corneal abrasions consists of: (1) cycloplegia, using two drops of either scopolamine hydrochloride 0.25-0.5%, cyclopentolate hydrochloride 1-2%, or homatropine hydrobromide 5%; (2) instillation of ophthalmic antibiotic solution or ointment; and (3) application of a tight patch to insure immobility of the eyelid. The patch can usually be discontinued in 24-36 hours, but repatching for another 24-36 hours may be necessary for larger abrasions. Lack of progressive improvement necessitates referral to an ophthalmologist. The use of topical anesthesia for other than facilitating vision testing, examination, or instrumentation is contraindicated. Repeated installation inhibits healing. Topical steroids or steroid antibiotic combinations are likewise contraindicated. Steroids are unnecessary and will cause rapid progression of a dendritic ulcer, including corneal perforation, should this lesion exist or supervene. Fungal superinfection and glaucoma may also result from injudicious use of topical steroids.

MAJOR INJURIES

Division Area—The management of ophthalmic injury begins as far forward as possible. Only first aid, including foreign body removal as previously discussed, is administered in these forward areas, and all significant casualties are evacuated to facilities where a physician is assigned. Early identification of ocular injury is an urgent matter. Serious eye injuries are second in priority of evacuation only to life-threatening wounds. In severe injury to the globe, inadvertent delay in ophthalmologic care can mean the difference between salvage and loss of the eye.

Any abnormality in the appearance of the eye injured by blast or fragmentation weapons, or by severe blunt trauma, demands the following course of action preparatory to evacuation:

1. Instruct the patient not to squeeze his eyelids.

2. Do not remove any penetrating foreign body protruding from the globe or the conjunctival fornices, as ocular contents may be extruded.

3. Occlude both eyes, but avoid any pressure directly on the eyes. The battle dressing tied around the head suffices.

4. Give systemic analgesics for moderate to severe pain.

5. Evacuate immediately as a supine litter patient to a forward

hospital, preferably with ophthalmology capability.

Where penetrating injury to the globe is suspected, the patient's eye can be protected from his own reflex lid squeezing by administration of a Nadbath block as follows: 1.0 cc of 2% xylocaine is injected using a 23 to 27 gauge needle no longer than 10mm. The area immediately behind the ear is palpated, and the needle is placed perpendicular to the anterior surface of the mastoid in the triangular space formed by the ear anteriorly, the mandible inferiorly, and the mastoid process posteriorly. The needle is advanced to the hub, delivering the anesthetic to the facial nerve as it exits the region of the stylomastoid foramen.

Ocular burns are usually first seen in the division area. Ultraviolet, thermal, and non-alkali chemical burns are treated as for corneal abrasions, However, non-alkali chemical burns require initial irrigation with tap water or saline solution for 10-15 minutes under topical anesthesia.

With white phosphorous burns of the eye, instillation of 0.5% copper sulfate solution identifies particles, which are otherwise presumptively located by foci of smoke or by darkening the particles. Larger particles may require removal with a needle or spud. The particles should be continuously irrigated to retard their further oxidation (reignition) and resultant tissue damage. These patients urgently require treatment by an ophthalmologist, in whose hands continuous irrigation with ophthalmic antibiotics in Ringer's solution may be performed by a percutaneous, indwelling, superior fornix angiocatheter, since severe edema of the lids often prevents the conventional administration of topical medication. Alkali burns may result from exposure to sodium hydroxide, lye, quick lime, ammonia, and agents often found in degreasing solvents. These burns represent an ocular emergency! Chemical penetration is so rapid that irrigation with copious volumes of water or sterile saline must be initiated within seconds. This irrigation must be continuous for at least 60 minutes. Irrigation should be continued until the pH remains below 8.0 for at least five minutes after irrigation ceases. An alkali burn is potentially devastating and prognosis may be poor, especially if the cornea appears cloudy or the conjunctive blanched. Atropine sulfate 1% and chloramphenicol ointments should be applied 3-4 times a day. Phenylephrine, which will further constrict blood vessels and worsen limbal ischemia, should not be used. Steroid ointment should be used only in the most severe burns and only during the first three days, as its use later may promote stromal melting. In an effort to reduce erosion of the corneal stroma when evacuation must be delayed beyond three days, N-acetyl-L-cysteine (MUCOMYST) may be applied by dropper in a 20% solution as frequently as each hour. Prompt evacuation is necessary.

Forward Hospital—In the absence of an ophthalmologist, treatment of major ocular injuries in forward hospitals normally is managed by the general surgeon and ideally is limited to interim measures aimed at prevention of infection within the eye. Systemic antibiotics and tetanus prophylaxis should be instituted at the earliest opportunity in the preoperative period.

Lid and conjunctival debris should be carefully irrigated away. Any sterile irrigating solution, including water, is acceptable. This should be followed by generous topical application of fresh solutions of an ophthalmic antibiotic (gentamycin sulfate, chloramphenicol or neomycin sulfate-polymixin B sulfate) and atropine sulfate 1%. A sterile, four-by-four-inch gauze strip is applied to keep the area clean, and additional protection is afforded by taping a Fox (or similar type) shield over the injured eye. A pressure dressing should be avoided as it may cause serious damage by expressing intraocular contents through a penetrating wound. Since patching also helps provide an excellent culture medium for bacteria, particularly *Pseudomonas*, topical antibiotic solution is carefully reinstilled every four hours, and a fresh, sterile gauze patch reapplied twice daily. Sterile irrigation of mucopurulent secretions from the lid margins and conjunctiva should be carried out when the gauze dressing is changed. The uninjured eye should be patched to reduce unwanted ocular motion.

No ocular surgery should be performed. Particularly, no attempt should be made to remove protruding or penetrating foreign bodies or to repair corneal or scleral lacerations. Preferably, no repair should be undertaken for lacerations involving the lid margin or the nasolacrimal apparatus. Even an eye which appears grossly irreparable may have surgery deferred, utilizing the same regimen of sterile gauze dressings and antibiotics.

Until recently, the selection of systemic antibiotics has been beset with two problems: (1) many drugs do not pass the blood-aqueous and blood-retina barriers to give adequate intraocular tissue concentrations, and (2) earlier drugs have had limited bactericidal spectra, especially for strains of *Pseudomonas aeruginosa*. When ophthalmologic care must be delayed, the following initial antibiotic regimen may be used if infection is suspected and the wound is of such size and location that extrusion of intraocular contents is not a risk:

Subconjunctival: Gentamycin 40mg
                 Cephaloridine 100 mg
                        or
                 Gentamycin 40mg
                 Methicillin 100 mg

Topical: Gentamycin 9mg/cc
                 Bacitracin 5,000u/cc

Systemic: Cephaloridine, 1gm stat, I.V. then 500mg q 6 hr.
                        or
                 Methicillin 2gm, I.V., q 8 hr.

Subconjunctival injection is best accomplished using topical proparacaine (0.5%) anesthesia, a small-volume syringe (2.5cc) and a short (5/8″) 27 gauge needle. The bulbar conjunctiva is engaged near the upper or lower fornix with the bevel facing the globe, and the needle is advanced toward the fornix, the injection being given while the needle tip is visible through the conjunctiva. Subconjunctival injections are contraindicated if the wound is of such size and location as to risk extrusion of intraocular contents. In such cases, only the topical and systemic routes should be used, as noted above.

While ideally handled by an ophthalmologist, many of the following ocular injuries can be managed well by surgeons or general medical officers:

1. Eyelid laceration, with and without margin involvement.
2. Deeply embedded corneal foreign bodies.
3. Ocular burns.
4. Ocular contusion injuries.

If evacuation or ophthalmologic care is delayed, repair of lid lacerations by a non-ophthalmologic surgeon may be necessary. Evaluation of any lid injury must include an evaluation for coexisting injury to the eyeball and penetrating injury to the intracranial contents. Lacerations and avulsions near the medial canthal tendon necessitate a careful examination for interruption of the canaliculus. In the repair of any lid injury, it is necessary to respect the complex anatomy of the lid, exact anatomical realignment being necessary (Figure 31). It is especially important that the levator muscle, the tarsal plate, and the medial canthal tendon be precisely reapproximated, or severe functional and cosmetic disabilities may ensue. Adequate coverage of the cornea is of critical importance. The repair of lid injuries requires a knowledge of the anatomy of the lid, fine ophthalmic instruments and sutures, and magnification provided by either loupes or an operating microscope. Lid tissue should be preserved wherever possible. Only tissue that is clearly necrotic should be debrided. Totally avulsed lid segments should be reattached after cleansing. Lacerated lids should be extensively irrigated and all foreign bodies removed.

Lid lacerations should be repaired in the following manner. Lacerations through the skin horizontal to the lid margin can be repaired with 6-0 black silk sutures. Lacerations that involve the lid margin itself must be repaired precisely: 4-0 black silk suture should be used to approximate the tarsal plates elsewhere and 6-0 black silk should be used to approximate the anterior and posterior borders of the lid margin and the skin of the lid elsewhere. Lid margin sutures should stay in for ten days. The lid should be placed on stretch using the long arms of the 4-0 black silk sutures for at least three days after the repair of the injury. A light pressure dressing should be placed over the eye after the instillation of an antibiotic ointment. The cornea must be checked each day. No elaborate reconstruction of the lids should be performed in a combat zone, though every effort should be made to preserve and reapproximate lid tissues at the time of the primary repair.

Lacrimal Secretory System. It is necessary to recognize a prolapsed orbital lobe of the lacrimal gland, distinguishing it from normal orbital fat. The orbital lobe of the lacrimal gland is pinkish-gray in contrast to the creamy-yellow color of orbital fat. The prolapsed orbital lobe should be irrigated and reposited in its fossa by means of a 4-0 chromic suture passed through the lobe and the periosteum lining the fossa.

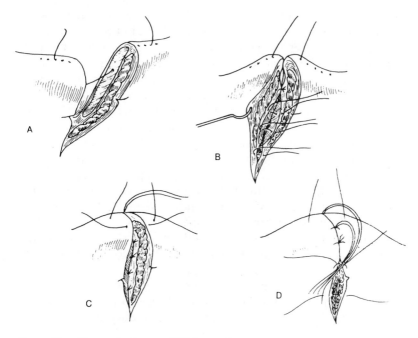

FIGURE 31.—Closure by layers of lid lacerations.

Lacrimal Excretory System. It is critically important to identify lacerations of the canaliculi so that they may be repaired
properly at the time of wound repair. The canaliculi must be
stented, preferably with silicone tubing. If silicone is not available,
fine silver wire (e.g. 3-0 or 4-0 Bowman probe) can be bent in the
form of a Johnson lacrimal rod and used as a stent. In cases of midface trauma where the nasolacrimal duct may have been interrupted, the entire lacrimal excretory system should be stented with
silicone tubing.

Orbit. A careful examination of the globe is mandatory in all
cases of injury to the orbit. The globe is significantly injured in
25% of orbital fractures. Retrobulbar hemorrhage must be
detected and treated if it is producing marked elevation of intraocular pressure and/or decreased visual acuity. If so, a lateral
canthotomy and cantholysis of the inferior crus of the lateral canthal tendon should be performed. If these maneuvers do not produce an improvement in intraocular pressure (i.e., decreasing it)

and vision, the hemorrhage must be released by an incision through the conjunctiva and Tenon's capsule between the lateral rectus and the inferior rectus muscle into the muscle cone. The incision should be made with sharp scissors, and blunt tip scissors should be used to gently spread the orbital fat within the muscle cone to permit the escape of blood. Pressure on the globe and optic nerve during any surgery upon the orbit and its contents must be avoided. Blindness can result from prolonged retraction pressure on the globe and nerve. Intraorbital extraocular foreign bodies are best left undisturbed unless they are large (greater than 1 cm in largest diameter) or are producing globe or optic nerve dysfunction. Radiographic evaluation of orbital fractures should include a stereo Waters' view and computerized tomography with coronal and sagittal reformatting. The latter is especially important in the evaluation of fractures of the optic canal. Blowout fractures of the orbital floor in general do not require immediate repair. Forced duction testing should always be performed before resorting to surgical repair. If surgery is performed, ductions of the globe should be tested intraoperatively to help prevent incarceration of tissues incident to surgical manipulation.

Enucleation. Under no circumstances should an eye be excised by a general surgeon in a forward unit unless the globe is completely disorganized.

In the unlikely circumstance that a patient with a severe ocular injury cannot be evacuated within several days to a facility that has an ophthalmologist and the ophthalmologist cannot be brought to the forward facility, primary enucleation should be considered if the patient has no light perception using the brightest available light source. Such a severe injury would most likely be an extensive corneoscleral laceration with either prolapse or loss of intraocular contents. However, even in the face of a severely damaged eye with no light perception, cosmetic function may remain; therefore, consultation with an ophthalmologist should be sought before such a definitive procedure is undertaken.

Be assured that this policy of delay is perfectly safe as it relates to sympathetic ophthalmia. Sympathetic ophthalmia (involvement of the uninjured eye) never develops until at least ten days after trauma, and only very exceptionally develops before 21 days. There is sufficient time for the patient to reach an ophthalmologist.

If the decision is made to remove the eye, the conjunctiva is incised at the limbus to separate it from the globe. Using a combination of blunt and sharp dissection, the four rectus muscles are exposed from their insertions as far posteriorly as possible (usually
10-15mm). Tenon's capsule (the connective tissue surrounding the
globe) is separated from the globe in the four quadrants between
the rectus muscles. The extraocular muscles are then cauterized
and severed 2mm from their insertions on the globe.

Traction should be exerted on the globe in the anterior direction as a curved Halsted clamp is placed behind the globe as deeply into the orbit as possible. By blunt dissection, the optic nerve
is isolated, clamped to crush the central retinal vessels, and cut
distal to the clamp. The globe is removed from the orbit. Before
the Halsted clamp is removed, hemostasis should be achieved by
direct cautery of the nerve stump. If available, it is most important to place a silicone sphere no larger than 16mm in diameter
in the position occupied previously by the globe. The sphere
should be placed within the muscle cone, posterior to the
posterior layer of Tenon's capsule, and a careful closure of
posterior Tenon's and anterior Tenon's, using interrupted 4-0
chromic catgut sutures, is completed. The conjunctiva is closed
horizontally with interrupted 5-0 plain catgut sutures. If available,
a ring conformer should be placed between the bulbar and
palpebral conjunctiva to prevent obliteration of the conjunctival
cul-de-sacs which impairs the patient's subsequent wearing of a
prosthesis. A scleral ring, rather than a scleral shell type of conformer, is preferred because the ring eliminates direct pressure
on the conjunctival suture line.

In the event that the patient still retains light perception or even
better vision in the face of a corneal or scleral laceration, primary
closure of the wound should be performed by the non-
ophthalmologist physician if the patient cannot be treated by an
ophthalmologist within a few days. The guiding principle is
meticulous wound closure without debridement, except for the
excision of prolapsed intraocular tissue.

Magnification of any type will be of great assistance. Instruments should not be introduced through the wound into the
eye. If the laceration involves both the cornea and sclera, the cornea should be repaired first. The smallest (7-0) silk suture material
available and the finest available instruments should be used. The
first suture should not be placed until the edges of the wound

are carefully aligned. Close attention to the limbal landmarks will assist in proper alignment. The curved needle is introduced almost perpendicularly into the tissue about 2mm from the wound edge, and is taken to midstromal depth (the cornea is less than 1mm thick in most areas) from where it is directed horizontally to the edge of the wound. The needle should penetrate the other edge of the wound at midstromal depth, and exit the cornea 2mm from the wound edge. The interrupted sutures should be placed every 2mm.

Scleral wounds should be closed similarly, using meticulous technique and midstromal depth placement of sutures. Non-colored sutures are usually used on the scleral wound, since these will remain buried after the conjunctiva is closed.

As a final note, all individuals rendering care for ophthalmic injuries must be aware of the frequent occurrence of combined neurosurgical and maxillofacial injuries when the eye and orbit are involved. Optimal treatment in these cases depends upon a well-coordinated team effort.

CHAPTER XXV

Laser Injury of the Eye

INTRODUCTION

Military application of laser devices will most certainly, in the future, generate casualties with laser injuries of the eye. The energy output of currently deployed rangefinders, for example, is sufficient to produce significant eye injuries at ranges up to a kilometer. High-energy output laser weapons with considerably greater potential for injury to the eye have not, to date, appeared on a battlefield.

LASER PRINCIPLES

1. Basics. A laser produces a beam of coherent light which travels at 186,000 miles per second, the speed of light. This beam can vary in wave length throughout the electromagnetic spectrum and can be visible or invisible. The common wavelengths of laser rays correspond approximately to the wavelengths of colors in the spectrum, specifically, the ultraviolet (below 400 nm), the visible (400–700 nm) , and the infrared spectra (above 700 nm). These various wavelengths of energy are absorbed by different layers within the eye.

a. Ultraviolet. Lasers utilizing the ultraviolet spectrum (below 400 nm) are absorbed in the anterior segments of the eye, primarily by the cornea, as well as by the lens.

b. Visible. Laser radiations in the visible spectrum (400–700mm) are absorbed primarily within the retina by the pigment epithelium and the choroid. Penetration depth is greater for the longer wavelengths (red) than with shorter wavelengths (blue).

c. Infrared. Absorbtion of lasers in the infrared spectrum (above 700 nm) occurs in two areas of the eye. Lasers at the lower end of the infrared spectrum (1000 nm) damage the retina and

the choroid, whereas the cornea is damaged by lasers at the top
end of the infrared spectrum (3000 nm).

TABLE 14.—*Typical lasers and their wavelengths*

Krypton	350 nm	ultraviolet
Argon	514 nm	visible
Ruby	694 nm	visible
CO_2	10,600 nm	infrared

2. Continuous versus Pulsed Waves. Continuous wave lasers, as
the name implies, are constantly emitted. These continuous wave
lasers vary in energy output from fractions of a watt up to the
kilowatt range. In contrast, pulsed lasers deliver lower energy levels
(10–50 microwatts), but nevertheless exhibit a higher potential for
eye injury. The greater destructive power of the pulsed laser lies
in the very short time interval (billionth of a second, ns) over which
the energy is delivered. On a comparative basis, a 20 mj pulse
delivered over a 20 ns time period is comparable in power to one
million watts of continuous laser emission.

3. Collimation. To collimate is to make parallel. The beams
emitted from a laser, although not perfectly collimated, are very
close to being parallel. The converse is true of the beams of light
emitted from an ordinary incandescent light bulb, which diverge
in all directions. As a result of this small divergence of laser beams,
the entire silhouette of a soldier or the entire optical system of
a battle tank can be covered by a single laser source six kilometers
away.

4. Irradiance. Irradiance refers to the concentration of energy
applied per unit area. Irradiance is expressed in watts per square
centimeter. The energy output of a particular laser is a constant
feature of that laser, whether it be the continuous or pulsed variety.
Laser beams can be focused onto a small target or defocused by
beam divergence to cover a larger area, the energy per unit area
correspondingly increasing or decreasing according to the square
of the target size. For example, because of divergence, the area
covered by a beam at six kilometers is greater than the area covered
by the same beam at one kilometer; however, the energy impacted
per unit area (irradiance) is greater at one kilometer. Therefore,
the "energy dose" received by the human eye at six km is less than
at one km. On the other hand, optical devices such as binoculars,

periscopes, and weapons-sighting devices all gather light and laser waves and magnify by converging the rays onto a smaller surface area within the eye, thereby increasing the potential for damage.

5. Tissue Effects. The biological effects produced by lasers are different for continuous and pulsed lasers. Continuous wave lasers produce primarily a thermal effect, photocoagulation. Eye examination may reveal superficial and deep burns of the cornea with opacification and tissue loss, or areas of retinal burns and necrosis. Pulsed lasers, on the other hand, produce injury faster than thermal conductivity principles would predict. Pulsed lasers produce mechanical effects, acoustic shock waves, ultrasonic waves, and high energy fields. The end result is tissue disruption (manifested as retinal tears) hemorrhage of the retina and the vitreous, and subsequent necrosis of the retina and the vitreous.

SPECIFIC LASERS

1. Carbon Dioxide Laser. The CO_2 laser, with a wavelength of 10.6 microns, is not visible. It is highly absorbed by water, glass, plastics, all biological tissues (cornea and skin), most organic substances, and all fabrics. A high-energy, continuous wave CO_2 laser will in one second char skin, destroy the cornea, opacify optical lenses, shatter glass, craze windshields, incinerate uniforms, and ignite fuels six kilometers distant from the source of emission. A similar laser operating in a pulsed mode can, in a single nanosecond pulse, ablate the corneal epithelial surface. These effects, plus the fact that this laser is not visible, can produce devastating effects on troop morale and combat effectiveness.

2. Noedymium:YAG (Nd:YAG) Laser. This laser, with a wavelength of 1064 nm, operates near the infrared wavelength spectrum. This wavelength is not visible. It is employed most commonly in the pulsed mode, producing retinal tears and hemorrhage within the retina and vitreous, and later retinal detachment and necrosis.

3. Lasers in the Visible Spectrum. The principal lasers employed in a military setting in this category are the pulsed ruby (red, wavelength 694 nm), the frequency doubled Nd:YAG (green, wavelength 532 nm), and the continuous wave argon (blue-green, wavelength 514 nm). They all produce retinal thermal burns. The presence of flash blindness, retinal burns, and retinal vitreous

hemorrhage may indicate exposure to pulsed laser.

4. Ultraviolet. Lasers operating in this region of the spectrum are currently generally encountered in a laboratory setting. Their biological effect is one of inducing a photochemical reaction. However, a pulsed ultraviolet laser may produce tissue burns. The cornea and the skin are the organs most affected.

MEDICAL CONCERNS

1. Index of Suspicion. Reports by combatants of observing bright flashes of light, of experiencing sudden eye discomfort or poor vision, or of feeling focal heat should alert the medical officer to the possibility of laser exposure and injury. Obvious lesions such as corneal burns, retinal tears, and hemorrhage or skin burns confirm one's suspicions. Conceivably, one might confuse the use of invisible lasers with chemical agent exposure which also irritates the eyes and skin. Spontaneous fires and unexplained damage to optical instruments further corroborate laser exposure.

2. Physical Examination. Surface and deep burns of the cornea and the skin indicate that a high energy CO_2 laser has been used. Retinal hemorrhage probably implicates use of pulsed laser in the visible or near-infrared portion of the spectrum. Isolated retinal burns probably indicate exposure to a visible laser in the continuous wave mode.

3. Therapy. At the present time there is no definitive treatment for laser injury of the eye. Corneal burns are treated the same as ocular burns from other traumatic agents, specifically topical antibiotics, patches, and frequent examinations to monitor epithelial healing. It should also be borne in mind that the likelihood of an isolated corneal burn, especially of only one eye, is very small. Generally, there will be burns of both eyes as well as burns about the face and mouth. The general principles of treatment of facial burns and airway maintenance apply.

a. Soldiers who sustain laser injuries of the retina only should not be treated the same as those with corneal burns of the eye. Their injuries may range from small retinal spot burns to complete detachments and vitreous hemorrhages. Eye patches should be used sparingly in these cases, since eye patches only serve to magnify the soldier's visual impairment and increase his dependency for the basic needs of survival on others.

b. Panic and hysteria may be the major difficulty encountered. The fear of blindness and the witnessing of blinding injuries in comrades can cause a major disruption of combat effectiveness. Although the long-term disability for these casualties is great, their near-term medical requirements are small. They do not require a large expenditure of resources and should not be allowed to overburden the medical evacuation system if other more critically wounded require those resources. The tactical situation and the availability of surface or aeromedical evacuation assets will determine when these patients are moved to the rear. Retinal burns and vitreous hemorrhage cases can be delayed. Corneal or other surface burns receive standard first aid measures and are evacuated. For those with lesser injuries, an assessment of visual function and the presence of pain will determine how useful a soldier can be to his unit and whether or not he should be evacuated.

4. Prevention. For CO_2 lasers, ordinary spectacle lenses will protect the eyes and ordinary visors will protect the face. When struck by the laser beam, one's spectacles and visors may become opaque or burned, thereby impeding vision. For visible laser protection, narrow-band filters for the elimination of lasers of specific or multiple wavelengths are currently undergoing development. The ideal protector will filter out only the deleterious wavelengths while allowing the remaining visible light to pass. Use of these wavelength filters may cause some tinting of one's vision. The use of several different wavelength filters may impair vision, particularly at night and during the hours of dusk and twilight due to their dark color.

CHAPTER XXVI

Wounds and Injuries of the Ear

Injuries of the ear are common in combat. Such injuries may be confined to the external ear in the form of contusions, lacerations, or avulsions. Blast injuries of the middle or inner ear may cause deafness which may be permanent. These wounds often are overlooked or relegated, to a low priority of treatment in a busy aid station or field hospital. However, such injuries, if not appropriately treated, may result in prolonged morbidity or permanent disability.

Patients who have sustained injuries to the ear that include impairment of hearing should be protected from additional acoustic trauma until maximum recovery is assured. Temporary or permanent reassignment of duty may be necessary.

THE EXTERNAL EAR

Trauma to the auricle is usually quite obvious and, unless treated promptly, may result in considerable cosmetic deformity. Among the more common injuries are lacerations, avulsions, contusions, or thermal injury.

In simple lacerations, the auricle should be debrided carefully with minimum excision of only the devitalized tissues. The physician then should close the laceration in layers, being careful to realign cartilage with absorbable suture material and the skin and subcutaneous tissues with a fine, atraumatic suture. All cutaneous sutures should be removed in 3-5 days.

If the auricle is partially avulsed, careful surgical debridement and reapproximation should be accomplished as soon as possible. In those instances when a portion of the auricle is missing, approximation of the anterior and posterior layers of skin over the exposed cartilage should be accomplished. Fragments of the auricle which are still present should not be sutured out of their normal anatomical alignment. In instances of total avulsion, the cartilage should be debrided of all overlying tissue and buried sub-cutaneously in the abdominal wall (or other suitable area) so that it may be used for reconstruction at a later date.

When there is a hematoma of the auricle, the hemorrhage is usually subperiochondral in origin. Such hematomas are evacuated surgically and a sterile pressure dressing is applied. The dressing should be removed at least every 48 hours and the wound inspected for recurrence of the hemotoma.

Thermal injury should be treated by careful cleansing and application of topical antibacterial agents such as mafenide (Sulfamylon) on fine mesh gauze. Asepsis is critical. Suppurative chondritis can be prevented by careful attention to the avoidance of further trauma. A mesh dressing can be used to protect the entire head. No pillows are used.

In all of the cited injuries, systemic coverage with broad spectrum antibiotics, tetanus toxoid booster, and aseptic technique are essential.

If a laceration of the external auditory meatus is recognized early, precise initial suture repair is indicated. However, lacerations of the external auditory canal or fractures through its bony portion are less obvious and may be overlooked. Thus, they often do not become apparent until secondary infection has occurred. The external canal should be cleansed as aseptically as possible and a cotton or gauze wick impregnated with broad-spectrum antibiotic ear drops placed in the canal. Such patients should then be referred to the care of an otolaryngologist because of the strong possibility of stenosis as the canal heals.

The problems of external otitis, especially in tropical and subtropical climates, is well known to combat physicians. As innocuous as this entity may seem, it has caused considerable morbidity. In such circumstances, the skin of the external canal becomes macerated, affording an excellent culture medium for secondary infection. The organisms most commonly encountered are various species of *Pseudomonas* and *Proteus* with an occasional *Staphylococcus*. Thus, thorough cleansing plus broad-spectrum topical (and at times systemic) antibiotics are the treatment. A wick placed into the swollen canal allows topical medicines to be more effective. Water precautions are instituted. Such infections are often extremely painful, requiring analgesics.

THE MIDDLE EAR

Injury of the tympanic membrane, which is common, is often associated with other much more serious injuries of the middle ear. The damage may be caused by direct penetration of a missile, by a fracture of the base of the skull involving the tympanic ring, or by sudden compression of the air in the external auditory meatus as the result of blast. A blast injury may cause a small hemorrhage in the substance of the membrane, rupture of the outer fibers, or a linear tear; or it may result in complete disintegration. The great risk is secondary infection, with possible deafness likely to be the end result.

Injury of the middle ear often does not present clear-cut symptoms. When it is suspected, the ear should be examined under aseptic precautions, with good illumination.

If rupture has occurred, instrumentation, drops, and syringing are all contraindicated. Wax is left in situ unless pain, deafness, or both require its removal. This is seldom necessary in a forward hospital. Eighty percent of these perforations will close spontaneously.

Treatment in the forward area consists of simple protection of the ear with a sterile dressing or a loose packing of sterile cotton. If the pinna is also damaged, the meatus should be packed with sterile cotton while the outer ear is being cleansed.

Until the ruptured tympanic membrane has healed, every precaution is taken to avoid nasopharyngeal infection. The patient is warned not to blow his nose. If suppuration occurs, it must be vigorously treated by ear drops and other standard measures to prevent chronicity. Delayed cholesteatoma formation is common in blast injuries.

BAROTRAUMA

Barotrauma is often encountered in flying personnel. Symptoms usually occur on descent, when edema of the eustachian tube mucosa prevents equalization of pressure within the middle ear. This can result in symptoms varying from mild pain and slight hearing loss to severe pain and extreme vertigo. When it occurs, topical and systemic nasal decongestants, coupled with frequent Valsalva maneuvers, often will reverse the process. On occasion, a myringotomy may be required. Prompt recognition and treatment will often sharply decrease the associated morbidity. The condition is more prone to occur in those with upper respiratory infections.

THE INNER EAR

Trauma to the inner ear may occur in combination with the above injuries or as an isolated injury secondary to blunt trauma. Such injury may be accompanied by total hearing loss, severe vertigo, high-pitched tinnitus, or facial nerve palsy. These injuries should be treated symptomatically and evacuated to the care of an otolaryngologist. If a basilar skull fracture is suspected, the use of antibiotics (usually penicillin) is mandatory. In all of these instances the patient should be cautioned against blowing his nose.

CHAPTER XXVII

Wounds and Injuries of the Neck

Wounds of the neck, because of the large number of vital structures within a compact area, are frequently complicated injuries which demand prompt surgical care. A single wound may damage multiple systems, involving the larynx, trachea, pharynx, esophagus, major vessels, multiple nerves, the spinal cord, and the cervical spine. Asphyxia and severe hemorrhage commonly occur. Pharyngeal and esophageal wounds that communicate with the mediastinum via the fascial planes of the neck may result in bacterial contamination of the mediastinum and subsequent mediastinitis. Foreign bodies carried through these soft tissues may cause further contamination. Small injuries to the skin and fascia may be associated with more severe injuries of deeper structures. Neck wounds are often associated with oral and intrathoracic injuries. These injuries may initially be occult but will demand attention. The hallmarks of good management of neck wounds are adequate incisions, generous exposure, and careful debridement followed by wide drainage. Antibiotics should be given to all patients with deep neck wounds.

IMMEDIATE LIFE THREATENING INJURY, MAJOR BLEEDING, AND AIRWAY OBSTRUCTION

Severe and even fatal external hemorrhage can occur from innocuous-appearing wounds of the neck. Probing or blind clamping of an open, bleeding neck wound rarely controls hemorrhage and frequently causes further injury. The hemorrhage in many severe neck injuries is venous in origin and can be controlled by external pressure. Airway compromise may result from direct trauma, from endotracheal blood and blood clots, from laryngotracheal edema, or from nerve injury. Endotracheal intubation in these cases may be impossible, particularly in patients with extensive bleeding from wounds of the mouth or pharynx. When airway obstruction persists in the patient who cannot be intubated orally, cricothyroidotomy provides rapid and safe airway control. This should be viewed as a temporizing life-saving procedure which will be replaced by a tracheostomy under controlled circumstances if one anticipates the requirement for airway control lasting more than 48 hours.

WOUNDS OF THE LARYNX AND TRACHEA

Serious wounds of the larynx and trachea may present in the following ways:

1. Asphyxia. Asphyxia results from serious laryngotracheal obstruction. The obstruction may be caused by destruction of the larynx, the fragments of which form obstructing flaps; by hemorrhage, which blocks the airway with blood or clots; or by traumatic laryngotracheal edema. Restlessness observed in these patients, if secondary to cerebral hypoxia, heralds impending asphyxia.

2. Dyspnea. Dyspnea may result from lesser damage to the larynx or trachea. The cause of asphyxial injuries is usually immediately apparent, whereas injuries causing dyspnea can often be found only by careful examination. The most common symptoms and signs of airway injury, in addition to dyspnea, are dysphonia, laryngeal cough, hemoptysis, dysphagia, and excess mobility of the larynx. Roentgenologic examination of the laryngeal and tracheal cartilages, which are always ossified to some degree in adults, and preoperative laryngoscopy are of diagnostic assistance.

3. Subcutaneous emphysema of the face and neck. Retropharyngeal swelling, although infrequently detected on physical examination, is readily demonstrable on biplanar soft-tissue X-ray films by narrowing or distortion of the air column.

All injuries of the trachea and larynx are serious. Diagnosis is confirmed by laryngoscopy or bronchoscopy, which should be performed at the slightest suspicion of injury. These examinations are often done at the time of airway control, following which an endotracheal tube may be inserted. The early use of this procedure often precludes the performance of a hasty tracheostomy. On the other hand, emergency tracheostomy may be necessary when the injury crushes or distorts the larynx or hypopharynx such that intubation cannot be accomplished. In such cases, urgent decompression of the deep subfascial space may also be necessary to relieve pressure on the airway. In the presence of a functioning tracheostomy, laryngeal injuries can go undiagnosed, with subsequent serious loss of function, much of which may have been prevented by early diagnosis and appropriate treatment.

Careful and conservative debridement of laryngotracheal injuries is emphasized. Following debridement, the fragmented larynx or trachea should be reapproximated and an intraluminal stent utilized to maintain the anatomical architecture. Late tracheal and laryngeal stenosis from injudicious and excessive removal of tissue, particularly cartilage and mucosa, must be prevented. Care must be taken to identify associated wounds of adjacent structures, such as esophagus, pharynx, and major vessels.

Airway control via either endotracheal intubation or tracheostomy requires constant aftercare to avoid sudden obstruction with resultant asphyxia. Proper tube size is important. Too small a tube can result in gradual respiratory insufficiency, leading to hypoxia and cardiac arrest. Overinflation of "hard" endotracheal tube balloons must be prevented to avoid damage to tracheal tissue.

WOUNDS OF THE PHARYNX AND ESOPHAGUS

The pharynx and esophagus are often involved in injuries of the neck, with resultant high likelihood of contamination of the deep fascial planes of the neck and the mediastinum. Small lesions of the posterior pharynx and esophagus are often overlooked in the presence of other neck injuries and can lead to severe morbidity and death. Examination must be thorough and includes endoscopy. Any penetrating injury, however small, must be suspect. Soft-tissue X-ray films may be useful as previously described. Radiopaque contrast media may demonstrate leaks not apparent by other means.

Management is based on surgical exploration, both to identify lesions and to debride and close lacerations of the mucosa and muscularis of the pharynx and esophagus. Double-layer closure of defects is the treatment of choice, followed by adequate external drainage. Wide wounds of the pharynx or esophagus which cannot be closed require either marsupialization or wide drainage. Nasogastric intubation is necessary early on to minimize wound contamination secondary to regurgitation and later on for feeding purposes.

VASCULAR INJURIES

Injury of major neck or mediastinal vascular structures is often fatal. Venous injuries have the added risk of air embolism. Serious vascular injuries may be masked by the severe shock state in the patient with multiple injuries. These may become apparent only after resuscitation has begun. The severity of blood loss may be masked when neck wounds communicate with the pleural space (hemothorax). Suspicion of vascular injury requires early exploration. Anterior thoracotomy in the third interspace on the involved side permits immediate intrathoracic access to the great vessels. Bleeding sites can be controlled with direct pressure and packs while developing definitive exposure. Definitive exposure of this region is then provided by median sternotomy. This exposure also can be obtained by extending the neck incision into a full median sternotomy incision.

The following points regarding the management of vascular injuries are emphasized:

1. The mortality from uncontrolled hemorrhage is second only to asphyxiation in wounds to the neck. Airway control and hemostasis are, therefore, the initial steps.

2. Serious vascular injury often presents as a gradually enlarging hematoma, which can encroach upon the airway. Airway encroachment is produced by hematoma which expands within the triple-layered, closed, deep fascial compartments of the neck. The fascial arrangement also prevents outward expansion of extravasating blood, sometimes making the diagnosis of vascular injury difficult.

3. Penetrating wounds of the neck, because of the possibility of vascular injury, require definitive surgical exploration. Exploration should include the carotid and internal jugular systems. Should vascular repair be required, adequate exposure with proximal and distal control is the cardinal technical consideration in vascular surgery.

4. Lateral repair or end-to-end anastomosis after debridement of the injured wall of any artery is preferred. If this is not possible, an autogenous vein graft may be used to bridge an arterial defect.

The use of an internal or external shunt to maintain cerebral circulation during repair is preferred. The importance of adequate
oxygenation and maintenance of blood volume cannot be
overemphasized.

5. The external carotid system may be ligated without morbidity. Ligation of the internal carotid artery may be the safest procedure for patients with an injury to this vessel when there is an
already established neurological deficit.

6. Ligation of the internal jugular system is indicated when
lateral repair is not possible.

NERVE INJURIES

Nerve injuries should be identified and recorded for possible
later repair. In general, immediate repair of traumatic nerve
defects is not recommended, except for isolated injuries of the
facial and spinal accessory nerves. Even when ideally treated by
delayed neurorrhaphy, the proximal location of the nerve injury
in the neck precludes significant success. High-velocity missile
wounds of the neck involving the spinal cord are almost always
fatal.

EMERGENCY TRACHEOSTOMY

Tracheostomy as a lifesaving procedure has proven its worth
many times over (Figure 32); however, tracheostomy requires a
thorough knowledge of anatomy and must be performed many
times before it can be done both quickly and safely.

Adequate lighting is essential. Positioning is also very important in tracheostomy. The patient lies supine, with the shoulders
elevated by sandbags or folded towels, so that the neck is extended. Local anesthesia is usually utilized. The incision may be
longitudinal or transverse. The transverse incision will insure a
better cosmetic result, but the longitudinal incision is almost
bloodless and there is more rapid exposure of the trachea with
it. It is made in the midline, through the skin and platysma, from
the cricoid cartilage to the suprasternal notch. The strap muscles
are separated in the midline by blunt dissection. When they are
retracted, the trachea is exposed. If the isthmus of the thyroid is
encountered, it is displaced upward or downward. Local

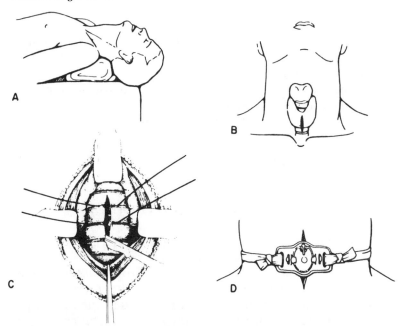

FIGURE 32.—Technique of tracheostomy. A. Position of the patient with neck hyperextended. B. Location of the incision. C. Thyroid isthmus elevated, pretracheal veins separated, vertical incision in trachea. D. Tracheostomy tube in place.

anesthesia, in the amount of 1-2 cc, is injected into the tracheal lumen to reduce the cough reflex. The pretracheal fascia is incised and stripped laterally as necessary to expose the underlying cartilages.

The ideal level at which to incise the trachea is at the level of the second, third, and fourth tracheal rings. The trachea is retracted with a hook between the cricoid and first ring while a vertical incision is made through three tracheal rings. The incision should be made long enough to accommodate the diameter of the tube to be inserted. A heavy silk suture, passed through each side of the incised trachea, may later be used as a retractor and guide to facilitate early tracheostomy tube changes. The adult male trachea can easily accommodate a size 6-9 tracheostomy tube. Smaller tubes cause airway resistance and can lead to hypoxia. Position and secure the tube. The skin incision does not require closure.

Suction should be available at operation to remove secretions from the trachea. If it is not available, the head should be lowered as soon as the trachea has been opened.

Complications associated with tracheostomy are more frequent than realized and should be mentioned:

1. Asphyxia from dislodged or occluded tubes.
2. Immediate or delayed severe hemorrhage from innominate, subclavian, and carotid vessels.
3. Subcutaneous emphysema with possible pneumomediastinum or pneumothorax.
4. Tracheoesophageal fistula.
5. Tracheal and laryngeal stenosis.

TECHNIQUE FOR CRICOTHYROIDOTOMY

As previously mentioned, in extreme airway emergencies or when the medical officer has had no experience with endotracheal intubation or tracheostomy or lacks the appropriate equipment, a cricothyroidotomy should be performed. The inferior border of the large, prominent thyroid cartilage is identified by palpation. The cricoid cartilage, which is the smaller protuberance just below, is similarly identified. The taut membrane which separates the thyroid cartilage from the inferiorly located cricoid cartilage is relatively superficial. After adequate skin incision, the space between these cartilages, which is avascular, is incised transversely and the tracheal lumen is readily entered through the incision. A small endotracheal tube, no. 5 or no. 6, should be rapidly inserted and the balloon inflated. If no tube is available, a clamp may be used temporarily to keep the incision open. The cricothyroidotomy should be relied upon for only 48 hours. If airway management is anticipated for greater than 48 hours a conventional tracheostomy should be accomplished under controlled circumstances as soon as possible.

CHAPTER XXVIII

Wounds and Injuries of the Chest

About 15% of combat injuries sustained during conventional land warfare will involve the thoracic viscera and/or the chest wall. In two-thirds, the thoracic wound will be the principle injury. The spectrum of injury ranges from casualties with grossly mutilating blast injuries to those with only tiny superficial fragment wounds. The great majority of chest casualties will have penetrating trauma. After excluding the approximately 10% with only soft tissue wounds, the remainder can be categorized into two populations: about two-thirds will have missile wounds of the heart, great vessels, or pulmonary hilum; and the others will have missile wounds of the pulmonary parenchyma. It is unusual for casualties in the former category to present as treatment problems, since the vast majority exsanguinate before reaching a medical treatment facility. By way of contrast, casualties with wounds of the lung usually survive to reach medical treatment, which in most instances involves no more than the insertion of a chest tube. About 5% of the total thoracic casualty population will have sustained blunt trauma, more often than not occurring when an armored fighting vehicle is damaged by a mine. Viewed from the historical perspective, the principal function of thoracic surgery in wartime has not been the performance of emergency life-saving surgery, but rather the management of chronic complications such as clotted hemothorax and empyema. Whether better field resuscitation, more rapid evacuation from the battlefield, and the availability of surgeons trained in the management of thoracic trauma will change the role of thoracic surgery is unclear.

ANATOMICAL AND PHYSIOLOGICAL PATHOLOGY

Shock and hypoxia, the pathophysiological derangements by which chest trauma kills, result from decreased venous return or inadequate alveolar gas exchange. Decreased venous return is usually a manifestation of exsanguination, thus the paramount importance of controlling bleeding. Inadequate alveolar gas exchange can result from such factors as loss of the usual negative intrapleural pressure, leading to collapse of the lung, and obstruction of the smaller air passages by secretions or blood. The therapeutic goal is to restore normal physiology and thereby to restore cardiac and pulmonary function. Thus is true not only in the immediate post-injury phase, but also later in the course when the surgeon is faced by such chronic complications as trapped lung or the need to reconstruct the chest wall. Salient aspects of common battlefield thoracic problems are considered below.

PNEUMOTHORAX

The presence of air in the pleural space results in the loss of the normal negative pressure gradient across the alveoli and the visceral pleura. The lung is no longer coupled to the parietal pleura and is collapsed by the recoil of its elastic tissue. Air no longer enters the collapsed alveoli which, however, remain perfused at least until hypoxia-mediated pulmonary vasoconstriction reduces flow. Perfusion of the nonventilated lung tissue results in a ventilation-perfusion inequality, which is apparent as desaturation of the arterial blood. The source of the intrapleural air is usually laceration of the pulmonary parenchyma. In a minority of casualties, the lacerated pulmonary tissue forms a flap valve which allows air to enter the pleural space, but not to exit. Intrapleural pressure may become so positive that the mediastinum is displaced to the opposite side and the uninjured lung severely compressed. The dire consequences of a tension pneumothorax are profound alveolar hypoventilation and decreased cardiac output, the latter probably being due to impeded venous return secondary to mechanical kinking of the great veins. Untreated, death may occur within minutes of injury. Pneumothorax may also result from air entering through a hole in the chest wall. Here the problem is not positive intrathoracic pressure, but the fact that, given a sufficiently large hole relative to the area of the airway, there will be less resistance to airflow into the pleural space than into the lung. Profound alveolar hypoventilation results. Open pneumothorax is not commonly seen in living casualties because the trauma necessary to produce a large defect usually causes a fatal intrathoracic injury.

HEMOTHORAX

Hemothorax is dangerous not only because it can lead to hypovolemic shock, but also because it may result in compression of the injured lung and thereby cause a reduction in vital capacity. Bleeding may arise from lacerated pulmonary parenchyma, from systemic arteries such as the intercostals or the internal mammaries, or from the heart and great vessels. Bleeding from the latter may be so massive as to create a rapidly fatal condition best characterized as a tension hemothorax.

HEMOPNEUMOTHORAX

About one-half of casualties with penetrating wounds of the lung will present with hemopneumothorax, a situation to be expected because of the propensity of a missile to lacerate contiguous structures, such as bronchioles and arterioles. A frequent concomitant injury is pulmonary "contusion." There is increasing evidence that the contusion around the missile tract is actually hematoma in a parenchymal laceration. Contusion remote from the permanent missile tract is due to intraalveolar blood which has entered the bronchial tree and is aspirated into the uninjured lung. A more severe manifestation of combined bronchial and arterial injury is seen in many fatally wounded thoracic casualties who quite literally drown in their own blood.

PERICARDIAL TAMPONADE

The great majority of missile wounds of the heart create a pericardial defect which allows blood from the lacerated myocardium to freely escape. Tamponade cannot occur and death results from exsanguination. Small fragment wounds are compatible with tamponade. As blood collects in the pericardial space, the transmural pressure gradient progressively falls, resulting in collapse of the great veins and displacement of the intraventricular septum to the left. As blood continues to collect, venous pressure rises and cardiac output and blood pressure fall. Because of the nonlinear pressure-volume characteristics of the pericardium, a point is ultimately reached at which a small additional increment of blood will result in sudden cardiovascular collapse and death.

BLUNT CHEST TRAUMA

The clinical syndrome associated with multiple rib fractures and a flail chest is the quintessential expression of blunt trauma and does not differ in its manifestations or treatment in combat casualties and civilian trauma victims. The severity of the injury is dependent upon the number and locations of the fractured ribs (which in turn determine the extent to which the chest wall is unstable), the presence of an underlying lung injury, whether a hemo/pneumothorax is present, and the magnitude of associated injuries to other thoracic viscera, such as an aortic disruption or a ruptured diaphragm. The unstable portion of the chest wall moves paradoxically with respiration, being drawn inward during inspiration and blown outward during expiration. The former results in decreased pulmonary ventilation, while the latter results in a weak cough and consequent retention of tracheobronchial secretions. Pulmonary contusion is frequently associated with flail chest and this, rather than the mechanical instability of the chest wall, may dominate the clinical picture.

TRAPPED LUNG/EMPYEMA

These chronic complications of thoracic trauma have the potential to become important sources of morbidity in future wars, unless the lessons learned in the past are remembered. Trapped lung results from incomplete early evacuation of blood from the pleural space with subsequent replacement of the fibrin clot by fibrous tissue, which, as it contracts, squeezes the lung into a nonfunctioning organ. Vital capacity is reduced and arterial hypoxemia may be apparent. Empyema, a frequent cause of death in World War I thoracic casualties, is another manifestation of inadequate evacuation of a hemothorax.

RETAINED MISSILE

Retained missiles may cause problems in two different ways. First, they may become the nidus of infection that results in an empyema or wound-tract sepsis. Second, they may on rare occasions enter the circulation by migrating from the lung or by being dislodged from a previously dormant state within a cardiac chamber. Then they may embolize in a quite unpredictable manner to other parts of the arterial tree.

DIAGNOSIS

Establishing a diagnosis of a thoracic injury in a combat casualty is exceedingly simple: there is a hole (or holes) in the chest, and the casualty usually complains of pain when be breathes. Often the casualty will be obviously dyspneic or be in frank respiratory distress, fighting for every breath. Those less severely injured will cough up bloody sputum, while gurgling breath sounds will be all too obvious in the dying. The casualty may have some of the more obvious clinical signs of shock: rapid and weak peripheral pulse, cold clammy skin, depressed sensorium, etc. Inspection may reveal a large hole in the chest wall from which frothy fluid is expelled with each exhalation. Certain clinical syndromes have stigmata which are so obvious that they may even be useful in spite of the chaotic conditions of the battlefield. With a tension pneumothorax, the trachea as felt in the neck is displaced to the side opposite to the injury, and the affected hemithorax may sound like a drum when it is percussed. When blunt injury has occurred, the medical officer will find tenderness to palpation and possibly bony crepitus in the traumatized area. He may notice that a portion of the chest wall, in size usually exceeding the area of the palm, appears to be moving out of sequence with the rest of the chest and abdomen.

Given the paucity of diagnostic imaging capabilities in the lower echelons providing combat casualty care, it is indeed fortunate that so much can be done with inspection and palpation. However, chest X-ray is useful if for no other reason than it allows the surgeon to determine that a chest tube has been placed where it should be placed. Furthermore, chest X-ray is helpful in establishing whether a small pneumothorax is present or whether a hemothorax has been adequately evacuated. A chest X-ray may also give some idea as to the likelihood of a cardiac injury, since the localization of a missile within the cardiac silhouette, especially when combined with shock, is suggestive of tamponade. Combat experience has shown that the classic physical findings of tamponade (muffled heart sounds, dilated neck veins, narrowed pulse pressure, a "paradoxical" decrease in systolic pressure of more than 10 mm Hg during inspiration, and enlarged heart to percussion), cannot be depended upon to establish this diagnosis.

TREATMENT

What therapeutic interventions can be undertaken is determined by the echelon of care. What echelons will be used depends in turn upon the pathway of evacuation. Casualties may be evacuated directly from the battlefield to surgical facilities, or they may pass through progressive echelons of increasingly sophisticated care. Regardless of the evacuation pathway, the medical officer at any echelon is unlikely to do any harm if he does the following:

REMOVE bloody secretions from the airway
SEAL chest wall holes
REMOVE air from the pleural space
REMOVE blood from the pleural space
RESTORE circulating volume deficits
REMOVE blood from the pericardial sac
REMOVE pus from the pleural space

Surgical and radiographic facilities are not available in battalion aid stations. Therefore, treatment of chest wounds at this echelon must be limited to first aid and lifesaving interventions. These are best addressed in terms of the Advanced Trauma Life Support (ATLS) course's priorities which are, of course, applicable to all echelons of care.

Relief of upper airway obstruction is assigned first priority. The great majority of combat casualties with upper airway obstruction have either massive trauma to the face or a severe brain injury. It is quite clear that both nasal and oral endotracheal intubation in the former population is likely to prove quite difficult. Thus, most casualties requiring airway control will need a surgical airway or an oral airway. A description of the technique for performing either a cricothyroidotomy or tracheostomy is found in the chapter on neck injuries. It is necessary at this point to comment about cervical spine control. Penetrating cervical cord wounds in salvageable combat casualties are quite unusual. It is essential that misplaced concern about aggravating a possible cervical cord injury should not interfere with life-saving care for real problems.

Second priority is accorded to correcting respiratory problems. At the unit level, this will mean first and foremost inserting an intercostal drainage tube by means of a closed thoracostomy or, much less commonly, dressing an open chest wound. The casualty with a tension pneumothorax is most expeditiously managed by first venting the hemothorax by inserting a large-bore needle (14 gauge) through the second intercostal space. A chest tube should then be inserted. The technique for inserting a chest tube is described in the chapter on multiple injuries. The essential feature is to make an incision in the chest wall sufficiently large to allow entrance of a finger. By so doing, one assures that the chest tube is in fact placed within the pleural space. The large hole also assures that a chest tube of optimal caliber (40–45 Fr.) can be inserted. Sites for insertion are usually the fifth intercostal space midaxillary line or the second intercostal space midclavicular line. A closed thoracostomy utilizing a trocar is a useful alternative to the above, although the size of the chest tube may be insufficient to allow adequate removal of blood and clot. A chest tube should not be inserted through the missile tract. The chest tube should be secured to the patient and connected to a flutter valve such as the Heimlich.

Third priority is assigned to the management of bleeding and shock. Little can be done for the thoracic casualty in shock at this echelon other than to start an intravenous infusion of crystalloid fluid through two or more large-bore catheters.

Given a tactical situation in which direct aeromedical evacuation from the battlefield to surgical treatment facilities is not possible, the fundamental contribution of the unit level to the medical care of the thoracic combat casualty will be to prepare the casualty for safe evacuation to a definitive care facility. From the practical standpoint, this means that casualties with penetrating missile wounds of the chest that are clearly not superficial should have chest tubes placed. Ancillary interventions must include the administration of a potent antimicrobal agent and relief of pain if indicated.

MANAGEMENT AT THE DIVISION LEVEL

Whatever could have been done at the unit level but was not done should be done by the divisional medical officer. Chest tubes should be connected to underwater seal and suction. X-ray will help determine whether additional tubes are needed. Antibiotic administration should be continued. The ability to infuse blood may make possible the salvage of occasional casualties who are exsanguinating. Perhaps the most important function of this echelon of care is triage. Two categories of casualties need to be recognized: those who need early surgical care and therefore need priority evacuation, and those casualties who stand a good chance of early return to duty. Thoracic casualties with little or no air leak or bleeding are good candidates for prompt return to duty and should be removed from the evacuation pathway.

MANAGEMENT AT THE
SURGICAL TREATMENT FACILITY

Emergency life-saving interventions may be necessary in casualties evacuated directly from the battlefield. However, more often than not, the important problem facing the surgeon will be to decide whether an operation beyond simple soft tissue wound care is indicated. The most common reason for performing a thoracotomy is massive or persistent bleeding. Since bleeding from most missile wounds of the lung parenchyma will stop when the lung is expanded, thoracotomy is seldom required. However, with the advent of more potent small arms, the surgeon is likely to encounter casualties with grossly destructive wounds of the lung, wounds which will not stop bleeding without surgical intervention. As a general rule, hemorrhage from chest wall arteries will require surgical ligation. Casualties with wounds of the heart or great vessels are much less common, constituting only 2–3% of the total thoracic population who survive to be evacuated from the battlefield.

The following are useful indications for performing a formal thoracotomy:

1. An opacified hemithorax on X-ray.

2. Initial drainage of 1,500 ml of blood followed by 500 ml or more in the next hour.

3. Drainage of 200–300 ml of blood per hour for more than 4 hours.

4. Massive airleak with continuous bubbling throughout the respiratory cycle.

5. X-ray evidence of massive pulmonary contusion or hematoma, with clinical and laboratory evidence of a life-threatening shunt or airway compromise secondary to pulmonary bleeding.

6. Physical signs of pericardial tamponade or suspicion of tamponade or shock, and X-ray evidence of a missile in proximity to heart.

Suspected wounds of the lungs are best approached through a formal posterior lateral thoracotomy made through the fifth or sixth interspace. Wounds of the heart are best approached through an anterior thoracotomy made in the fifth intercostal space on the side of the missile wound with extension across the sternum if necessary. A median sternotomy is less often employed if for no other reason than that appropriate instruments to divide the sternum may not be available. A pericardiocentesis should not be used as an alternative to thoracotomy. The need to be constantly vigilant for signs of recurrent tamponade, and the possibility that the operating room will have been preempted by a mass casualty situation just when it is obvious that conservative management has failed, speak against pericardiocentesis in a combat zone hospital.

Although it is usually said that the casualty should have received optimal resuscitation (correction of hypovolemia and acidosis, etc.) prior to going to the operating room, from the practical standpoint this is frequently not possible because operation is required for resuscitation. All thoracotomies should be done under general anesthesia with controlled positive pressure ventilation through a secure airway. Intraoperative management will usually involve debridement of partially detached lung, ligation of bleeding vessels, and oversewing of lacerated lung. If airleaks persist, if the parenchyma of one or more lobes has been shattered, or if the anesthetist reports persistence of copious tracheobronchial bleeding, a formal resection should be considered, Although unusual, there are case reports of life-saving lobectomies and pneumonectomies given such circumstances. Chest closure should follow standard practice. At least two chest tubes should be inserted, one high and anterior and one low and lateral. Antibiotic coverage, starting before the incision is made, is essential.

Wounds of the heart seen at operation are usually small, and hemorrhage can be controlled by digital pressure while bolstered mattress sutures are inserted. Care should be taken not to incarcerate an epicardial coronary artery in the suture; the suture can always be placed deep to the artery. A rare casualty will have a wound of an epicardial artery. Given the nonavailability of cardiopulmonary bypass, there is no alternative but to ligate the vessel and hope for the best.

Large open wounds of the chest wall require debridement and airtight closure of the musculofascial layer. Rib fragments should be removed and rib ends smoothed to prevent subsequent laceration of the lung. It is frequently possible to evaluate the lung and to evacuate the pleural space by extending the wound defect. Thus the casualty is spared a formal thoracotomy. This fact helps explain why fewer 20% of thoracic casualties have formal thoracotomies; many have de facto minithoracotomies as part of their chest wall wound management.

Clotted hemothorax and infected hemothorax are complications which may become apparent prior to evacuation from the combat zone. A clotted hemothorax should be surgically removed if it is less than 7–10 days old. Beyond that time, thoracotomy should be delayed for 4–5 weeks, after which a pleural decortication should be performed. During the decortication, care should be taken when performing the dissection where the parietal pleura reflects onto the lung posteriorly. If this "corner" is not turned properly, the dissection may enter the aorta or esophagus. The same problem exists when the dissection is carried into the diaphragm. If the procedure is delayed for months, the problem will be a trapped lung. Decortication is indicated if more than the equivalent of one lobe is nonfunctional. An infected hemothorax cannot be removed by tube drainage and will require decortication at whatever time it becomes apparent. Retained foreign bodies should be removed electively if they exceed 1.5 cm in size. Notwithstanding the experience of World War II, intracardiac foreign bodies should not be removed unless cardiopulmonary bypass is readily available.

Penetrating combat trauma involving the esophagus or trachea is rare. There is suggestive evidence that small penetrating injuries, especially of the membranous trachea, may be benign. If pneumo-mediastinum is apparent on X-ray, bronchoscopy is indicated. If no wound is apparent, observation is indicated. When an esophageal wound is found at the time of thoracotomy perform-ed for bleeding, more often than not a gross defect is found which can be treated only by defunctionalization. Use of a gastric patch to close a low esophageal war wound has been described. Another rare manifestation of penetrating chest trauma is post-traumatic pneumatocele. Lungs tolerate the temporary cavity produced by a high-energy transfer missile with much less damage than do solid parenchymal organs, such as the brain and liver, but occasional casualties will be seen who develop a cyst around the permanent tract. This should occasion some concern because such post-traumatic cysts may become infected or be the site of massive hemorrhage. If they do not promptly regress, they should be excised.

About 20% of the casualties with wounds of the trunk will have penetrating injuries of both the chest and abdomen. In about 50% of these casualties, the same missile is responsible for both com-ponents. Experience has shown that the abdominal component usually has the greatest injury severity, and that adequate treat-ment consists of laparotomy and insertion of a chest tube. The surgeon must not neglect to close the perforation of the diaphragm.

POSTOPERATIVE MANAGEMENT AND EVACUATION CONSIDERATIONS

The combat surgeon must not expect to find available the same spectrum of resources as are found in the civilian surgical inten-sive care ward. Nevertheless, survival of at least 90% of the chest casualties evacuated from the battlefield is to be expected. In the postoperative period, careful attention should be paid to the maintenance of adequate pulmonary ventilation and the removal of tracheobronchial secretions by coughing and suctioning. These interventions have been instrumental in lessening the incidence of the pulmonary edema-like syndrome known as "wet lung," which was so common in World War II casualties. Analgesia, preferably given by intercostal block, may lessen the need for suc-tion. However, the surgeon must not delay in resorting to suctioning or even bronchoscopic aspiration for the removal of secretions. Patients who cannot ventilate adequately will require the assistance of a volume cycled respirator. Surgeons should be aware that arterial blood gas determinations may not be available for guiding the management of such patients. Furthermore, reliance on clinical judgment rather than invasive monitoring will be necessary to minimize the possibility of fluid overload during the early postoperative period. Diuretic agents may be necessary to decrease pulmonary extravascular water. In a recent Israeli experience, as many as 25% of severely wounded casualties were inadvertently volume overloaded and needed diuretics or even phlebotomy. It is unwise to attempt to evacuate casualties who still require ventilatory support from the combat zone. Patients should not be evacuated by air until at least three days have elapsed following removal of chest tubes. In one series, about 20% of the Vietnam chest casualties evacuated by air developed a recurrent pneumothorax, and arterial hypoxia was a common finding.

CHAPTER XXIX

Wounds of the Abdomen

INITIAL EVALUATION

The goal of the initial evaluation is to allow the surgeon to determine the probability of an intra-abdominal injury. There is no overriding need for a more specific diagnosis. There are no clearly defined minimally acceptable standards for success. The surgeon must simply do the best that he can for the most patients under the existing circumstances. The "best" is defined as no missed intra-abdominal injuries with the fewest possible negative exploratory laparotomies.

The combat surgeon can consistently achieve this goal by consciously taking four actions. These actions are systematic evaluation of the patient, classification of the patient, consideration of extenuating circumstances, and preparation for operation. Each of these acts is of equal importance. They must be performed simultaneously.

SYSTEMATIC EVALUATION

Evaluation of the combat casualty differs from evaluation in civilian practice. First, there always is a possibility of early evacuation secondary to factors beyond the surgeon's control. The military surgeon cannot assume that he will be able to re-examine the patient at a later time. A decision must be reached each time the surgeon and patient are separated. Procrastination, reflection, and consultation are luxuries seldom enjoyed by the forward surgeon. Second, sophisticated studies, such as arteriography and CT scans, will generally not be available in the forward hospital. Third, the surgeon must deal with distractions such as multiple casualties, massive wounds, logistics breakdowns, the possibility of hostile fire, and the general confusion of war. He must maintain a high index of suspicion and an appreciation of the subtle nature of the signs of serious intra-abdominal injury. All of these casualties can be evaluated rapidly yet carefully if the examination is performed in a systematic manner. The surgeon must appreciate that rapid pulse, narrowed pulse pressure, lowered blood pressure, poor capillary refill, and decreased urinary output are evidence of hypovolemia. In the absence of external evidence of blood loss or evidence of intrathoracic blood loss, these signs are presumptive evidence of intra-abdominal injury.

The History

In war, few individuals have an appreciation of anything beyond their own immediate environment. These conditions produce wildly inaccurate and often contradictory reports of time of wounding, weapons used, and location of injuries. The surgeon is exposed to reports of local and strategic military activities that may or may not be true. It is wisest for the surgeon to believe only what can be seen or felt. The history is of value when the patient identifies the presence, absence, or the location of pain; allergies, and time of last meal. Any other information must be carefully evaluated before being seriously considered. The history is useful when received from other medical personnel, but this should be confined to clinical information.

Inspection

The casualty must be undressed. Mud and other material that can conceal a wound must be cleared. Illumination must be adequate. The surgeon must personally do the exam, but at least one person must assist him. The assistant must understand what the surgeon is trying to do. The surgeon must carefully inspect all of the abdomen from the nipples to the upper thigh, the flanks, the back, and the perineum. This cannot be done without turning the patient, abducting the lower extremities, and spreading the buttocks. The examining team must make allowances for other injuries while performing this examination.

Any evidence of a penetrating injury, no matter how innocuous, must be assumed to represent an intra-abdominal wound and treated accordingly. Missile tracts are unpredictable. Even though these wounds must be debrided, exploration of the wound itself is time consuming and more often than not reveals no definitive information. The surgeon must assume that a penetrating injury of the torso is evidence of an intra-abdominal wound unless the converse is proven. More discretion can be used if there is only evidence of blunt trauma.

Abdominal distension is abnormal in healthy soldiers and may be the only evidence of an intra-abdominal injury. The examining surgeon must consciously search for this most subtle of signs. Splinting of respiration is also abnormal and, excluding chest injury, should be considered strong evidence of intra-abdominal injury.

Palpation

Tenderness must be searched for systematically. This may be difficult to accomplish in an excited, apprehensive young soldier who might well have other painful injuries. The surgeon must be certain that he has the patient's attention and cooperation. Each abdominal quadrant should be examined separately. The presence of involuntary guarding confirms intra-abdominal injury, but this sign may be hard to define under these circumstances. Medial and lateral pressure on the iliac spine and pressure on the pubic symphysis are used to search for pelvic fractures. The presence or absence of femoral pulses should be noted. Abdominal tenderness is more often due to intra-abdominal injury than to abdominal wall trauma. If tenderness is present, the surgeon should reexamine the abdomen after a urinary catheter and a nasogastric tube are in place. Urinary retention and acute gastric dilation are not uncommon in these patients.

Auscultation

This is an essential part of the evaluation. Absent or significantly decreased bowel sounds are abnormal in a healthy young soldier and must be considered presumptive evidence of intra-abdominal injury.

SECONDARY EVALUATION

If there is any reason to suspect an intra-abdominal injury, secondary evaluation is necessary. The surgeon must convince himself that there is clear and unequivocal evidence that there is no intra-abdominal injury. If this is the case, attention can be directed to other problems.

Indwelling Urinary Catheter

If there is no evidence of urethral injury, an indwelling urinary catheter should be inserted and the absence or presence of blood in the urine noted.

Nasogastric Tube

A nasogastric tube should be passed and connected to some type of drainage. The absence or presence of blood in the aspirate should be noted.

Rectal Exam

A digital rectal exam is of critical importance in patients with a lower abdominal or perineal wound. The presence or absence of blood in the rectum is determined. The value of a more sophisticated exam, such as endoscopy or barium enema, is limited by the usual presence of stool in the rectum of most of these patients and the time needed to perform the exam. The position of the prostate should be noted.

Re-examination

The abdomen should be re-evaluated when these procedures are completed. An acutely distended urinary bladder or stomach can be the cause of abdominal pain or tenderness.

X-rays

Simple KUB and lateral films of the abdomen are of great assistance in the search for radiopaque fragments. The films are of value only if positive. Normal X-rays do not rule out injury. If exploratory laparotomy is contemplated, a "single shot" intravenous pyelogram is important to determine if there are two functioning kidneys and if there is evidence of extravasation of urine.

Further studies, such as angiography, are not likely to be available. Other studies, such as peritoneal lavage, often require more time than the surgeon has to devote to one patient.

It is best for the surgeon to base decisions on the information available at this point in the evaluation. Further studies can be valuable, but the forward surgeon in a mobile hospital must be able to function with the information obtained by this evaluation. The opportunity for more detailed and sophisticated evaluation should be used when available, but the dimension of time, the press of more casualties, and the resource limitations must be considered before resorting to these studies.

CLASSIFICATION OF THE PATIENT

The surgeon must classify the patient at specific points during examinations. This allows "weighing" of the data collected during the exam. This classification applies to the patient at hand. This is not triage, even though these actions can be similar to the decision-tree used by a triage officer who is sorting multiple casualties. Mandatory classification of the patient at specific points forces even the inexperienced surgeon to safely and rapidly collect as much information as is needed to care for the patient. This allows the surgeon to act decisively and quickly, but without carelessness.

As each step in the collection of information is completed, the patient should be unequivocally classified as:

Priority I   Definite intra-abdominal injury
Priority II   High probability of intra-abdominal injury
Priority III   Low probability of intra-abdominal injury

Priority I patients should be prepared for operation immediately. There is no need for further collection of data. Actions described as "Secondary Evaluation" (urinary catheter, nasogastric tube, rectal exam, and X-rays) must be completed.

Priority II patients should have "Secondary Evaluation" completed and then operated upon in most cases.

Priority III patients should be systematically examined according to the text, but secondary evaluation is seldom necessary. Any patient can be moved to a more urgent priority at any time. Each step in the evaluation must be used to prioritize these patients.

If there is evidence of hypovolemic shock and no other apparent injury, to include the chest, the patient is classified as Priority I. If there is hypovolemic shock and evidence of other injuries, no matter how sever, the patient is considered Priority II.

Inspection

If there is evidence of evisceration, omentum, stool, bile, or urine leaking from a penetrating wound or if there is loss of tissue from the abdominal wall, the patient is classified as Priority I.

If there is evidence of penetrating wounds. significantly contused tissue, or abdominal distension, the patient is a Priority II. Patients with altered mental states are Priority II. If the abdomen appears normal, the patient is classified as Priority III.

Palpation

A patient with significant tenderness, abdominal rigidity, or pelvic tenderness is Priority II.

Auscultation

A patient with absent or significantly decreased bowel sounds is Priority II.

Further Evaluation

A patient with bloody urine, bloody nasogastric aspirate, blood in the rectum, X-ray evidence of free air, or intra-abdominal foreign bodies is classified Priority I.

This simple approach to evaluation of the soldier with an intra-abdominal injury will ensure that each patient has the benefit of mature surgical judgment despite urgency and distractions.

The patient who is classified Priority II at the completion of the secondary evaluation presents a dilemma. There is no simple resolution; however, a third set of actions, namely, consideration of extenuating circumstances, may help the surgeon to decide whether or not to operate.

CONSIDERATION OF EXTENUATING CIRCUMSTANCES

The third action represents the greatest departure from civilian practice because the unique features of combat surgery are considered. The surgeon must maintain concentration and attention to detail in the care of the individual patient at the same time that these conditions are considered. Consideration of these rules often allows the surgeon to make a decision concerning the care of patients in the Priority II classification. The surgeon must keep several factors in mind:

1. There are no inviolable rules.

2. Any change in the patient's condition cancels all previous decisions.

3. The surgeon must know of the availability of blood or blood products. If they are not available or are available in limited supply, the surgeon should tend to classify the patients in a more urgent category. In other words, the surgeon should tend to operate earlier.

4. The surgeon must know the number of beds available for holding (re-evaluation) and postoperative care.

5. The surgeon must consider the available methods of evacuation. This may be prolonged surface evacuation or rapid movement by air.

6. The surgeon should be aware of the likelihood of movement of the hospital or the likelihood of the hospital coming under fire.

7. The surgeon must appreciate both the quality and quantity of anesthesia support.

8. Knowledge of the availability and sophistication of operative nursing support is critical.

9. The surgeon should know of the availability and sophistication of surgical assistance.

10. Knowledge of the availability of respiratory therapy support for the postoperative patient is essential.

11. Decrements in overall unit efficiency secondary to fatigue must be considered.

PREPARATION FOR OPERATION

Preparation of the patient for operation must be accomplished simultaneously with the other actions. Well-briefed and well-trained nursing personnel are invaluable. Simple routines that are understood by all hospital personnel must be established.

Two large-bore intravenous catheters should be inserted as soon as the patient arrives in the receiving area. Blood must be taken for typing and cross-matching. Antibiotics and tetanus toxoid should be administered as soon as the patient arrives in the receiving area.

An indwelling urinary catheter should be in place. The volume

and character (i.e., bloody or not) of the urine should be noted
at the time of catheterization and the time recorded so that
urinary output after catheterization can be determined later.

A nasogastric tube should be in place.

Associated injuries must be dealt with appropriately. This is
especially true in cases of intrathoracic injuries or massive blood
loss in which the patient's ability to survive the operation can be
affected. It is important to remember that these patients can spend
hours "out of sight" under operative drapes where significant extremity blood loss and the loss of distal pulses may go
unappreciated.

Endotracheal tubes must be in place and properly secured. The
neurological status must be known prior to induction of
anesthesia.

Finally, accurate but succinct notes must be recorded. The ever-
present possibility of evacuation makes this essential.

TREATMENT

Exploration

Before the operation begins, the surgeon should be certain that
illumination is as good as it can be. The surgeon must understand
the capabilities of the assistant. Mutual understanding between
the surgeon and the assistant must be reached before the operation begins. This understanding must consider the ability of the
assistant to obtain hemostasis as well as the assistant's understanding of anatomy, knowledge of general surgical principles, and
operative exposure. The surgeon should understand exactly how
much (or how little) suction will be available. The surgeon should
consider all of these factors when planning the operation.

The incision should be a long midline incision, generally from
the xiphoid to the pubic symphysis.

HEMOSTASIS

The surgeon and the rest of the operative team must have a plan
before the peritoneal cavity is entered. If there is a great deal of
free blood, it is best to use several large laparotomy pads to
evacuate the blood. Suction with irrigation is more effective after
the bulk of free blood has been removed. The surgeon must

quickly decide which area of the abdomen demands first attention. Generally, the amount of hemorrhage will be the determining factor. Direct pressure on individual vessels such as the splenic artery, the great vessels, or the descending thoracic aorta through a limited thoracotomy might be necessary at this time. The first assistant's experience and knowledge of anatomy are critical in the plan for these actions.

EXPOSURE

It is simpler to eviscerate the entire small bowel in complicated cases. The ligaments of the liver can be divided to obtain further exposure in the right upper quadrant. Access to the thoracic cavity should be obtained by extending the midline abdominal incision into a median sternotomy.

The surgeon must have a systematic plan to explore the abdomen. This is similar to an aviator's pre-flight checklist and serves the same purpose to insure that no important step is missed. The excitement and distractions of combat surgery dictate that no laparotomy is concluded until the entire abdominal cavity has been explored.

LEFT UPPER QUADRANT

Distal Esophagus, Diaphragm, Stomach, Spleen, and Kidney

The principles for dealing with injuries to organs in the left upper quadrant of the abdomen are simple. Careful exploration should assure integrity of the diaphragm, the anterior and posterior wall of the stomach, and the esophageal hiatus. The surgeon must palpate the kidney and search for a retroperitoneal hematoma. Perforations of the stomach should be closed primarily with minimal, if any, debridement. Injuries to the lower esophagus should be closed primarily after adequate mobilization. All injuries of the diaphragm should be closed with a single layer of interrupted heavy, nonabsorbable sutures. Large injuries to the diaphragm with herniation of abdominal contents should be repaired transabdominally after the abdominal viscera have been returned to their normal location. The most common error made in the treatment of diaphragmatic injuries is missed diagnosis. All patients with gastric injuries should be treated with nasogastric suction until normal bowel function returns. Enough gastric distention to disrupt a gastric repair is common in patients who are evacuated by air in the early postoperative period.

The diagnosis of renal injury depends on a high index of suspicion, hematuria, or evidence of fragments traversing the kidney. Penetrating injuries of the kidney should be explored and hemostasis obtained. In some cases, a nephrectomy is necessary to achieve hemostasis. Gerota's fascia, if intact, can effectively tamponade hemorrhage in the case of blunt injury to the kidney. In blunt trauma, this fascia should not be opened as hemorrhage is usually self limited.

The spleen should be inspected, but should not be mobilized unless there is evidence of bleeding. In civilian practice, the spleen is infrequently removed because of trauma. If hemorrhage can be controlled quickly and simply with confidence that it will not recur, the spleen can be preserved in combat surgery. If there is extensive injury to the spleen, the organ should be removed. The major difference between the management of civilian and combat injuries to the spleen is in the management of moderate injuries. If a moderate amount of effort is needed to secure hemostasis, it is best to remove the spleen of a combat casualty. The combat surgeon has neither the time required to preserve the moderately-injured spleen, nor the certainty of close personal postoperative observation required for such conservatism. Patients who have undergone splenectomy should be given antibiotic prophylaxis beginning at the time of surgery. This should be continued through the convalescent period. The patient should be vaccinated against those organisms which cause overwhelming sepsis as soon as possible.

RIGHT UPPER QUADRANT

Liver, Gallbladder, and Porta Hepatis

Injuries to the liver are usually trivial, but they can be difficult, complex, and fatal. The major concern in the treatment of liver injuries is hemostasis. Simple lacerations or perforations through the periphery of the liver that have stopped bleeding require no specific therapy. The surgeon must obtain hemostasis when treating deeper wounds of the liver that continue to bleed. If possible, the surgeon should ligate all bleeding vessels. Adequate

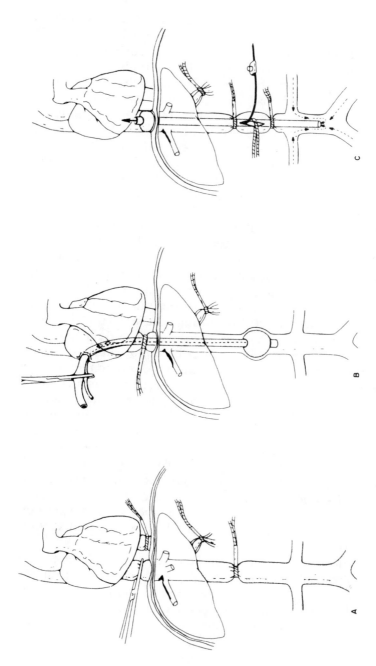

FIGURE 33.—Control of bleeding from caval and hepatic vein injuries associated with liver injuries. A. Four-clamp technique. B. Balloon tamponade via right atrium. C. Intracaval balloon catheter via the suprarenal vena cava.

suction and exposure are essential. Two suction units should be used. The cautery, clips, and ligature are equally effective. The surgeon should perform resectional debridement of significantly devitalized tissue. A formal hepatic lobectomy is never indicated. The Pringle maneuver, using a vascular clamp that will temporarily occlude the porta hepatis, might help control massive hemorrhage. This clamp may be applied for as long as 30 minutes with safety. The abdominal incision can be extended into the right chest to give better exposure of the retrohepatic cava or hepatic veins. Mobilization of the superior and anterior attachments of the liver allows mobilization of the organ. Only surgeons *with personal experience* in their use should consider using caval balloon catheters (Figure 33).

Hypothermia and coagulopathy frequently develop in patients with massive liver injury and hemorrhage. The liver pack can be lifesaving for these patients. Large absorbent pads are placed under tension behind, above, below, and in front of the liver. This maneuver allows the surgeon to explore and repair other areas of the abdominal cavity. Then the wound can be closed by placing a series of large towel clips through the skin and fascia with the packs left in place. A dressing is applied, and the patient is returned to the recovery room where his temperature is brought to normal and he is given appropriate blood component therapy and antibiotics. In 12-72 hours, the patient can be returned to the operating room where, under anesthesia, the abdomen is reopened, the packs are removed, and further hemostasis obtained if necessary. Frequently, bleeding will be found to have stopped.

Injuries to the gallbladder should be treated by cholecystectomy. Injuries to the hepatic artery or the portal vein should be repaired, if possible. Injuries to the common bile duct should be repaired over a small T-tube with a closed suction drain placed adjacent to the repair. The tissue surrounding all but the most innocuous injuries to the liver should be drained by use of closed suction (Figure 34).

Broad-spectrum antibiotics and blood component therapy to correct bleeding disorders should be given. Large mattress sutures in Glisson's capsule for deep liver injuries should not be used because hemobilia can develop later. A useful adjunct for hemostasis is the insertion of an intact vascularized pedicle of

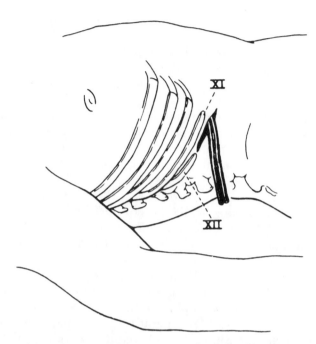

FIGURE 34.—Drainage of the abdomen. For adequate drainage of the abdomen, drains must be placed in the most dependent portion of the peritoneal cavity. This is best accomplished through the posterior flank utilizing sump drains.

omentum into a liver injury with loose closure of the liver over the omentum.

Duodenum and Pancreas

Injuries to the duodenum are easily overlooked. The surgeon should suspect duodenal injury if missiles or missile tracks are found in the region of the duodenum, if there is blood in the nasogastric tube and retroperitoneum, or if there is air in the region of the duodenum. All patients who have had blunt trauma, and all patients who have had penetrating trauma in the region of the duodenum must have both a generous Kocher maneuver to expose the duodenum and an opening into the lesser sac that will expose the anterior pancreas and duodenal sweep. Minimal debridement and repair should be done for perforations, lacerations, and partial or complete transections. These patients need closed-suction drainage adjacent to, but not in contact with, the anastomosis. When more extensive injuries of the duodenum require more extensive debridement, the biliary, pancreatic, and gastric flow must be preserved. Missed injuries to the duodenum are often fatal. They may present late with signs of retroperitoneal abscess.

Injuries to the pancreas always require drainage, generally closed-suction drainage. This may suffice for simple, superficial, blunt, or penetrating injuries of the pancreas, but deeper injuries, particularly those that involve the major pancreatic ducts, require more aggressive therapy. This may include resection of the distal pancreas. Transection or near-transection of the midbody of the pancreas can be treated by ligation of the distal end of the proximal duct and a Roux-en-Y anastomosis of the distal remnant into the gut. The choice to divert or resect the distal portion of the divided pancreas depends on the experience of the surgeon and the presence of associated injuries. If there is severe destruction of the head of the pancreas and duodenum, a pancreaticoduodenectomy may be required to save the patient. This situation is uncommon. Postoperatively, these patients frequently develop external fistulae. Closed-suction drain ensure that these fistulae are controlled. They may persist. The skin must be protected from the activated enzymes in the drainage. Fistula can lead to significant nursing problems. These can be limited by attention to details early.

MIDABDOMEN

Small Intestine

Simple perforations, lacerations, or tears of the small intestine should be minimally debrided and closed primarily with a single layer of interrupted sutures (Figure 35).

The surgeon must carefully search for multiple injuries by examining the small intestine in a systematic fashion, beginning at the ligament of Treitz and proceeding distally, looking at 10" segments of bowel on one side and then the other. The entire small bowel must be examined all the way to the cecum. The surgeon must carefully search for injuries to the mesentery at the edge of the bowel, since small tangential bowel perforations in the mesenteric surface may not be obvious on superficial exami-

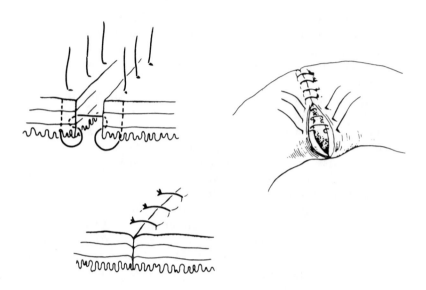

FIGURE 35.—An inverting single-layer suture technique is satisfactory for repair of small bowel injuries and anastomomosis of small bowel after resection.

nation. Use the "rule of twos" in treating penetrating injuries of the intestine and colon. Since fragments almost always perforate both walls of the intestine, they create an even number of injuries to the gut. Therefore, an even number of perforations can be expected. While this rule is not absolute, it is helpful in assuring that no injuries are missed. Rather than several individual repairs, a limited resection encompassing multiple injuries may be a safer and more expeditious approach in the patient with multiple injuries in close proximity. Injuries of the mesenteric vessels should be dealt with by ligation and bowel resection if there is nonviable or questionably viable bowel.

Injuries to the aorta and inferior vena cava are usually fatal. Those who survive to reach the hospital frequently require urgent laparotomy as part of their resuscitation. These patients will frequently deteriorate during resuscitation and transfusion. They must be identified, explored, and hemostasis must be achieved, if they are to survive. An occasional patient with a severe splenic or hepatic injury can present in a similar fashion and require urgent operation for hemostasis. In this sort of case, continued

transfusion and resuscitation in order to make the patient a better operative risk do not work, and death is the usual outcome.
A senior surgeon must diligently search for these patients in the
preoperative area and ensure early surgical intervention for
hemostasis.

The intraoperative management of these injuries includes
generous incisions, the obtaining of adequate proximal and distal
control and then appropriate repair of the injury. Frequently,
minimal debridement and primary closure will suffice.
Autogenous tissue (vein graft) is better than synthetic material in
the repair of the more extensive vascular injuries, but suitable vein
grafts may not always be available.

Helpful maneuvers to achieve hemostasis in these patients include the insertion of a balloon catheter into the proximal and
distal vessels through the injury site, use of a sponge stick to compress the aorta against the spine at the level of the diaphragm, and
control of the aorta with a vascular clamp above the diaphragm
via a limited thoracotomy.

Ureters

The ureters are infrequently injured. A ureteral injury usually
causes hematuria. If this is noted preoperatively, an intravenous
pyelogram will often provide a more secure diagnosis in these patients. Urine and blood will collect along the course of the ureter,
particularly if there was a penetrating injury. These collections
should prompt the surgeon to conduct a careful exploration of
the entire course of the ureter.

Ureteral injuries can be repaired with fine absorbable sutures
and closed-suction drainage close to, but not touching, the repair.
Internal stenting is not required in simple injuries. In more extensive injuries with significant tissue loss, repair will depend
upon the location and extent of the injury and the experience of
the surgeon. If the lower third of the ureter is injured, it may be
reimplanted into the dome of the bladder through a muscular tunnel. The kidney can be mobilized, if necessary, to provide some
additional length. Repairs should be done transversely or on a bias
to maintain the diameter of the lumen since strictures may otherwise result. Drainage of all urinary repairs is required. Closed suction is preferred.

Colon

Injuries to the colon frequently result from penetrating abdominal injuries. The basic rule is that combat injuries of the colon should not be closed. The majority of these patients should have either a loop colostomy which includes the injury, or resection of the injured colon and proximal diversion (Figure 36).

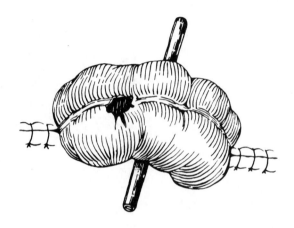

FIGURE 36.—Under certain circumstances, exteriorization of colon wound is acceptable. The loop of colon is exteriorized over a glass rod or a rubber catheter.

Major injuries of the right colon should be treated by right hemicolectomy, with creation of a proximal ileostomy and distal mucus fistula (Figure 37). The reason for such a didactic approach is that these patients have an unprepared colon, usually have associated injuries, and it is unlikely that the operating surgeon will be able to follow the patient through the postoperative period. These particular lessons have been learned and relearned at great expense in previous conflicts.

An option that is consistent with these guidelines is exteriorization of certain colon repairs. Injuries to the transverse and sigmoid colon may be repaired and then exteriorized in continuity for 6-10 days. If healing takes place, as is the case approximately 50% of the time, the repaired colon can be replaced into the abdomen at a second procedure. If the repair fails to heal, it can be converted to a loop colostomy with no particular danger to the patient. If this method is chosen, the opening in the abdominal wall must

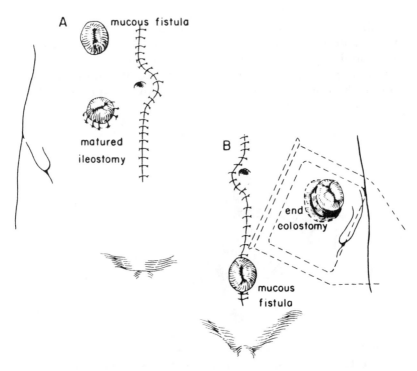

FIGURE 37.—A. Following severe injury to the right colon, especially with associated severe injury to contiguous organs, right colectomy is indicated. A matured ileostomy, which will accommodate an ileostomy appliance and the distal mucous fistula, are shown. B. The construction of an end colostomy and a distal mucous fistula that allows placement of an appliance over the proximal stoma is mandatory for diversion of the fecal stream in management of low sigmoid and rectal injuries.

be large enough to allow for the stool to progress into the repaired segment and back to the abdomen. This opening will be larger than that needed for the usual loop colostomy. Failure to allow for this can result in the buildup of pressure in the repaired segment that will cause failure of the repair.

Preoperative antibiotics are indicated when intestinal injuries are suspected; however, their postoperative use beyond 12 hours is questionable. As in suspected injuries of the small intestine, the surgeon must conduct a careful, methodical inspection of the colon from one end to the other. Again, it is appropriate to emphasize that injuries on the mesenteric surface of the colon are difficult to diagnose and must be searched for diligently, particularly in the presence of hematoma.

Pelvis

Injuries of the pelvis can be particularly difficult and frustrating. Hemorrhage from pelvic fractures or fragment injuries may not respond to the usual hemostatic techniques. A major advance in treatment of fracture dislocations of the pelvis associated with hemorrhage is the pelvic fixation device. This should be considered early in the management of these patients. Injuries of the bladder and rectosigmoid are easily overlooked. The surgeon must search for these carefully to avoid devastating complications.

Rectum

The surgeon must suspect a rectal injury in any patient who has suffered a penetrating wound of the pelvis or in whom fragments could have traversed the pelvis. Anteroposterior and lateral roentgenograms, interpreted with the knowledge of entrance and exit wounds, are particularly helpful in determining if a rectal injury is likely to be present. Digital examination of the rectum is required. Endoscopy to determine the presence of intraluminal blood is indicated in these patients.

Blood in the rectum should be assumed to be evidence of a transmural injury. A search for the specific location of the injury must be made. Rectal injuries are difficult to diagnose at the time of laparotomy. If no injury can be found in a patient with frank blood in the rectum, the surgeon must treat the patient as if a rectal injury has occurred.

The treatment of patients with rectal injuries includes four components: first, a proximal, totally diverting colostomy; second, thorough cleansing and irrigation of the distal rectosigmoid; third, repair of the rectal tear, if accessible; and fourth, drainage of the presacral space with soft drains of the closed-suction type (Figure 38).

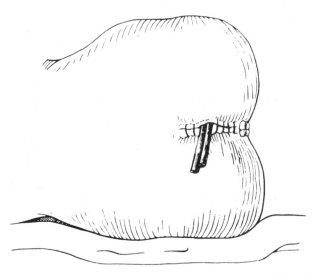

FIGURE 38.—Presacral drainage is best accomplished by direct vision through a posterior incision in a dependent position utilizing sump drains.

Bladder

Injuries of the bladder are usually associated with hematuria. The surgeon should suspect a bladder injury when the entrance or exit wound, the two-plane roentgenograms, or hematuria suggest that this is the case. A cystogram is the definitive test. It is obtained by the instillation of contrast into the bladder via an indwelling urethral catheter. Two roentgen views should be taken, one with the bladder full and the other after voiding. Extravasation indicates bladder perforation and requires operation.

These injuries should be repaired with two layers of absorbable sutures, insertion of an indwelling suprapubic catheter, and placement of a soft closed-suction drain into the region of the repair. Bladder injuries will heal if the edges of the wound are approximated and adequate bladder decompression is maintained for ten days.

Reproductive Organs

Conservation should be practiced in the management of injuries of the reproductive organs. Penetrating or crush injuries of the labia, penis, scrotum, and testicles are best treated by conservative debridement and primary repair, if practical. The scrotum should be drained with a soft rubber drain. Injuries to the uterus, ovaries, and fallopian tubes will require conservative debridement and repair. Drainage is seldom indicated.

POSTOPERATIVE CARE

Wound Closure

Reliability of the abdominal wound closure is of major importance. Patients are frequently moved in the early postoperative period. Generally speaking, a secure closure requires the use of a strong monofilament nonabsorbable suture which incorporates large "bites" of fascia. The closure may be interrupted or "running," but the latter is much more expeditious. Full-thickness retention sutures over bolsters are required in difficult closures and in most reoperative, complicated abdomens. When placed, they should be 2-3 cm apart and 3-4 cm from the edges of the wound. These sutures are usually left in place for three weeks. They may or may not be used in conjunction with a separate fascial closure. The skin and subcutaneous tissue in contaminated abdominal wounds should not be closed primarily. Delayed primary closure can be done in 4-5 days.

Stomas

Intestinal stomas require some care in the site selection. Anatomy and abdominal wall injuries will influence this choice. The future fitting of an appliance must be considered. Vascularity of the stoma must be preserved, since failure will require another laparotomy. The Brooke type of "turn-back" ileostomy stomas with 1.5-2 cm of elevation is preferred for stoma fitting and nursing management.

Colostomies for rectal injuries should always be a "diverting" type of end colostomy with a separate muscus fistula. The stomas may be flush. They should be matured at the primary operation by sewing the ends of the colon circumferentially to the skin. Loop colostomies are seldom needed in combat casualties, but they are simpler to construct and need not be opened for several days postoperatively. All stomas should have an adequate opening in the abdominal wall at all levels. They should be fixed to the fascia by several interrupted sutures superficially in the wall of the intestine or colon. A patient with a stoma should remain under the observation of the same surgeon to ensure the viability and satisfactory performance of the stoma. This also allows the surgeon the opportunity to explain to the patient the necessity for the procedure, the stoma's function, its care, and when the patient can expect the stoma to be closed.

Ileus

Postoperatively, the bowel undergoes a normal period of motor, but not secretory, inertia. This causes abdominal distention. The distention can be minimized by the use of nasogastric suction. Some patients may have a prolonged ileus. This may be due to contamination, bowel manipulation at operation, too rapid a resumption of feeding, an anastomotic leak, a missed injury, or intraabdominal infection. Systemic nonabdominal sepsis and spinal cord injuries can also cause ileus. Treatment consists of nasogastric suction and parenteral fluid, and electrolyte and nutritional support. A search for the specific cause of the ileus should be ongoing, particularly if other findings are present.

Records

Accurate and complete documentation is essential; it need not be wordy. Legible handwritten operation notes and hospital summaries performed by the surgeons should be concise and cover the important points. Important points include the indications for operation, the findings, what was done, what was not done, technical points if they represent a deviation from the usual or if likely to be relevant in the future care of the patient, how the patient did postoperatively, and what the management plan would be if the physician were to continue caring for him. Liberal use of sketches and diagrams are of value.

CHAPTER XXX

Reoperative Abdominal Surgery

Certain complications that arise after initial abdominal operation require abdominal reoperation. As the casualty progresses
rearward along the medical evacuation chain, medical personnel
must be ever vigilant in the early recognition of these complications. The U.S. Air Force, with its aeromedical evacuation responsibility, has a special interest and great experience in the recognition and treatment of these complications. During the Vietnam
conflict, one of every six casualties with abdominal wounds removed from the air evacuation system at Clark Air Force Base required
reoperation.

Because of the severity of their abdominal wounds and the high
frequency of associated injuries, these patients frequently present
confusing findings. The indications for reoperation are often not
well defined. To make matters even more difficult, these complications may not develop until the postoperative patient arrives at
a higher echelon hospital and comes under the care of surgeons
who were not involved in the primary operation. On occasion, the
medical records accompanying these patients may lack sufficient
detail regarding the injury and the details of the first operative
procedure to be helpful in subsequent evaluation. Given these circumstances, the surgeon must rely heavily on past experience for
guidelines in reoperation of abdominal war wounds. The inherent
problems of making a preoperative diagnosis in the most difficult
group of patients should not deter an aggressive approach. This
philosophy will prove much more rewarding than procrastination.
Practical points gained from such experience follow.

TIME OF REOPERATION

The greatest number of reoperations for intra-abdominal complications are performed in the first three weeks, with a peak incidence from the fourth to the eighth day. This further serves to

identify the timeframe during which the casualty should not be evacuated because frequent evaluation by experienced surgeons may not be available. If transfers are essential during this period, the transit time should be measured in hours rather than days. When a heavy casualty load makes early evacuation necessary, the least seriously injured patients should be selected rather than those with extensive intra-abdominal injury. This philosophy will allow for earlier diagnosis and treatment of those complications that are most likely to arise. The ideal status for evacuation of the patient with a postoperative abdominal wound is after he has become afebrile and alimentation has begun.

SPECIFIC REASONS FOR REOPERATIONS

Dehiscence

In addition to wound infection, two factors contribute to dehiscence: the failure to place retention sutures in war wounds, and the air evacuation of patients with postoperative ileus. The lowest incidence of dehiscence is achieved when the abdomen is closed with retention sutures, 2–3 cm apart, through all layers, in combination with closure of individual layers. Of the 626 casualties with abdominal wounds seen at Clark AFB, there were 26 with dehiscence (4.1%). Retention sutures had not been used in any of the 26 cases. Ileus is a factor in dehiscence because of the pressure exerted by distended bowel on the abdominal wound. Bowel gas expands by 15–30% of sea level volume at the usual cabin pressure of evacuation aircraft. The avoidance, therefore, of evacuation when ileus exists is desirable. The use of reliable nasogastric decompression minimizes this problem.

Retraction of Colostomy

Reoperation may become necessary in the early postoperative period because of retraction or necrosis of a colostomy or ileostomy. If the bowel has been exteriorized under tension, retraction may result. Tension becomes a problem when the bowel is not adequately mobilized by liberal incision in the lateral peritoneal reflections of the colon. The foregoing is especially applicable to fixed segments of the bowel, such as flexures and the descending colon. Failure to suture the mesenteric segment securely to the peritoneum also may contribute to retraction. Correction of this complication requires reoperation to perform the mobilization of the colon that should have been performed at initial operation. Construction of another stoma in more proximal bowel or within the retracted segment under no tension is then possible. If easy deliverance of the bowel to the abdominal wall is not possible even after such mobilization due to inflammatory shortening of the mesentery, performance of a more proximal colostomy in a mobile portion of bowel and resection of the bowel between the retracted colon and the new stoma must be carried out. In the case of ileostomy, immediate maturation of the stoma by eversion and mucosa-to-skin suture with fine absorbable suture prevents problems. In addition, mesentery-to-peritoneum suture is as necessary here as it is in the colon. If retraction of a ileostomy does occur, laparotomy is necessary to construct a new stoma in fresh bowel slightly more proximal to the original stoma.

Missed Intra-Abdominal Injury

Three factors influence the failure to identify and treat significant intra-abdominal injury: the adequacy of the operative incision, the necessity for complete systematic exploration, and the failure to explore by dissection the hidden areas of the abdomen when indicated. The operative incision must be adequate in size as well as in position. A generous midline incision is best for exposure because of the facility with which it can be made and closed. Quadrant incisions are generally not as good unless the course of the wounding agent is known with absolute certainty, a situation that seldom prevails. Systematic exploration requires an adequate incision. An incision that admits only one of the surgeon's hands into the abdomen is inadequate for complete exploration. Changes in the location of certain intra-abdominal organs during changes in body position and respiration may be responsible for injuries distant from the external wounds and are an additional reason for systematic, complete examination of all organs. The most commonly overlooked injuries at celiotomy are those of the retroperitoneal structures, the fixed portions of the colon, and the viscera bordering the lesser sac. These areas can be inspected adequately only by intraoperative dissection, which should be done when there is any likelihood that injury to these organs has occurred.

Intra-abdominal injury can be overlooked when a missile penetrates the abdomen through an entrance site other than the anterior abdominal wall. When the patient, who has undergone operative treatment of thigh, buttock, chest, or flank wounds, develops signs of peritonitis, an intraperitoneal wound must be suspected. Abdominal roentgenography may be of help by identifying free air or a previously unrecognized intra-abdominal metallic fragment. This examination should be done in all such cases to assure early detection of these hidden wounds.

Stress Ulcer Hemorrhage

Upper gastrointestinal hemorrhage in postoperative casualties is most often due to stress ulceration. The surgeon's most important priority in dealing with this problem is prevention, specifically with H2 antagonists and antacids. The mainstay and most readily available treatment uses antacids every 2 hours to titrate the gastric pH to greater than 5. Many burn and trauma units have found this condition a rarity since these aggressive preventive measures have been practiced.

Once developed, stress ulcers require vigorous evaluation and therapy. If endoscopy is available, it should be performed. Copious gastric lavage with iced saline, followed by maximum administration of H2 blockers and hourly antacids, may suffice. Transfusions are frequently necessary. Operation is usually indicated for hemodynamic instability or if more than five units of blood must be transfused. These ulcerations are frequently multiple. They may be gastric or duodenal, or both. The majority are gastric. Stress ulcers usually present in individuals with uncontrolled sepsis, in the intraperitoneal region or elsewhere. Generally, the nonoperative management of stress ulcers is not effective and lasting unless the sepsis is controlled. The choice of operative procedure for stress ulcer depends upon the experience of the surgeon. Generally, vagotomy, pyloroplasty, and oversewing of the bleeding ulcers suffice if the sepsis has been controlled. If the septic source has not been identified and addressed, then the surgeon should consider a major resectional procedure.

Intestinal Obstruction

Postoperative mechanical intestinal obstruction, when present, usually develops within the first two weeks after injury. Early operative treatment has been employed with success; the use of long intestinal tubes having been less helpful. Adhesions and intraloop abscesses are the usual causes of obstruction in these cases. It should be stressed that this complication occurs relatively late and should not be confused with prolonged ileus in the earlier postinjury period. Water-soluble radiopaque iodine compounds such as Gastrografin can be employed to differentiate these two conditions. When administered orally, the contrast material fails to traverse the intestinal tract in mechanical obstruction. In the unobstructed case, the contrast material passes through the intestinal tract within a few hours, as evidenced by serial abdominal roentgenograms or by the initiation of bowel movements.

Intra-Abdominal Hemorrhage

Late hemorrhage in abdominal wounds is seen when an infectious process erodes a blood vessel of significant size. This occurs most often in the retroperitoneum when a hematoma was not explored. When it results from a missile wound, the area is contaminated and cellulitis or abscess formation reactivates bleeding by clot resolution or vessel erosion. Undetected wounds in the fixed portion of the colon, duodenum, pancreas, and retroperitoneum (with eventual infection) and hemorrhage from the lumbar venous plexus are most troublesome and may be fatal. Since such hemorrhage is usually profuse, operation, although mandatory, may not be effective.

Intra-Abdominal Abscesses

The drainage of abscesses accounts for the greatest number of reoperations in abdominal wounds. When this complication presents relatively early in the postinjury period, it is most often associated with other complications, such as stress bleeding, fistula formation, and intestinal obstruction. Abscesses may also be chronic and present much later, with low-grade fever and inanition.

Treatment involves evacuation of the abscess, collapse of the cavity, and prevention of recurrence. Closed-suction drains help to achieve these objectives. If the cavity is not well formed, irrigation may disseminate organisms to other intraperitoneal sites.

Judgment, therefore, must be exercised regarding the use and volume of irrigating solutions. Drains should be dependently positioned to achieve the maximum effect of gravity.

Large Abdominal Wall Defects

When a considerable portion of the abdominal wall has been lost as a result of a wound or necessary debridement, the surgeon must consider the effects of initial treatment on the subsequent course. If a primary closure is attempted, strangulation of tissue by undue tension may cause necrosis of wound edges. A too-tight closure can lead to limitation of diaphragmatic excursion and respiratory compromise. If small intestine is allowed to become the base of a granulating wound, fistula formation and intestinal obstruction may result. Both of these situations may require reoperation. The most successful form of treatment in these cases, at initial operation or reoperation, has been the insertion of a Marlex mesh prosthesis, sewn to the undersurface of the remaining viable abdominal wall. As it is becoming encased in granulation tissue, the mesh should be covered with a dressing soaked in saline. Once the base of the wound is covered by healthy granulation tissue, it can be covered by a split-thickness skin graft or a sliding pedicle graft. An occasional patient, without abdominal wall loss, may require this type of closure due to tension.

In the austere situation where Marlex or other stock prostheses are not available, the surgeon may have to improvise. Recent experimental studies have shown that these defects can be successfully covered with polyvinyl chloride (Via Flex). This is the material from which Ringer's lactate and blood bags are made. Experimental use of these bags in animals to close defects has been very encouraging.

Fistulae

A well-formed fistula, regardless of source, may be treated by high-volume suction. This suction may be directed at the gut above the fistula, the fistula itself or both. Closure usually occurs when distal obstruction is not present. When it is associated with abscess or peritonitis, operative intervention is indicated. Closure with adequate drainage, resection, exteriorization, repair, and proximal diversion, singly or in combination, should be employed as the local situation dictates. Healing of fistulae always requires adequate nutrition. Nutritional support should be vigorously pursued, either enterally or parenterally.

CHAPTER XXXI

Wounds and Injuries of the Genitourinary Tract

INTRODUCTION

Genitourinary tract injuries in a combat zone constitute approximately 5% of the total injuries encountered. With the exception of the external genitalia, these wounds invariably will be associated with serious visceral injury and, as a result, are generally managed in areas where there are major surgical and roentgenographic capabilities. The treatment of urologic injuries does not vary from established surgical principles: hemostasis, debridement, and drainage. In contrast to intraperitoneal injuries, preoperative evaluation, utilizing appropriate urographic diagnostic procedures, is simpler and more expedient than an extensive retroperitoneal exploration at the time of laparotomy. Preoperative urologic contrast studies are particularly rewarding when an unsuspected injury, anomaly, or absence is discovered.

WOUNDS OF THE KIDNEY

Renal injuries, except for renal pedicle injuries, are usually not life threatening; however, if not diagnosed or treated properly, they may cause significant morbidity. The diagnosis of renal injury should be suspected based upon the type of trauma sustained, the physical examination, and the urinalysis. Microscopic or gross hematuria is usually present; however, the absence of hematuria does not exclude renal trauma. Renal injury must be suspected in the presence of associated findings such as multiple rib fractures, vertebral body or transverse process fractures, crushing injuries of the chest of thorax, or any penetrating injury to the flank or upper abdomen.

The primary radiographic study used to diagnose renal trauma is the intravenous pyelogram (IVP). This study will usually define

380

renal anatomy, showing injury to the affected kidney. Of equal importance, the IVP should also confirm the presence and functional status of the contralateral kidney and the presence or absence of congenital anomalies, such as horseshoe or congenital single kidney. Delayed films may be necessary to visualize contrast extravasation. If the functional status of the unaffected kidney is not ascertained prior to surgical exploration, an intravenous pyelogram must be performed on the operating table prior to any attempt at exploration of the injured kidney. It has been a generally accepted practice to perform preoperative IVPs on all individuals with abdominal wounds who require laparotomy.

Renal trauma, either blunt or penetrating, may be classified according to the degree or extent of anatomical damage to the kidney. Minor injuries consist of renal contusions or shallow cortical lacerations. Major injuries are comprised of deep cortical lacerations, shattered kidneys, renal vascular pedicle injuries, or total avulsion of the renal pelvis.

Some renal injuries will be minor and may be managed nonoperatively with hydration and bedrest. Major injuries usually require operative intervention with debridement of nonviable renal tissue (partial nephrectomy), closure of the collecting system, and drainage of the retroperitoneal area. In some instances, total nephrectomy may be required. Since there is an 80% incidence of associated visceral injuries with major renal trauma, most cases will require a laparotomy for evaluation and repair of intraperitoneal injuries. Hemodynamically significant injuries are addressed first. If control of hemorrhage requires exploration of the renal space, it is imperative to first gain vascular control of the renal pedicle prior to opening the perirenal fascia and releasing the relatively hemostatic tamponade. Vascular control is obtained by using a periaortic approach to the renal vascular pedicle. The small intestine is retracted superiorly and the posterior peritoneum is incised over the aorta. Since the left renal vein crosses anterior to the aorta, over the origin of both the right and left renal arteries, it must be mobilized to gain control of the origin of either renal artery. After applying atraumatic vascular clamps to the appropriate renal artery and vein, the respective colon may then be mobilized and reflected medially. The perirenal fascia is then opened and the renal wound evaluated.

Operative treatment consists of hemostasis, local debridement and suture, total nephrectomy, or rarely, partial nephrectomy. Urinary diversion in the form of tube nephrostomy or a ureteral stent is recommended in the presence of associated injuries of the duodenum, pancreas, or large bowel. If the tactical situation rules out immediate surgical treatment for major renal injury and the patient is hemodynamically stable, he should be supported with intravenous fluids until evacuation.

WOUNDS OF THE URETER

Ureteral injuries are rare and are frequently overlooked. The diagnosis is made only if the possibility of such an injury is considered in all cases of retroperitoneal hematoma and injuries of the fixed portions of the colon, the duodenum, and the spleen. Ureteral injuries are diagnosed preoperatively by the IVP. Intraoperative location of the ureteral injury, if required, is facilitated by intravenous injection of indigocarmine.

Surgical repair is based upon three factors: the anatomical segment of the traumatized ureter, other associated injuries, and the clinical stability of the patient. Debridement, hemostasis, and drainage are key factors in any successful repair, especially with high-velocity missile injuries.

If a small segment of ureter in its upper or middle segment is damaged, the proximal and distal segments may be spatulated for 1 cm and a ureteroureterostomy performed using interrupted 4-0 absorbable sutures. In the injury near the bladder, a ureteroneocystostomy should be performed. Upper and midureteral injuries in which a large ureteral segment has been damaged may require a temporizing cutaneous ureterostomy with stent placement or transureteroureterostomy. In the presence of duodenal, pancreatic, large bowel, or rectal injuries, proximal urinary diversion with a nephrostomy tube and internal ureteral stent management are required. When a distal ureteral injury is associated with a rectal injury, a ureteral reimplantation is not recommended, and a transureteroureterostomy should be performed. Adequate retroperitoneal drainage is always employed using soft rubber or silicone drains.

If the ureteral injury is not diagnosed initially and manifests itself at a later date, diversion with a nephrostomy tube is performed and ureteral repair should be delayed for 3–6 months.

WOUNDS OF THE BLADDER

Bladder wounds are common and should always be considered in patients with lower abdominal wounds, gross hematuria, or an inability to void following abdominal or pelvic trauma. These tears may be intraperitoneal or extraperitoneal. After insuring urethral integrity in appropriate cases (see "Wounds of the Urethra" *infra*), the diagnosis is made radiographically. Cystography is performed by retrograde filling of the bladder via a urethral catheter with radiopaque contrast medium elevated 20–30 cm above the level of the abdomen. An X-ray of the full bladder is taken, and another X-ray is taken after draining the bladder by unclamping the urethral catheter. Small extraperitoneal areas of extravasation may be apparent only on the postevacuation film.

Penetrating injuries and blowout perforations of the bladder dome due to blunt lower abdominal trauma of a full bladder are most often intraperitoneal. Cystography reveals contrast medium interspersed between loops of bowel. Management consists of exploration, multilayer repair of the injury with absorbable sutures, suprapubic tube cystostomy, and drainage of the perivesical extraperitoneal space.

Extraperitoneal injuries to the bladder are most often the result of laceration by bony fragments of a pelvic fracture. Cystography reveals a flame-like extravasation of contrast medium on the postevacuation film. Extraperitoneal injuries may be repaired primarily as above; however, they usually heal with 10–14 days of Foley catheter drainage without the need for primary repair.

WOUNDS OF THE URETHRA

Injuries to the male urethra should always be suspect in patients with blood at the urethral meatus. Urethral catheterization is contraindicated until integrity has been established by retrograde urethrography. After sterile prepping of the penis, retrograde urethrography is performed by inserting the end of a cathetertip syringe into the urethral meatus with gentle retrograde instillation of 15–20cc of a water-soluble contrast medium. An X-ray is taken during injection. Urethral injury will be represented by extravasation of the contrast material. Contrast must be seen flowing into the bladder to ascertain urethral integrity proximal to the urogenital diaphragm.

The urethra is divided into anterior and posterior (prostatic) segments by the urogenital diaphragm. Posterior urethral disruption commonly occurs following pelvic fracture injuries. Rectal examination reveals the prostate to have been avulsed at the apex. Improved continence and potency rates are attained when suprapubic tube cystostomy is used as the initial management. No attempt at reapproximation of the urethral edges should be made, as such attempts increase the risk of impotency, release the tamponade of the pelvic hematoma, and too often result in an infected hematoma. With expectant observation virtually all these injuries will heal with an obliterative prostatomembranous urethral stricture, which can be repaired secondarily in 4–6 months after reabsorption of the pelvic hematoma. Initial exploration of the pelvic hematoma is strictly reserved for patients with concomitant transmural rectal injury.

Anterior urethral injuries may result from blunt trauma, such as results from falls astride an object (straddle), or from penetrating injuries. Blunt trauma resulting in minor nondisruptive urethral injuries may be managed by gentle insertion of a 16 French foley catheter for 7–10 days. If any difficulty in passing the catheter is encountered, or if the blunt trauma has an associated perineal or penile hematoma indicating more than a minor mucosal injury, the urethra is not instrumented and suprapubic tube cystostomy is performed. Suprapubic urinary diversion is maintained for 10–14 days and urethral integrity is confirmed radiographically prior to removal of the suprapubic tube. Healing may occur without stricture formation. If a stricture develops, it is readily managed by direct vision urethrotomy or open urethroplasty at a later procedure.

Penetrating wounds of the anterior urethra should be managed by exploration and debridement. Small, clean lacerations of the urethra may be repaired primarily by reapproximation of the urethral edges using interrupted 4-0 chromic catgut sutures. Most penetrating urethral injuries, however, will be associated with devitalized margins requiring debridement. One should refrain from the temptation to mobilize the entire urethra for a primary anastomosis, as the shortened urethral length in the pendulous urethra will invariably result in ventral chordee and an anastomosis under tension. Instead, the injured urethral segment should be marsupialized by suturing the skin edges to the cut edges of the urethra. Marsupialization should be performed until healthy urethra is encountered both proximally and distally. Closure of the marsupialized urethra is subsequently performed at six months to reestablish urethral continuity.

WOUNDS OF THE EXTERNAL GENITALIA

The management of wounds of the penis, scrotum, testes, and spermatic cord consists of control of hemorrhage, debridement (which should always be as conservative as possible), and repair, as early as possible, to prevent deformity.

In injuries of the penis, tears of Buck's fascia should be sutured. When denudation has been extensive, the penis may be placed in a scrotal tunnel until plastic repair can be carried out in an appropriately equipped facility.

The scrotum has a good blood supply, and extensive debridement is therefore not necessary. In complete avulsion, the testes can be placed in protective pockets in the thighs.

It is essential, when dealing with testicular wounds, to conserve as much tissue as possible. Herniated parenchymal tissues should be replaced and the tunica albuginea closed by mattress sutures. The testicle is placed in the scrotum or in a protective pocket in some adjacent structure. A testicle should never be resected unless it is hopelessly damaged and its blood supply destroyed.

CHAPTER XXXII

Wounds and Injuries
of the Hand

The hand is constantly subject to serious trauma. Even though minor injuries may be incapacitating, the hand has remarkable recuperative powers. It can be trained to compensate for much of its lost function. Hand injuries should never be taken lightly, even those that appear to be relatively minor. Appropriate early management will yield the maximum possible return of function.

Injuries of the hand, in themselves, seldom result in shock or fatality. The casualty with a hand wound who presents in shock should therefore be evaluated for other more significant wounds. Those life-threatening wounds should be given treatment priority prior to attending to the hand wound. When other priorities dictate delay in treatment of the hand injury, hemostasis and further injury to the hand are prevented by dressing and immobilizing the hand.

CARE IN THE DIVISION AREA

Care of the wounded hand in the division area is limited to control of hemorrhage and immobilization by a compressive dressing (Figure 39). The immobilized extremity is elevated. Antibiotic therapy is initiated and the wounded soldier evacuated to a facility with roentgenographic and surgical capabilities.

Should the tactical situation preclude early evacuation, the following additional measures are recommended:

1. Wrist watches and rings are removed. The hand is thoroughly cleansed with soap and water. The combatant's fingernails, which in combat are usually filthy, are clipped and cleaned.

2. Shreds of obviously dead tissue are excised. Amputation of digits is rarely indicated. If amputation appears necessary, it is done later, after the opportunity for more careful evaluation and planning.

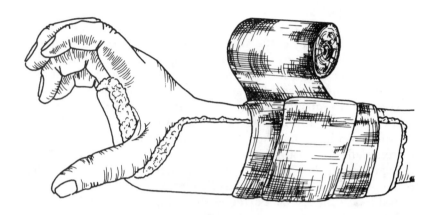

FIGURE 39.—Immobilization of injured hand and forearm in position of anatomical function.

3. Oozing is controlled by the application of a generous gauze dressing. Petrolatum-impregnated gauze and grease in any form should be avoided. The hand is immobilized in the position of function.

INITIAL WOUND SURGERY

Anesthesia

Both general anesthesia and conduction (nerve) blocks are satisfactory for surgical management of the wounds of the hand. Local anesthesia does not provide satisfactory anesthesia. Adrenalin is not injected into hands or fingers, since any additional perfusion compromise, coupled with already marginal perfusion, can result in irreversible ischemic changes.

Debridement

Ideally, the surgeon works with an assistant, a good light, and adequate time. The surgeon should operate while seated, with the draped extremity extended and the hand resting on a suitable support. Necessary instruments include fine tissue forceps, skin hooks, straight and curved ophthalmic scissors, small knife blades, and fine needles. Some sort of magnification is essential.

Cleansing of the surgical field prior to operation is of paramount importance. Since the combatant's hand is usually filthy, attention to detail at the time of the initial cleansing under anesthesia is invaluable in diminishing subsequent sepsis. The preparation extends from the distal edge of the tourniquet to the tips of the trimmed fingernails.

Hemostasis must be complete. It is accomplished with the aid of intermittent application of the tourniquet. The tourniquet should never be kept inflated for longer than two hours. It should be released prior to application of the dressing to allow identification and control of bleeding points. Injuries of the radial or the ulnar artery can usually be safely ligated, since both have rich terminal anastomoses. *Both* arteries should not be ligated.

Trimming of the wound edges should not be routinely carried out. The removal of even a few millimeters of normal skin may necessitate later skin grafting. Contused skin and dirt-tattooed skin is preserved for delayed closure. Only devitalized skin is excised.

The deep structures of the hand should be explored thoroughly to determine the full extent of the injury and to allow adequate debridement. Care must be exercised during wound exploration and debridement to prevent damage to previously undamaged structures. The carpal tunnel may be opened to locate and protect the median nerve and its branches during debridement. Incision of the transverse carpal ligament, in addition to decompressing the median nerve, will improve tendon function in the severely damaged hand. In certain injuries associated with massive swelling of the hand, decompression of the intrinsic muscles may be indicated. Incision of the intermetacarpal fascia through small dorsal incisions reduces the possibility of developing intrinsic contracture.

Dead muscle, tissue, bloodclot, readily accessible foreign bodies, and other debris are removed. Bone fragments that are not grossly contaminated are preserved. Severely damaged and useless tendons should be excised. Every bit of viable tissue should be preserved. During the procedure, the wound is copiously irrigated with physiologic salt solution.

Only digits which are irretrievably damaged are amputated. Amputation of the thumb is a last resort, and is performed only after repeated evaluation. It is sometimes possible to preserve a skin pedicle from a finger that must be amputated, to provide later coverage for the remainder of the hand. In digital amputations, the tendons should be removed with the bone, but the digital vessels and nerves should be retained. Tendon repair, including tendon grafts, should not be performed by the forward surgeon.

Nerves which are traumatically divided are usually disrupted over a considerable distance and should not be primarily repaired. However, nerves which can be approximated in relatively healthy tissue without any tension should be approximated with one or two sutures of nonabsorbable suture material. This will prevent retraction, thereby facilitating future neurorrhaphy. Digital nerves are an exception and when possible should be repaired primarily, with the expectation of avoiding a painful neuroma.

WOUND CLOSURE

Delayed closure of the wound is performed several days after the initial debridement. In this way, one can be sure that the wound is free of sepsis and necrotic tissue prior to closure. Although it is possible to perform primary closure in certain wounds of the hand, the possibility of deep sepsis and wound breakdown does not justify the risk of primary closure in the combat situation.

At the time of wound closure (i.e., within 3–5 days post-debridement), unstable fractures or dislocations may be stabilized with small Kirschner wires. Stability thus achieved results in a hand which can be actively moved in the post-wound period, lessening the development of later deformity. Internal fixation other than small Kirschner wires should not be used by the forward surgeon.

Dressing

The dressing consists of well-fluffed gauze, applied evenly and snugly over a layer of fine-mesh gauze. Petrolatum-impregnated gauze impedes healing and should not be used. The deeper parts of the wound must not be plugged. The fingers are spread without tension, with the thumb in opposition. Padding is placed between the fingers. An attempt is made to align all fractures while applying the dressing.

The dressing should cover the entire wound, but should not

constrict it. It is reinforced with layers of sterile absorbent cotton covered by a firm pressure bandage. Only fractured fingers are splinted. Unaffected digits are left free to move. Whenever possible, the tips of all fingers are left exposed allowing periodic inspection to determine the adequacy of distal perfusion.

Splinting

The hand is supported in the position of function on a molded volar plaster splint with the wrist dorsiflexed approximately 30°, the metacarpophalangeal joints at 70°, and the interphalangeal joints at 10° flexion. The slightly-flexed thumb should be placed in 45° of palmar abduction. This is the position of the hand holding a water glass.

Postoperative Management

After operation, the hand and arm are elevated. Movement of all uninvolved joints is enforced.

CHAPTER XXXIII

Wounds and Injuries of the Spinal Column and Cord

INTRODUCTION

Combat injuries of the spinal column, with or without associated spinal cord injury, differ from those generally encountered in civilian practice. Whereas the majority of civilian spinal column and cord trauma is closed, most combat injuries are open, contaminated, and usually associated with other organ injuries.

Management of the casualty with spinal column or cord injury is initially the same as for all casualties. Regardless of whether the wounds are single or multiple, open or closed, and involve one or multiple organ systems, medical intervention must be prioritized. The first priorities remain: A-airway, B-breathing, and C-circulation, followed by evaluation and management of less compelling problems. After the ABCs have been addressed, management of the spinal cord injury takes on a high priority.

From the prognostic standpoint, the greater the initial function retained, the better the neurological outcome. Data from both military and civilian spinal cord injury sources reveal that in those injuries presenting with immediate loss of motor and sensory function (complete injury), the likelihood of neurological recovery is minimal and will not be influenced by surgical intervention. On the other hand, operation may be neurologically beneficial in the incomplete injury in which there is evidence of neurological deterioration—and a potentially reversible cause of the deterioration. Even though the neurological outcome of the open, complete injury is not likely to be influenced by surgical intervention, operation is generally indicated to debride the wound so as to minimize the risk of CNS sepsis.

CLASSIFICATION

Four discriminators must be considered in the classification of spinal cord injuries: (1) the *TYPE* of injury (open or closed); (2) the *EXTENT* of the injury (complete versus incomplete); (3) the *LOCATION* of the injury (cervical, thoracic, lumbar or sacral); and (4) the *DEGREE* of bony and ligamentous disruption (stable versus unstable).

To insure optimal preservation of neurological function during extrication and evacuation of the victim, several questions must be considered during the initial assessment. Might there be a spinal cord or column injury present? Does any neurological function persist below the level of the anatomical injury? What is the neurological level of the injury? Is it changing? Is the vertebral injury mechanically stable or unstable? If these questions cannot be answered and a spinal injury is suspected, the patient must be managed as if one existed.

MECHANICAL INTEGRITY OF THE VERTEBRAL COLUMN

The vertebral column is composed of three structural columns (Table 15). Loss of integrity of two of the three columns results in instability of the spine. Instability is common following closed mechanical injury of the vertebral column, but is not usually the case with gunshot or fragment wounds of the vertebral column. Instability of the vertebral column is documented on the lateral radiograph by demonstrating 3.5 mm or greater displacement or translation of one vertebral element on another, or by an interspinous, sagittal vertebral column angulation of 11° or more on the lateral view. Should questions exist regarding neck stability, lateral extension and flexion radiographs should be obtained under the direct supervision of a medical officer. Computerized tomography is effective in demonstrating spinal instability, but will not be available in forward hospitals.

TABLE 15.—*Support of the Spinal Column*

Column	Bony Elements	Soft Tissue Elements
ANTERIOR	Anterior two thirds of vertebral body	Anterior longitudinal ligament; Anterior annulus fibrosus
MIDDLE	Posterior one third of vertebral body; Pedicles	Posterior longitudinal ligament; Posterior annulus fibrosus
POSTERIOR	Lamina; Spinous processes; Facet joints	Ligamentum flavum; Interspinous ligaments

Because instability may not be immediately confirmed following trauma, any patient who complains of a sense of instability (holds his head with his hands), has unexplained vertebral column pain, has tenderness to percussion along the vertebral column, or has neurological injury without evidence of skeletal injury should be suspected of an injury to the spine. Similarly, any trauma victim who is unconscious or confused, or has evidence of trauma above the clavicles, should be managed as though cervical spinal injury were present.

Injury of vertebral supporting structures (Table 15), with or without bony involvement, makes the spinal cord vulnerable to secondary injury. Proper emergency stabilization of the spine during extrication and transfer of the victim is crucial in order to prevent neurological complications in this group of patients. Ligamentous injuries, in contrast to bony injuries, frequently do not heal without surgical stabilization. Typically, bony injuries of the spine heal in 12 weeks, the recommended period for protecting spine fractures. After three months, flexion-extension X-rays should be obtained to assess stability. Evidence of instability or progressive loss of alignment are indications for operative stabilization.

PATHOPHYSIOLOGY OF INJURY TO THE SPINAL CORD

Injury of the spinal cord results from the following mechanisms: (1) compression, (2) contusion, (3) edema, (4) ischemia and (5) physical transection. Usually an aggregate of two or more of these mechanisms is responsible. When the injury is complete and the cord is physically intact, the term physiological transection is used, as opposed to anatomical transaction where there is physical loss of continuity.

In physiological transections, the fundamental cause of irreversible damage to the spinal cord is loss of blood supply. The blood supply of the spinal cord is tenuous, especially in the thoracic region. Injury to the anterior spinal artery is the most common cause of spinal cord ischemia. Damage to the microcirculation, especially that of the central gray matter, is associated with compression-type injuries and edema formation. Closed trauma tends to cause vascular injuries. Axial loads are associated with displacement of bone elements or herniated disc material, with resultant compression injury. High-velocity missile wounds in the paravertebral area, even in the absence of direct contact, can cause neurological injury. The missile need not pass directly through neural tissue to induce injury. The pathological events which lead to injury at some distance from the actual projectile track are tissue contusion and/or hemorrhage produced by either radial stretching of the tissue around the missile's path during formation of the temporary cavity or fragmentation of the projectile and bone resulting in multiple secondary missiles. The destructive nature of high-velocity missiles explains the futility of decompressive laminectomy in the management of these wounds.

ANATOMICAL CONSIDERATIONS

Cervical Spine

Injury to the upper cervical spinal cord between C-1 and C-4, the level from which the cervical plexus and the phrenic nerves are derived, can result in the loss of both voluntary and involuntary diaphragmatic motion, the loss of chest wall muscle function, and the loss of function of the cervical strap muscles, which serve as accessory muscles of ventilation. A complete injury at this level, in the absence of some method of immediate assist, results in cessation of ventilation and death. When the cervical cord is injured below this level, the level of the cord injury is determined by assessment of motor and sensory function (Figure 40 and Table 16). The presence of any neural function below the level of the bony injury, to include the preservation of motor or sensory activity within the perianal (S-2, S-3) sacral dermatomes (sacral sparing), indicates an incomplete cord injury and is a favorable prognostic sign.

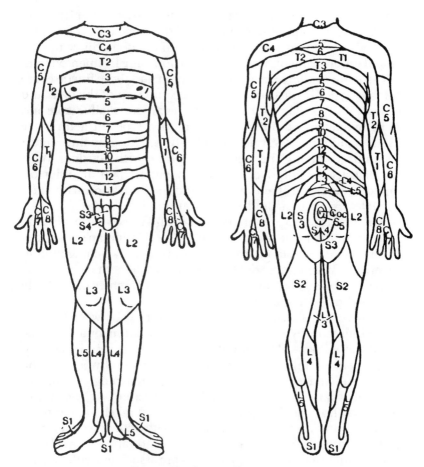

FIGURE 40.—Sensory Dermatomes

Axial loading (compression) injuries of the upper cervical spine can cause disruption of the ring of C-1 (Jefferson fracture). This fracture is rarely accompanied by cord damage because of the width of the neural canal at the C-1 and C-2 levels.* A C-1 fracture is usually stable and can be managed nonoperatively in the absence of other fractures or signs of instability. An associated fracture of C-2 must always be ruled out when fractures of C-1 are present. In this case, management depends on the type of injury present at C-2. Odontoid process (dens) fractures involving C-2

*One-Third Rule: At this level one-third of the spinal canal is occupied by the spinal cord, one-third by the odontoid process, and one-third is free space.

occur along the process in one of three locations. Type I fractures pass through the uppermost portion of the dens. Type II fractures of the odontoid pass through the base of the dens. Since the upper and lower segments are attached to opposing ligamentous and bony structures, there usually is separation and these fractures are unstable. Type III fractures occur at the junction of the dens and body of C-2. Type I and Type III fractures are normally stable and can be managed with immobilization only. Type II fractures are unstable and require surgical stabilization. These fractures must be stabilized during the assessment phase with Gardner Wells skeletal traction followed, in time, by either halo or other orthopedic apparatus, fixation or surgical stabilization with early internal wire, or plate and screw fixation.

Axial load forces applied to the head and upper cervical spine may disrupt the posterior elements of C-2 (Hangman's fracture). This is a relatively stable fracture and is usually managed nonoperatively. When fracture of the posterior elements of C-2 is accompanied by displacement, dislocation, or fracture of the body of C-2, surgical stabilization is indicated.

Fractures or dislocations of the cervical spine between C-3 and C-7 are caused by hyperflexion, axial load, rotation, or a combination of these forces. Typically these injuries result in instability. Hyperextension injuries to the cervical spine usually occur at the C-6, C-7 interspace, but produce complete neurological injuries less often than do flexion injuries. The extent of the injury depends on how much ligamentous and vertebral element integrity (two column integrity) is lost. The severity of the skeletal injury and the resulting neurological deficit do not always correlate.

Facet joint fractures and dislocations are associated with flexion-rotation injuries. They are often difficult to demonstrate on the initial anterior-posterior and lateral radiographs. For this reason, tomographic studies may be necessary. Thirty percent displacement of one vertebra on another indicates unilateral facet dislocation, whereas 50% displacement indicates bilateral facet disruption. Unilateral facet disruption is usually stable. In the absence of neurological findings, this injury can be managed nonoperatively. If it does not reduce with traction, this injury should be surgically reduced and stabilized. Bilateral facet dislocations are always unstable and require surgical stabilization. Complete neurological injury normally accompanies this injury.

TABLE 16.—*Assessment of Spinal Cord Injuries*

Level	Sensory Deficit	Motor Deficit	Reflex
C-2,3	Neck; back of head	Diaphragm; Accessory respiratory muscles.	—
C-4	Shoulders	Diaphragm, Shoulder shrug	—
C-5	Anterolateral side of arm	Elbow flexion	Biceps
C-6	Radial side of forearm; thumb	Wrist extension	Branchioradialis
C-7	Mid palm; long finger	Interior finger flexor; wrist flexion; elbow	triceps
C-8	Ulnar side of hand; wrist	Interior finger flexors	—
T-1	Ulnar side of forearm	Hand intrinsics	—
T-3	Above nipples	—	—
T-4	Nipple level	—	—
T-5	Below nipples	—	—
T-9, 10	Above umbilicus	Abdominal flexors	Umbilical
T-11, 12	Below umbilicus	—	Umbilical
L-1	Suprapubic	—	—
L-2	Anterior thigh	—	—
L-3	Around the knee	—	—
L-4	Medial side of leg	Knee extension	Knee
L-5	Lateral side of leg	Foot dorsiflexion	—
S-1	Lateral foot, soles and heels	Ankle plantar flexion	Ankle
S-2, 3, 4	Perianal; scrotum	Rectal sphincter	Bulbocavernosus; cremasteric

Thoracic and Lumbar Spine

The vascular supply of the spinal cord is most vulnerable between T-4 and T-6, where the neural canal is most narrow. Even minor degrees of vertebral column malalignment in this region result in neurological injury. Thoracic cord injury usually results from a combination of flexion, axial loading, and rotation forces. These stress forces are seen with parachute jumps and pilot ejections from high-performance aircraft. While the thoracic rib cage contributes to the rotary stability of the thoracic spine, wedge compression (flexion) fractures of the upper thoracic vertebral column are not uncommon. The most common site for a compression fracture is at L-1 and L-2. When not accompanied by other elements of injury, anterior wedge compression fractures of 25–30% can be considered stable. Greater degrees of compression and associated displacement require surgical stabilization.

Most axial-loading burst fractures in the lumbar region occur between L-2 and L-4 and are unstable. These fractures often cause extrusion of bone into the spinal canal and/or progressive angular deformity. Surgical stabilization and, occasionally, removal of bone fragments that compress the spinal cord constitute the definitive management of these injuries.

MANAGEMENT CONSIDERATIONS IN THE COMBAT ENVIRONMENT

The medical officer must realize that there are certain fundamental differences between the civilian practice of medicine and the compelling realities of the battlefield. If this were not the case, handbooks such as this one, dealing with military surgery, would be redundant and unnecessary. One such difference is exemplified in the initial management of the casualty with a possible spinal column or cord injury where there is an ongoing and immediate threat to the life of both the casualty and combat medic who comes to his aid.*

Current Advanced Trauma Life Support (ATLS) guidelines concerning spinal column and cord injury or *potential* injury state that "any patient sustaining injury above the clavicles or a head injury resulting in an unconscious state should be suspected of having an associated cervical spinal column injury which should be immobilized with a properly applied spine board, and a semirigid cervical collar." U.S. Army field manuals present similar guidelines with regard to neck injuries and suspected fractures of the neck. Proper immobilization of the spine and movement of the casualty requires two or more people, a spine board and semirigid cervical collar. These guidelines are appropriate for the civilian

---

*The reader should bear in mind that the differences which follow apply only to the active battlefield where there is immediate and ongoing threat to the life of the casualty and those who come to his aid.

sector, the peacetime military, and for secure military areas, but not for battlefields. The realities of war can make the ideal management of casualties unrealistic. If ATLS guidelines were strictly adhered to, one could envision the first day of a NATO-Warsaw Pact conflict with thousands of casualties strapped to long boards and wearing cervical collars while waiting to have their spines "cleared." Simple logistics would preclude idealized management of this number of potential spinal injuries. Common sense must prevail.

On the active battlefield, during a fire fight or when one leaves his hole during an artillery or mortar barrage, the objective is to bring the casualty out of the line of fire, into a hole, or behind cover, where the basic fundamentals of casualty care (the ABCs) can be applied. The longer the casualty and the medic remain exposed, the greater the likelihood of additional wounds and additional casualties. Under conditions such as these, the prime consideration is preservation of the lives of both the wounded and the rescuers.

Additional insights regarding immediate battlefield management of the casualty with possible cervical injury is provided by the WDMET (Wound Data and Munitions Effectiveness Team) data from the Vietnam experience. Only 1.4% of all casualties with penetrating wounds of the neck, who survived long enough to become candidates for cervical immobilization, might have benefitted from such treatment. These data do not support the use of cervical collars and spine boards for penetrating and perforating neck wounds on the battlefield. Also noteworthy in the WDMET data on cervical injuries is that 13 of those killed in action, and 7 of those wounded in action, were providing battlefield care for others when they were hit. The conclusion from the WDMET data is that battlefield splinting of the cervical spine was of very little value in preventing neurological injury, while it materially increased the risks to the casualty and the provider.

INITIAL MANAGEMENT

Initial management of the individual with suspected injury of the cervical spine entails preservation of the airway, maintenance of ventilation, control of hemorrhage, and the preservation of residual neurological function. Movement of the head and neck must be minimized. When the injured individual presents in the prone position, he should be log-rolled into the supine position with the most experienced person present maintaining the neck in the neutral position. Once the victim is in the supine position, the airway should be maintained with the chin lift maneuver. The neck should never be hyperextended in these situations. If a surgical airway is required, cricothyroidotomy is the method of choice. Stabilization of the neck during transport is provided by a stiff cervical collar or sand bags. Then the head should be taped to whichever extraction device is utilized (Figures 41, 42).

When injury to the spine is suspected, spinal alignment must be maintained when the victim is moved. Table 17 summarizes extrication techniques for suspected spine injuries. This can be accomplished by log-rolling onto a stretcher or, where two-man assistance is available, the two-man arm carry is an appropriate method of initial transport to a rigid surface (Figure 43). This

TABLE 17.—*Extrication Techniques for Suspected Spinal Column Injuries**

Technique	Cervical	Thoracic and Lumbar	Comment
Spine board with semi-rigid collar	YES	YES	Recommended technique; see figures 41, 42
Two-Man Arm Carry	NO	YES	Conscious or unconscious victims; see figure 43.
Three-Man Arm Carry	YES	YES	Third man protects the cervical spine.
Pistol Belt Drag	NO	YES	Use these three on the battlefield if no other alternatives exist.
Shirt Drag	NO**	YES	″ ″
Neck Drag	NO	YES	″ ″

*The following carries are not recommended for extricating casualties with suspected spine injuries.
  1. Pack-strap carry
  2. Fireman's carry
  3. One-man arm carry
  4. Cradle drop drag
  5. Two-man fore & aft carry
  6. Two-hand seat carry

**Extenuating circumstances where victim and rescuer must maintain low profile.

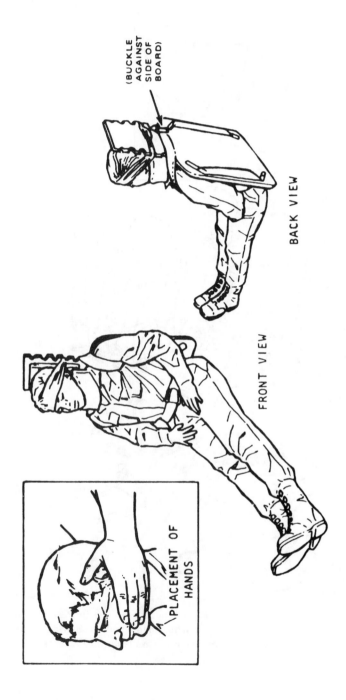

FIGURE 41.—Fractures of the cervical spine can be immobilized by either a "short" or "long" spine board. Fractures of thoracic-lumbar spine are best immobilized on a long board. One person always maintains control of the head and neck, while others rotate and properly position the patient on the spine board.

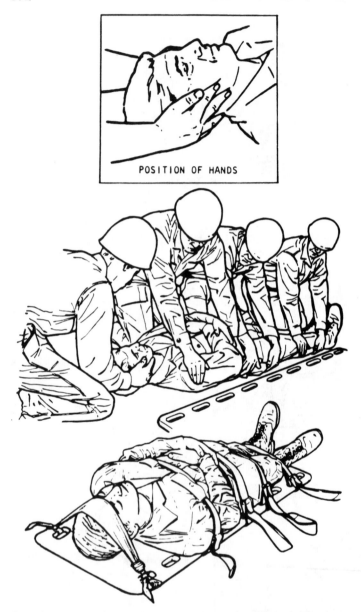

POSITION OF HANDS

FIGURE 42.—Spinal immobilization using a long board. The bearers should assemble the required items: long spine board, four 6-foot patient securing straps, cravat, and four pieces of padding. If an item is not available, the bearers should improvise it from available materials.

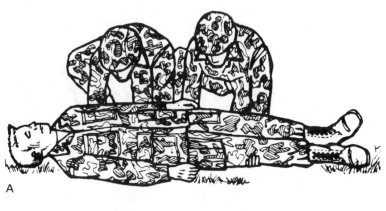

A

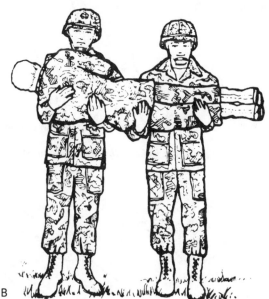

B

FIGURE 43.—Under more stable battlefield conditions, where assistance of another individual is available, in the absence of other alternative methods of stable spine support, the two-man arm carry is appropriate for suspected thoracic-lumbar spine injuries.

technique does not protect the cervical spine; therefore, if cervical spine injury is also suspected, the victim should not be moved until a semirigid collar and spine board are available. In the absence of back boards and stretchers, makeshift litters can be fashioned from doors, lumber, or poles and clothing. (Figure 44).

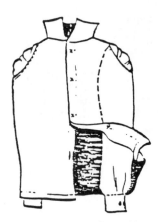

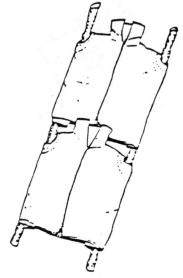

A   Button two or three shirts or jackets and turn them inside out, leaving the sleeves inside.

B   Pass poles through the sleeves.

Litter made with poles and jackets (Illustrated A and B).

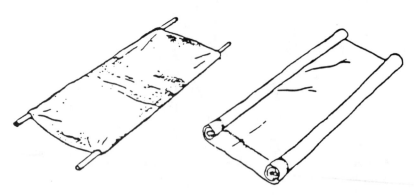

Litters made by inserting poles through sacks and by rolling blanket.

FIGURE 44.—Field-expedient litters.

RECEIVING AREA

Protection of the cervical spine must continue until that area is radiographically cleared. The first X-ray to be obtained is a lateral view of the cervical spine. The entire cervical spine, C-1 to the C-7, T-1 junction, must be visualized. If the C-7 vertebra cannot be visualized, either the arms can be pulled towards the feet by an assistant standing at the foot of the stretcher, or a "swimmers view" (lateral X-ray of the cervical spine with one arm at the side and other elevated alongside the head) can be taken. If questions remain about interpretation of the cervical spine films and if the techniques to improve visualization are unsuccessful, protection of the neck must continue throughout the stabilization phase and the casualty must be transferred to a facility where either tomography or computerized tomography capabilities are available. Immobilization can be discontinued only after all seven cervical vertebrae, including the ring of C-1, the odontoid, and the soft tissues anterior to the cervical spine are visualized and cleared. After the cervical spine has been evaluated, the remainder of the spine can be examined physically and radiographically. The medical officer should palpate the spinous processes in order to disclose areas of tenderness or malalignment. The search for malalignment is particularly important in the evaluation of the unresponsive patient.

When complex wounds involving the head, thorax, abdomen, or extremities coexist with vertebral column injuries, lifesaving measures take precedence over the definitive diagnosis and management of spinal column and cord problems. During these interventions, secondary injury to the unstable spine must be prevented by appropriate protective measures.

INITIAL CLOSED REDUCTION AND STABILIZATION OF CERVICAL INJURIES

Skeletal traction using Gardner-Wells skull tongs is the treatment of choice for the reduction and stabilization of cervical spine injuries (Figure 45, Table 18). While a halter or chin strap may be temporarily utilized during the initial evacuation, they are not satisfactory for long-term use.

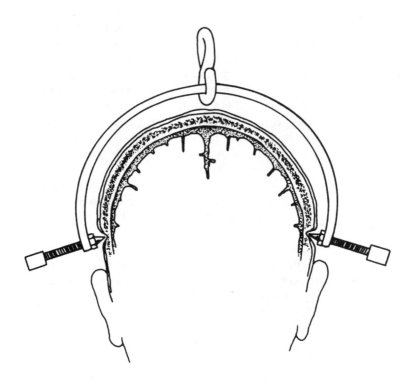

FIGURE 45.—Gardner-Wells tongs. See Table 18 for application.

When cranial tongs are used for traction, the rule of thumb for determining the amount of weight to be applied to the tongs for fracture reduction is 5 lbs. per level of injury. For example, to reduce a C-5 fracture, you would begin with 25 lbs. of weight. If this is insufficient weight to achieve reduction, appropriate additional increments of weight can be successively applied every 20–30 minutes under radiological control until reduction is attained. The maximal amount of weight that can be safely applied to properly placed Gardner-Wells tongs is 80–90 lbs.

TABLE 18.—*Application of Gardner-Wells Cranial Tongs*

Step	Procedure	Comment
1	INSPECT INSERTION SITE: Select a point just above apex of each ear.	Rule out depressed skull fracture in this area.
2	SHAVE & PREP PIN INSERTION SITE	
3	INJECT LOCAL ANESTHETIC: Inject 2–3 cc of 1% xylocaine or equivalent agent one centimeter above each ear in line with the external auditory meatus.	May omit if patient is unconscious.
4	ADVANCE GARDNER-WELLS TONG PINS: Insert pins into skull by symmetrically tightening the knobs.	A spring loaded device in one or the two pins will protrude when the pins are appropriately seated. (A data plate on the tongs provides additional information.)
5	APPLY SKELETAL TRACTION: Use a pulley fixed to the head of the litter or frame to direct horizontal traction to the tongs.	Use 5 lbs. rule (i.e. 5 lbs. of weight for each level of injury, (see text). High cervical fractures usually require minimal traction to reduce. Monitor with series X-rays. The tong-pin site requires anterior or posterior positioning to adjust for cervical spine flexing or extension as indicated.
6	ELEVATE HEAD OF LITTER: Use blocks in order to provide body-weight counter traction.	The knot in the cord should not be permitted to drift up against the pulley. Should this occur, traction is no longer being applied.
7	DECREASE TRACTION WEIGHT: When X-rays confirm that reduction is adequate, decrease traction to 5–15 lbs.	Unreducibile or unstable fractures should be maintained in moderate traction until surgical intervention. If neurological deterioration occurs, immediate surgical intervention must be considered.

TABLE 18.—*Application of Gardner-Wells Cranial Tongs (continued)*

Step	Procedure	Comment
8	DAILY PIN CARE	Cleanse tracts with saline and apply antibiotic ointment to the pin sites. Maintain pin force (see Step 4) by tightening as necessary to keep spring-loaded device in the protruded position.
9	TURN PATIENT APPROPRIATELY: Use Stryker, Foster, or similar frame and turn patient every four hours.	When initially proned, obtain X-rays to ensure that the reduction is maintained. If reduction is not maintained when the patient is proned, rotate the patient only between the 30° right and left quarter positions. The use of a circle electric bed is contraindicated with injuries of the spinal cord or column.
10	IF SATISFACTORY ALIGNMENT CANNOT BE OBTAINED, FURTHER WORKUP IS NECESSARY.	Consider myelogram, CT scan, tomograms, and neurosurgical/ orthopedic consultations.

INITIAL MANAGEMENT OF THE THORACIC-LUMBAR REGIONS

Casualties with thoracic-lumbar spine injuries should always be transported on long spine boards and evacuated to a center capable of managing spine injuries. The thoracic-lumbar junction is notoriously unstable following injury. Short spine boards are unsatisfactory for evacuation because they provide insufficient thoracic-lumbar spine protection. Closed reduction of thoracic-lumbar spinal injuries above L-2 in the neurologically intact should not be attempted.

MYELOGRAPHY

The use of metrizamide myelography is indicated in the following situations:

1. Patients with incomplete injuries who demonstrate neurologic deterioration upon serial reassessment.
2. Patients with an incomplete neurological injury who require surgery for spine stabilization or other procedures.
3. Patients with incomplete injuries who fail to improve following closed reduction.
4. Patients with progressive neurological improvement followed by the sudden appearance of a neurological plateau.
5. Patients with neurological injury without evidence of vertebral column injury.

Myelography is not advisable in neurologically complete injuries. If performed, and found abnormal in the patient with absent neurological function below the level of injury, a tendency exists for the obstruction to be surgically "relieved." Neurological improvement seldom follows operation and may contribute to mechanical instability of the spine. Thus, knowledge of an obstruction to the flow of contrast material serves no beneficial function.

EMERGENCY SURGERY IN CLOSED INJURIES OF THE CORD AND COLUMN

Emergency surgery is indicated in the following closed injuries of the spinal cord: 1) the spinal-cord-injured patient with an incomplete lesion who deteriorates neurologically, and 2) the neurologically intact or incomplete patient with an unreducible dislocation of the vertebral column. Where vertebral body fracture results in neural canal compromise, an anterior decompression is the indicated route in order to minimize anterior spinal artery compromise. However, consideration must be given to the mechanics of the spinal column injury so that a stable column is not rendered unstable by the decompression. The operative approach is directed to the site of neurological compromise and to the level of spine instability. Consideration should be given to stabilizing the spine at the time of decompression. Rarely in the presence of a complete neurological injury, when subdural or extradural hematomas or extrinsic masses resulting from fracture or soft-tissue fragments are decompressed, will neurological improvement occur. Individual nerve roots, in contrast to the spinal cord, frequently demonstrate recovery, with or without surgery. Some recovery of function can also be anticipated from injuries to the cauda equina, since this structure is also made up of peripheral nerves.

EMERGENCY OPERATIONS IN PENETRATING INJURIES OF THE CORD AND COLUMN

High-velocity missile wounds of the spine, especially those with dural disruption, require immediate debridement. Low-velocity missile injuries of the spinal cord require less extensive debridement. The operative approach to the management of open wounds of the spine includes exploration of the path of the missile, assessment of the nature and extent of the anatomical disruption, and management of other concurrent surgical problems. Missiles that pass through the esophagus or colon, before striking the vertebral column, can cause osteomyelitis of the spine or disc-space infection. Consequently, when the colon or esophagus and the vertebral column are sequentially injured by a missile, both structures must be managed surgically. Intravenous antibiotic administration (a combination of first-generation cephalosporin and an aminoglycoside is recommended) and tetanus prophylaxsis should be started immediately. Where cerebral spinal fluid (CSF) leakage from the wound is identified following debridement, the wound can be closed loosely and a compression dressing applied. Continued subcutaneous spinal fluid collection or persistent leakage is an indication for wound exploration and dural repair.

In the presence of extensive open wounds of the spine, every attempt should be made to repair muscle and skin, and to perform a watertight closure of the dura within the first 6–12 hours post–injury. If logistics make it impossible to manage an open spine wound during the first 48 hours, it is preferable to debride and loosely pack the open wound. If there is no CSF leakage, the wound may be left open for 3–5 days followed by delayed closure, or allowed to heal by second intention. In those injuries with complete anatomical disruption of the spinal cord, the dural sack can be ligated to prevent CSF leak. Although not optimal, tissue deficits may require dural repairs or "patch" grafts to be left uncovered. Instrumentation for spinal stabilization and fusion (i.e., rods, etc) is contraindicated in the presence of an open wound.

PHARMACOLOGIC TREATMENT

The value of pharmacological agents in the management of spinal cord injuries remains questionable. Attempts to prevent the deleterious effects of trauma on the nervous system or to restore lost neurological function have led some to use steroids (50 mg of Decadron initially, followed by 10 mg qid on a reducing scale over a four or five day period), and 20% mannitol (500 cc by rapid IV infusion). Benefit from either drug, employed singularly or in combination, has not been demonstrated. Hyperbaric oxygen therapy, which can reduce edema and hyperoxygenate tissues, may be of value in the incomplete injury if initiated within a few hours of injury.

GENERAL MANAGEMENT

Traumatically-induced sympathectomy seen with injuries to the vertebral column above T-6 produce bradycardia, hypotension, and hypothermia. Ringer's lactate may be required to maintain adequate vascular volume and maintain a reasonable blood pressure. Atropine (0.4–0.6 mg every four hours) may improve blood pressure levels by maintaining the cardiac rate above 40/min. Hypotension in the complete spinal cord injury is to be anticipated, due to marked decrease in peripheral vascular resistance.

The use of a nasogastric tube is always indicated in the acute spine-injured patient. Its use reduces the chance of emesis, and allows earlier diagnosis of stress ulcer hemorrhage. Cimetidine (300 gm by IV infusion every six hours) is utilized during the first 7-10 days post injury, along with the installation of aluminum hydroxide gel (Amphogel, 30 cc) and a magnesium hydroxide (Mylanta II, 15 cc) into the nasogastric tube every two hours to prevent stress ulceration. The use of this combination tends to counteract the diarrhea caused by one and the constipation brought on by the other. The use of a nasogastric tube, connected to low suction, also reduces the effects of paralytic ileus, which often follows injury of the thoracic and lumbar spine.

A major concern following spine and spinal cord injury is the

occurrence of deep venous thrombosis. The most appropriate prophylactic measures include: (a) awareness, (b) adequate fluid hydration, (c) thigh-length compression hose (changed two to three
times daily to evaluate the skin and check for edema), and (d) subcutaneous heparin (5,000 units twice a day). This dose of subcutaneous heparin during the immediate post-trauma period is
not likely to cause intraspinal bleeding.

The bladder is emptied by intermittent catherization. Frequently, for the female patient, this is not possible and an indwelling
catheter is required. In the combat situation, for logistics reasons,
it may be necessary to leave an indwelling catheter in place. Failure
to decompress the bladder can lead to a hypertensive crisis severe
enough to cause bleeding into the brain (autonomic hyperreflex-
ia). The use of prophylactic urinary antibiotics is not advised.
Liberal fluid intake (2,000 cc daily) and the use of an acidifying
agent (e.g., cranberry juice) to reduce the occurrence of urinary
calculi is recommended. Bowel training includes the use of
suppositories.

Decubitus ulcers must be prevented. Patients are instructed in
prevention techniques. Where self care is not appropriate, patient
care and turning must be provided by attendants. For the recum-
bent patient, all pressure points are carefully padded and frequently observed. The skin is kept dry and powered. All bony prominences are inspected daily. Physical therapy is started immediately to minimize contracture and disuse atrophy. All joints
incapable of being actively mobilized by the patient require daily
ranging through their full arc of motion. Foot supports prevent
contractures of the ankle and pressure decubiti of the heel.

APPENDIX A

Glossary of Drugs With National Nomenclatures

ANTIBIOTICS

United States	Germany	Netherlands	France
Ampicillin U.S.P.	Amblosin	Ampicilline	Ampicilline.
Bacitracin U.S.P.	Bacitracin	Bacitracine	Bacitracine
Cefazolin	Cefazolin	Cefazolin	Cefazolin
Cefoxitin	Cefoxitin-Natrium	Cefoxitin-Natrium	Cefoxitine
Ceftazidime	Ceftazidim	Ceftazidime	Ceftazidime
Cefuroxime	Cefuroxim	Cefuroxime	Cefuroxime
Cephapirin	Cefapirin-Natrium	Cefapirine-Natrium	Cefapirine
Chloramphenicol U.S.P.	Chloramphenicol DAB 7	Chooramfenicol	Chloramphenicol
Clindamycin	Clindamycin	Clindamycine	Clindamycine
Erythromycin U.S.P.	Erythromycinum Ph. Int.	Erythromycine	Erythromycine
Gentamicin sulfate U.S.P.	Gentamicine	Gentamicine sulfaat	Gentamycine
Kanamycin U.S.P.	Kanamycin	Kanamycine	Kanamycine
Methicillin U.S.P.	Methicillin-Natrium	Methicilline	Methicilline
Metronidazole	Metronidazol	Metronidazol	Metronidazole
Mezlocillin	Mezlocillin	Mezlocilline	Mezlocilline
Nafcillin	Nafcillin-Natrium	Nafcilline-Natrium	Nafcilline
Neomycin sulfate U.S.P.	Neomycin	Neomycine sulfaat	Neomycine
Polymyxin B sulfate U.S.P.	Polymyxini B-sulfas Ph. Int.	Polymyxine B Sulfaat	Polymyxine B
Potassium penicillin G, U.S.P.	Penicillin G-Kalium DAB 7	Kalium penicilline B	Penicilline
Potassium phenoxymethyl penicillin U.S.P.	Potassium phenoxymethyl penicillin	Kalium fenoxymethyl penicilline	Phenoxymethylpenicilline

ANTIBIOTICS (continued)

United States	Germany	Netherlands	France
Streptomycin sulfate U.S.P....	Streptomycinsulfat DAB 7 ..	Streptomycine sulfaat	Streptomycine sulfate
Sulfisoxazole	Sulfisoxazol	Sulfisoxazol	Sulfafurazol
Tetracycline U.S.P.	Tetracyclinum Ph. Int.	Tetracycline	Tetracycline
Ticarcillin	Ticarcillin	Ticarcilline	Ticarcilline
Tobramycin	Tobramycin	Tobramycine	Tobramycine
Trimethoprim/	Trimethoprim mit	Trimethoprime met	Trimethoprime +
sulfamethoxazole	sulfa-methoxazol	sulfa-methoxazol	sulfamide
Vancomycin	Vancomycin	Vancomycine	Vancomycine

ELECTROLYTIC AND WATER BALANCE

United States	Germany	Netherlands	France
Calcium chloride injection U.S.P.	Kalziumchlorid-Losung	Calciumchlorideoplossing ..	Chlorure de calcium injectable
Calcium gluconate injection U.S.P.	Calcium gluconicum 10% ..	Calcium gluconaat injectie .	Calcium levulinate
Dextrose injection U.S.P.	Traubenzuckerlosung 10% ..	Glucose injectie	Solution injectable de glucose, isotonique
Ethacrynic acid U.S.P.	Etacrynsaure	Ethacryne zuur	Acide etacrynique
Furosemide U.S.P.	Furosemid	Furosemide	Furosemide
Lactated Ringer's injection U.S.P.	Ringer-Lactat-Losung	Ringer lactaat injectie	Lactate de calcium
Mannitol U.S.P.	Mannit	Mannitol	Mannitol
Potassium acetate injection U.S.P.	Kaliumazetat-Losung	Kaliumacetaatoplossing voor injecties	Injection d'acetate de potassium
Potassium chloride injection U.S.P.	Kaliumchlorid-Losung	Kaliumchlorideoplossing voor injecties	Chlourue de potassium injectable

ELECTROLYTIC AND WATER BALANCE (continued)

United States	Germany	Netherlands	France
Probenecid U.S.P.	Probenecid	Probenecide	Probenecide
Ringer's injection U.S.P.	Ringer-Losung	Ringer injectie	Solution de Ringer
Sodium chloride injection U.S.P.	Natriumchloridlosung, isotonisch, pyrogenfrei steril (DAB 7)	Natrium chloride injectie	Solution injectable de chlorure de sodium, isotonique
Sodium polystyrene sulfonate	Kationen-Austauscherharz	Natrium polystyreen sulfonaat	Sulfonate de sodium polystyrenique

MISCELLANEOUS DRUGS

United States	Germany	Netherlands	France
Acetazolamide Injection	Acetazolamid-natrium	Acetazolamide	Acetazolamide
Acetylcysteine	Acetylcystein	Acetylcysteine	Acetylcysteine
Acetylsalicylic acid U.S.P.	Acetylsalicylsaure DAB 7	Acetylsalicyl zuur	Acetylsalicylique acide
Amitriptyline	Amitriptylin	Amitriptyline	Amitriptyline
Amyl nitrite N.F.	Amylnitrit	Amyl nitriet	Nitrite d'amyle
BAL; Dimercaprol	Dimercaprol	Dimercaprol	Dimercaprol
Carbamazepine	Carbamazepin	Carbamazepine	Carbamazepine
Chlorpromazine U.S.P.	Chlorpromazini hydro-chlorridum Ph. Int.	Chloorpromazine	Chlorpromazine
Dexamethasone sodium phosphate	Dexamethasonnatrium-phosphat	Dexamethason Natrium fosfaat	Phosphate de sodium dexamethasone
Digoxin U.S.P.	Digoxinum Ph. Int.	Digoxine	Digoxine
Diphenhydramine	Dipphenhyddramin	Difeenhydramine-hydrochloride	Diphenhydramine
Droperidol	Dehydrobenzperidol	Droperidol	Droperidol

MISCELLANEOUS DRUGS (continued)

United States	Germany	Netherlands	France
Fluoresceine	Fluorescein	Fluoresceine	Fluoresceine
Heparin	Heparin	Heparine	Heparine
Hydralazine	Hydralazin	Hydralazine	Hydralazine
Hypertonic glucose	Hypertonische glukose	Hypertonische glucose	Glucose hypertonique
Hydrocortisone acetate	Hydrocortisonacetat	Hydrocortison Acetaat	Acetate d'hydrocortisone
Hydrocortisone sodium succinate injection U.S.P.	Hydrocortisonnatrium-succinat	Hydrocortison natrium succinaat injectie	Hydrocortisone succinate de sodium
Indigocarmine injection	5,5'-Indigodisulfonsaure dinatriumsalz ampullen iv	Indigokarmijnoplossing voor injecties	Injection de carmin d'indigo
Methylprednisolone sodium succinate	Methylprednisolonnatrium-succinat	Methylprednisolon natrium succinaat	Succinate de sodium methylprednisolone
Naloxone	Naloxon	Naloxon	Naloxone
Oxygen U.S.P.	Sauerstoff	Zuurstof	Oxygene
Regular Insulin	Altinsulin	Normale insuline	Insuline ordinaire
Sodium nitrite U.S.P.	Natriumnitrit DAB 7	Natrium nitriet	Nitrite de sodium
Sodium thiosulfate U.S.P.	Natriumthiosulfat DAB 7	Natrium thiosulfaat	Hyposulfite de sodium

DRUGS AFFECTING SYMPATHETIC NERVOUS SYSTEM AND NERVE ENDINGS

United States	Germany	Netherlands	France
Albuterol	Salbutamol	Salbutamol	Salbutamol
Atenolol	Atenolol	Atenolol	Atenolol
Atropine sulfate U.S.P.	Atropinsulfat DAB 7	Atropine sulfaat	Atropine sulfate
Cyclopentolate hydrochloride U.S.P.	Cyclopentolathydrochlorid	Cyclopentolaat hydrochloride	Cyclopentolate
Dobutamine	Dobutamin	Dobutamine	Dobutamine
Dopamine	Dopamin	Dopamine	Dopamine

DRUGS AFFECTING SYMPATHETIC NERVOUS SYSTEM AND NERVE ENDINGS (continued)

United States	Germany	Netherlands	France
Ephedrine	Ephedrine	Efedrine	Ephedrine
Epinephrine U.S.P.	Adrenalin DAB 7	Adrenaline	Adrenaline
Homatropine hydrobromide U.S.P.	Homatropinhydrobromid DAB 7	Homatropine hydrobromide	Homatropine bromhydrate
Isoproterenol U.S.P.	Isoprenalini hydrochloridum Ph. Int.	Isoprenaline	Isoprenaline
Levarterenol bitartrate U.S.P.	Noradrenalinhydrogentartrat DAB 7	Levarterenol bitartraat	Noradrenaline
Mephentermine	Mephentermin	Mefentermine	Mephentermine
Metaproterenol	Orciprenalin		Orciprenaline
Metaraminol	Metaraminol	Metaraminol	Metaraminol
Methoxamine	Methoxamin	Methoxamine	Methoxamine
Phenylephrine	Phenylephrin	Fenylefrinehydrochloride	Phenylephrine
Physostigmine salicylate U.S.P.	Physostigminsalicylat DAB 7	Fysostigmine salicyclaat	Physostigmine
Pralidoxime chloride U.S.P.	Pralidoximi methiodidum Ph. Int.	Pralidoxime chloride	Pralidoxime
Propranolol	Propranolol	Propranololhydrochloride	Propranolol
Scopolamine U.S.P.	Scopolaminhydrobromid DAB 7	Scopolamine U.S.P.	Scopolamine

GENERAL ANESTHETICS

United States	Germany	Netherlands	France
Cyclopropane U.S.P.	Cyclopropan	Cyclopropane	Cyclopropane
Enflurane	Enfluran	Enfluraan	Enfluran
Etomidate	Etomidat	Etomidaat	Etomidate
Fentanyl	Fentanyl	Fentanyl	Fentanyl
Halothane U.S.P.	Halothan	Halothaan	Halothane
Isoflurane	Isofluran	Isofluraan	Isoflurane
Ketamine	Ketamin	Ketamine	Ketamine
Midazolam	Midazolam		Midazolam
Nitrous oxide U.S.P.	Distickstoffoxide, Lachgas	Lachgas, distikstofoxide	Protoxyde d'azote
Thiopental sodium U.S.P.	Thiopental-natrium	Thiopental-natrium	Penthiobarbital injectable

LOCAL ANESTHETICS

United States	Germany	Netherlands	France
Bupivacaine	Bupivicain	Bupivicainehydrochloride	Bupivicaine
Chloroprocaine N.F.	Chloroprocain	Chloroprocaine	Chloroprocaine
Cocaine hydrochloride U.S.P.	Cocainhydrochlorid DAB 7	Cocaine hydrochloride	Cocaine chlorhydrate
Dyclonine	Dycloninhydrochlorid	Dycloninhydrochloride	Dyclonine
Lidocaine hydrochloride	Lidocainii hydrochloridum	Lidocaine hydrochloride	Lidocaine
Mepivacaine hydrochloride N.F.	Mepivacainhydrochloride	Mepivacainehydrochloride	Mepivacaine
Prilocaine hydrochloride N.F.	Prilocainhydrochlorid	Prilocainehydrochloride	Prilocaine
Procaine hydrochloride	Procainhydrochlorid DAB 7	Procaine hydrochloride	Procaine
Proparacaine hydrochloride U.S.P.	Proxymetacainhydrochlorid	Proparacaine hydrochloride	Proxymetacaine
Tetracaine hydrochloride U.S.P.	Tetracainhydrochlorid DAB 7	Tetracaine hydrochloride	Tetracaine

MUSCLE RELAXANTS

United States	Germany	Netherlands	France
Atracurium			besilate d'Atracurium
Curare	Dimethyltubocurarinium-chlorid	Curare	D-Tubocurarine
Pancuronium bromide	Pancuroniumbromid	Pancuronium bromide	Bomure de Pancuronium
Succinylcholine U.S.P.	Succinylcholin	Succinylcholine	Succinylcholine
Tubocurarine chloride U.S.P.	D-Tubocurarini chloridum Ph. Int.	Tubocurarine chloride	Tubocurarine

ANALGESICS

United States	Germany	Netherlands	France
Alfentanil	Alfentanil	Alfentanil	Alfentanil
Butorphanol	Butorphanol	Butorphanol	Butorphanol
Codeine phosphate U.S.P.	Codeinephosphate DAB 7	Codeine fosfaat	Codeine
Meperidine hydrochloride U.S.P.	Pethidini hydrochloridum Ph. Int.	Pethidine hydrochloride	Pethidine chlorhydrate
Methadone hydrochloride U.S.P.	Methadoni hydrochloridum Ph. Int.	Methadon hydrochloride	Methadone
Morphine sulfate U.S.P.	Morphini sulfas Ph. Int.	Morfine sulfaat	Morphine
Nalbuphine	Nalbuphinhydrochlorid	Nalbuphinhydrochloride	Nalbuphine
Sufentanil	Sufentanil	Sufentanil	Sufentanil

TOPICAL AGENTS

United States	Germany	Netherlands	France
Copper Sulfate	Kupfer-sulfat	Kopersulfaat	Sulfate de cuivre
Mefinide	Mafenid	Mafenide	Mafenide
Petrolatum U.S.P.	Petrolatum	Petrolatum	Petroleine
Silver nitrate U.S.P.	Silbernitrat DAB 7	Zilvernitraat	Nitrate d'argent
Silver sulfadiazine	Sulfadiazin-silber	Zilversulfadiazine	

CHOLINERGIC MUSCLE STIMULANTS

United States	Germany	Netherlands	France
Edrophonium	Edrophoniumchlorid	Edrophoniumchloride	Edrophonium
Neostigmine	Neostigmin	Neostigminebromide	Neostigmine

GASTROINTESTINAL DRUGS

United States	Germany	Netherlands	France
Bisacodyl	Bisacodyl	Bisacodyl	Bisacodyl
Cimetidine	Cimetidin	Cimetidine	Cimetidine
Glycerine	Glycerol	Glycerol	Glycerol
Metoclopramide	Metoclopramid	Metoclopramide	Metoclopramide
Ranitidine	Ranitidin	Ranitidine	Ranitidine
Sorbitol	Sorbit	Sorbitol	Sorbitol

SEDATIVES, HYPNOTICS AND ANXIOLYTICS

United States	Germany	Netherlands	France
Amobarbital U.S.P.	Amobarbitalum Ph. Int	Amobarbital	Amobarbital
Diazepam	Diazepam	Diazepam	Diazepam
Paraldehyde U.S.P.	Paraldehyd DAB 7	Paraldehyde	Paraldehyde
Pentobarbital U.S.P.	Pentobarbital	Pentobarbital	Pentobarbital
Secobarbital U.S.P.	Quinalbarbitone	Secobarbital	Secobarbital

PLASMA EXPANDERS

United States	Germany	Netherlands	France
Dextran	Dextran	Dextran	Dextran
Fresh Frozen Plasma	Gefrierfrischplasma	Vers ingevroren plasma	Plasma frais congele
Normal human serum albumin U.S.P.	Humanalbumin 20%	Norman humaan albumine uit serum	Albumine humaine
Plasma protein fraction U.S.P.	PPL, Humanalbumin 5%	Protein fractie uit plasma	Plasma

VACCINES AND ANTITOXINS

United States	Germany	Netherlands	France
Gas gangrene antitoxin, pentavalent	Gasodem-Antitoxin, polyvalent	Gas gangreen-antitoxine pentavalent	Serum antigangreneux polyvalent
Tetanus immune globulin (human) U.S.P., Hyper-immune human antitetanus	Tetanum-immunglobulin, Hyperimmunglobulin gegen tetanus	Tetanum-immuno globuline Serum tegen tetanus	Serum antitetanique (menselijk)
Tetanus toxoid U.S.P.	Tetatoxoid	Tetanus vaccin	Vaccin antitetanique

ANTISEPTICS

United States	Germany	Netherlands	France
Alcohol U.S.P.	Aethanol DAB 7	Alcohol	Alcool ethylique
Hexachlorophene U.S.P.	Hexachlorophen WHO	Hexachlorophene	Exophene
Povidone Iodine Solution ...	Polyvidon-Iod	Povidon-ioodoplossing	Polyvidone iodee

APPENDIX B

Useful Tables

TABLE 1.—*Atomic weights, valences, and equivalent weights of certain elements*

Element	Atomic weight	Valence	Equivalent weight
Sodium	23.0	1	23.0
Potassium	39.0	1	39.0
Magnesium	24.0	2	12.0
Calcium	40.0	2	20.0
Chlorine......................	35.5	1	35.5
Phosphorus	31.0	3	10.3
Sulfur	32.0	2	16.0

TABLE 2.—*Millequivalent per gram of certain elements and compounds*

Element or compound	Milli-equivalent	Element or compound	Milli-equivalent
Sodium	43.5	Potassium chloride:	
Potassium	26.0	Potassium	13.5
Magnesium	85.0	Chloride	13.5
Calcium..........	50.0	Sodium lactate:	
Chloride	29.0	Sodium	9.0
Sodium chloride:		Lactate..........	9.0
Sodium	17.0		
Chloride	17.0		

TABLE 3.—*Normal range of concentration of serum constituents*

Constituent	Concentration per 100 milliliters	Milliequivalent per liter	Millimoles per liter
Sodium . . . . milligram	310-340	135-148	135-148
Potassium . . . . milligram	13.6-20.7	3.5-5.3	3.5-5.3
Magnesium . . . . milligram	1.8-3.0	1.5-2.5	1.5-2.5
Calcium. . . . . milligram	9.6-11.0	4.8-5.4	4.8-5.4
Chloride . . . . milligram	348-383	98-108	98-108
Urea nitrogen. . . . . milligram	8-18		3-6.5
Carbon dioxide	101-132	23-30	23-30
Total Protein . . . . gram	6.0-8.2		
Albumin . . . . gram	3.8-5.0		
Globulin . . . . gram	2.3-3.5		

TABLE 4.—*Normal range of concentration of whole blood gases and pH value*

Constituent	Concentration torr[1]	kPa[2]
pO2 —Arterial	75-105 torr	10-14
Venous	30 torr	4
pCO2—Arterial	33-44 torr	4.5-5.9
Venous	38-49 torr	5.1-6.6
pH	7.35-7.45	

1. One torr = 1 mm Hg at sea level.
2. One Kilo Pascal (kpa) = 7.5 mm Hg = 7.5 torr.

TABLE 5.—*Equivalent United States and imperial weights and measures*

Unit of measurement	Abbreviation	United States measure	Imperial measure
1 milligram	mg	0.015432 grain	0.015432 grain.
1 gram	g	15.432 grains	15.432 grains.
1 kilogram	kg	35.274 ounces (avoirirdupois)	32.150 ounces (apothecary).
		32.150 ounces (apothecary)	35.274 ounces (apothecary).
1 grain	gr	0.0648 gram	0.0648 gram.
		64.8 milligrams	64.8 milligrams.
480 grains	gr	31.1035 grams	31.1035 grams.
		437.5 grains	437.5 grains.
1 ounce	oz	28.350 grams	28.350 grams.
1 milliliter	ml	16.23 minims	16.894 minims.
1 liter	l	33.814 fluid ounces	35.196 fluid ounces.
1 minim	min	0.0616 milliliter	0.0592 milliliter.
1 fluid ounce	fl. oz.	29.573 milliliters	28.412 milliliters.
1 pint[1]	pt.	473.17 milliliters	568.25 milliliters.

[1]Sixteen fluid ounces, U.S. measure; 20 fluid ounces, imperial measure.

TABLE 6.—*Approximate equivalent metric and imperial doses*

Milliliters	Minims	Grams	Grains	Milligrams	Grains
0.1	1 ½	0.1	1 ½	0.1	1/600
0.12	2	0.12	2	0.125	1/480
0.15	2 ½	0.15	2 ½	0.25	1/240
0.2	3	0.2	3	0.3	1/200
0.25	4	0.25	4	0.5	1/120
0.3	5	0.3	5	0.6	1/100
0.4	6	0.4	6	1	1/60
0.5	8	0.5	8	1.5	1/40
0.6	10	0.6	10	2	1/30
1	15	1	15	2.5	1/24
1.3	20	1.3	20	3	1/20
2	30	2	30	5	1/12
3	45	3	45	8	1/8
4	60	4	60	9	3/20
5	75	5	75	10	1/6
6	90	6	90	12	1/5
8	120	8	120	16	1/4
10	150	10	150	20	1/3
15	225	15	225	25	2/5
20	300	20	300	30	1/2
25	375	25	375	50	3/4
				60	1
				75	1 ¼

TABLE 7.—*Equivalent avoirdupois and metric weights*

Pounds	Kilograms	Pounds	Kilograms
100	45.359	155	70.306
105	47.627	160	72.574
110	49.895	165	74.842
115	52.163	170	77.110
120	54.431	175	79.378
125	56.698	180	81.646
130	58.966	185	83.914
135	61.234	190	86.182
140	63.502	195	88.450
145	65.770	200	90.718
150	68.038		

TABLE 8.—*Equivalents of centigrade and Farenheit thermometric scales*

Degrees C	Degrees F	Degrees C	Degrees F	Degrees C	Degrees F
-10	14.0	31	87.8	72	161.6
-9	15.8	32	89.6	73	163.4
-8	17.6	33	91.4	74	165.2
-7	19.4	34	93.2	75	167.0
-6	21.2	35	95.0	76	168.8
-5	23.0	36	96.8	77	170.6
-4	24.8	37	98.6	78	172.4
-3	26.6	38	100.4	79	174.2
-2	28.4	39	102.2	80	176.0
-1	30.2	40	104.0	81	177.8
0	32.0	41	105.8	82	179.6
1	33.8	42	107.6	83	181.4
2	35.6	43	109.4	84	183.2
3	37.4	44	111.2	85	185.0
4	39.2	45	113.0	86	186.8
5	41.0	46	114.8	87	188.6
6	42.8	47	116.6	88	190.4
7	44.6	48	118.4	89	192.2
8	46.4	49	120.2	90	194.0
9	48.2	50	122.0	91	195.8
10	50.0	51	123.8	92	197.6
11	51.8	52	125.6	93	199.4
12	53.6	53	127.4	94	201.2
13	55.4	54	129.2	95	203.0
14	57.2	55	131.0	96	204.8
15	59.0	56	132.8	97	206.6
16	60.8	57	134.6	98	208.4
17	62.6	58	136.4	99	210.2
18	64.4	59	138.2	100	212.0
19	66.2	60	140.0	101	213.8
20	68.0	61	141.8	102	215.6
21	69.8	62	143.6	103	217.4
22	71.6	63	145.4	104	219.2
23	73.4	64	147.2	105	221.0
24	75.2	65	149.0	106	222.8
25	77.0	66	150.8	107	224.6
26	78.8	67	152.6	108	226.4
27	80.6	68	154.4	109	228.2
28	82.4	69	156.2	110	230.0
29	84.2	70	158.0		
30	86.0	71	159.8		

Index

427

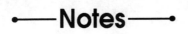

Notes

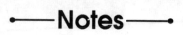

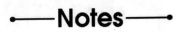

Notes

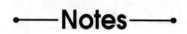
Notes

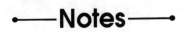
Notes

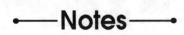

Notes

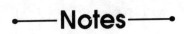

Notes

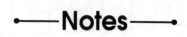

Notes

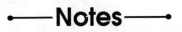

Other Books Available From Desert Publications

001	Firearms Silencers Volume 1	$9.95
003	The Silencer Cookbook	$9.95
004	Select Fire Uzi Modification Manual	$9.95
005	Expedient Hand Grenades	$16.95
007	007 Travel Kit, The	$8.00
008	Law Enforcement Guide to Firearms Silencer	$8.95
009	Springfield Rifle, The	$11.95
010	Full Auto Vol 3 MAC-10 Mod Manual	$9.95
012	Fighting Garand, The	$11.95
013	M1 Carbine Owners Manual	$9.95
014	Ruger Carbine Cookbook	$11.95
015	M-14 Rifle, The	$9.95
016	AR-15, M16 and M16A1 5.56mm Rifles	$11.95
017	Shotguns	$11.95
019	AR15 A2/M16A2 Assault Rifle	$8.95
022	Full Auto Vol 7 Bingham AK-22	$9.95
027	Full Auto Vol 4 Thompson SMG	$9.95
030	STANAG Mil-Talk	$12.95
031	Thompson Submachine Guns	$13.95
033	H&R Reising Submachine Gun Manual	$12.95
035	How to Build Silencers	$6.95
036	Full Auto Vol 2 Uzi Mod Manual	$9.95
049	Firearm Silencers Vol 3	$13.95
050	Firearm Silencers Vol 2	$9.95
054	Company Officers HB of Ger. Army	$11.95
056	German Infantry Weapons Vol 1	$14.95
058	Survival Armory	$29.95
060	Survival Gunsmithing	$9.95
061	FullAuto Vol 1 Ar-15 Mod Manual	$8.95
064	HK Assault Rifle Systems	$27.95
065	SKS Type of Carbines, The	$16.95
066	Private Weaponeer, The	$9.95
067	Rough Riders, The	$24.95
068	Lasers & Night Vision Devices	$29.95
069	Ruger P-85 Family of Handguns	$14.95
071	Dirty Fighting	$9.95
072	Live to Spend It	$29.95
073	Military Ground Rappelling Techniques	$11.95
074	Smith & Wesson Autos	$27.95
080	German MG-34 Machegun Manual	$9.95
081	Crossbows/ From 35 Years With the Weapon	$11.95
082	Op. Man. 7.62mm M24 Sniper Weapon	$7.95
083	USMC AR-15/M-16 A2 Manual	$16.95
084	Urban Combat	$21.95
085	Caching Techniques of U.S. Army Special Forces	$19.95
086	US Marine Corps Essential Subjects	$16.95
087	The L'il M-1, The .30 Cal. M-1 Carbine	$14.95
088	Concealed Carry Made Easy	$14.95
089	Apocalypse Tomorrow	$14.95
090	M14 and M14A1 Rifles and Rifle Marksmanship	$16.95
091	Crossbow As a Modern Weapon	$11.95
092	MP40 Machinegun	$11.95
093	Map Reading and Land Navigation	$9.95
094	U.S. Marine Corps Scout/Sniper Training Manual	$16.95
095	Clear Your Record & Own a Gun	$14.95
096	Sig Handguns	$16.95
097	Poor Man's Nuclear Bomb	$19.95
098	Poor Man's Sniper Rifle	$14.95
100	Submachine Gun Designers Handbook	$16.95
101	Lock Picking Simplified	$8.50
102	Combination Lock Principles	$8.95
103	How to Fit Keys by Impressioning	$9.95
104	Keys to Understanding Tubular Locks	$9.95
105	Techniques of Safe & Vault Manipulation	$9.95
106	Lockout -Techniques of Forced Entr	$11.95
107	Bugs Electronic Surveillance	$10.00
110	Improvised Weapons of Amer. Undergrnd	$10.00
111	Training Handbook of the American Underground	$10.00
114	FullAuto 8 M14A1 & Mini 14	$9.95
116	Handbook Bomb Threat/Search Procedures	$8.00
117	Improvised Lock Picks	$9.95
119	Fitting Keys by Reading Locks	$17.00
120	How to Open Handcuffs Without Keys	$9.95
121	Electronic Locks Volume 1	$8.00
122	With British Snipers, To the Reich	$24.95
125	Browning Hi-Power Pistols	$9.95
126	P-08 Parabellum Luger Auto Pistol	$9.95
127	Walther P-38 Pistol Manual	$9.95
128	Colt 45 Auto Pistol	$9.95
129	Beretta - 9MM M9	$11.95
130	FullAuto Vol 5 M1 Carbine to M2	$9.95
132	Ranger Handbook	$16.95
133	FN-FAL Auto Rifles	$13.95
135	AK-47 Assault Rifle	$9.95
136	Uzi Submachine Gun	$9.95
139	USMC Battle Skills Training Manual	$24.95
140	Sten Submachine Gun, The	$9.95
141	Terrorist Explosives Handbook	$6.95
142	U.S. Army Counterterrorism Training Manual	$14.95
143	Sniper Training	$24.95
144	The Butane Lighter Handgrenade	$9.95
146	The Official Makarov Pistol Manual	$12.95
147	Official Makarov 9mm Pistol Manual	$12.95
148	Unarmed Against the Knife	$9.95
149	Black Book of Booby Traps	$14.95
151	Militia Battle Manual	$18.95
152	Glock's Handguns	$14.95
153	Heckler and Koch's Handguns	$17.95
154	The Poor Man's R. P. G.	$14.95
155	The Poor Man's Ray Gun	$9.95
156	The Anarchist Handbook Vol. 2	$11.95
157	How to Make Disposable Silencers Vol. 2	$16.95
158	Modern Day Ninjutsu	$14.95
159	The Squeaky Wheel	$12.95
160	The Sicilian Blade	$13.95
162	The Anarchist Handbook Vol. 1	$11.95
163	How to Make Disposable Silencers Vol. 1	$16.95
164	The Anarchist Handbook Vol. 3	$11.95
165	How to Build Practical Firearm Silencers	$14.95
180	Build Your own AR-15	$14.95
182	How to Build Flash/Stun Grenades	$14.95
183	The Black Book of Arson	$14.95
200	Fighting Back on the Job	$11.95
202	Secret Codes & Ciphers	$9.95
204	Improvised Munitions Black Book Vol 1	$14.95
205	Improvised Munitions Black Book Vol 2	$14.95
206	CIA Field Exp Preparation of Black Powder	$8.95
207	CIA Field Exp. Meth/Explo. Preparat	$8.95
209	CIA Improvised Sabotage Devices	$12.00
210	CIA Field Exp. Incendiary Warfare	$9.95
211	Science of Revolutionary Warfare	$9.95
212	Agents HB of Black Bag Ops.	$9.95
216	Electronic Harassment	$11.95
217	Improvised Rocket Motors	$6.95
218	Impro. Munitions/Ammonium Nitrate	$8.95
219	Improvised Batteries/Det. Devices	$8.95
220	Improvised Explosives for Detonators	$7.95
221	Evaluation of Imp Shaped Charges	$8.95
222	American Tools of Intrigue	$8.00
225	Impro. Munitions Black Book Vol 3	$23.95
228	Poor Man's James Bond Vol 2	$24.95
229	Explosives and Propellants	$11.95
230	Select Fire 10/22	$9.95
231	Poor Man's James Bond Vol 1	$24.95
232	Assorted Nasties	$19.95
234	Full Auto Modification Manual	$18.95
240	L.A.W. Rocket Systems	$8.00
241	Clandestine Ops Man/Central America	$11.95
250	Mercenary Operations Manual	$9.95
260	Improvised Shaped Charges	$8.95
262	Two Component High Expl. Mixtures	$8.95
263	Survival Evasion & Escape	$13.95
300	Infantry Scouting, Patrol, & Sniping	$13.95
301	Engineer Explosives of WWI	$9.95
303	Brown's Alcohol Motor Fuel Cookbook	$13.95
306	How to Build a Junkyard Still	$11.95
310	Alcohol Distillers Handbook	$7.95
350	Brown's Book of Carburetors	$11.95
367	MAC-10 Cookbook	$9.95
400	Brown's Lawsuit Cookbook	$8.95
401	Hand to Hand Combat	$5.95
404	USMC Hand to Hand Combat	$7.95
409	US Marine Bayonet Training	$7.95
410	Camouflage	$7.95
412	Guide to Germ Warfare	$13.95
414	Emergency War Surgery	$24.95
415	Homeopathic First Aid	$9.95
416	Defensive Shotgun	$7.95
420	Hand to Hand Combat by D'Eliscue	$5.95
424	999 Survived	$6.00
425	Sun, Sand & Survival	$6.00
432	USMC Sniping	$16.95
435	Prisons Bloody Iron	$9.95
436	Napoleon's Maxims of War	$9.95
437	Invisible Weapons/Modern Ninja	$11.95
438	Cold Weather Survival	$10.00
440	Homestead Carpentry	$9.95
442	Construction Secret Hiding Places	$11.95
443	US Army Survival	$29.95
444	Survival Shooting for Women	$11.95
447	Survival Medicine	$9.95
448	Can You Survive	$12.95
454	Canteen Cup Cookery	$9.95
456	Leadership Hanbook of Small Unit Ops	$11.95
457	Vigilante Handbook	$11.95
470	Shootout II	$14.95
500	Guerila Warfare	$14.95
504	Ranger Training & Operations	$14.95
507	Spec. Forces Demolitions Trng HB	$16.95
510	Battlefield Analysis/Inf. Weapons	$9.95
511	US Army Bayonet Training	$7.95
542	Desert Storm Weap. Recog. Guide	$9.95
544	Professional Homemade Cher Bomb	$10.95
552	Combat Loads for Sniper Rifles	$12.00
610	Take My Gun, If You Dare	$10.95
C-002	Aunt Bessie's Wood Stove Cookbook	$7.50
C-011	Trapping & Destruc. of Exec. Cars	$7.50
C-020	How To Open A Swiss Bank Account	$6.95
C-023	Defending Your Retreat	$9.95
C-029	Methods of Long Term Storage	$8.95
C-038	Federal Firearms Laws	$6.95
C-040	M1 Carbine Arsenal History	$6.50
C-050	Hw To Build A Beer Can Morter	$4.95
C-052	Criminal Use of False ID	$11.95
C-175	Surviving Doomsday	$11.95
C-386	Beat the Box	$9.00
C-679	Self-Defense Requires No Apology	$11.95
	M16A1 Rifle Manual Cartoon Version	$6.95
FP-9	Micro Uzi Select Fire Mod Manual	$9.95

PRICES SUBJECT TO CHANGE WITHOUT NOTICE

DESERT Publications

215 S. Washington Ave.

870-862-2077

El Dorado, AR 71730-1751 USA

$5.95 shipping & handling